T0375221

GALEN: ON DISEASES AND SYMPTOMS

Galen's treatises on the classification and causation of diseases and symptoms are an important component of his prodigious *oeuvre*, forming a bridge between his theoretical works and his practical, clinical writings. As such, they remained an integral component of the medical teaching curriculum well into the second millennium. In these four treatises (only one of which has been previously translated into English), Galen not only provides a framework for the exhaustive classification of diseases and their symptoms as a prelude to his analysis of their causation, but he also attempts to establish precise definitions of all the key terms involved. Unlike others of his works, these treatises are notably moderate in tone, taking into account different views on structure and causation in a relatively even-handed way. Nonetheless, they are a clear statement of the Dogmatic position on the theoretical foundations of medicine in his time.

IAN JOHNSTON was born at Collaroy, New South Wales, in 1939. An eminent neurosurgeon, he was appointed a member of the Order of Australia (AM) in 2000 for services to medicine. Throughout his medical career he has also pursued a lifelong passion for ancient languages, completing degrees in Greek and Latin, and in classical Chinese at the Universities of New England and Sydney. His translations of Chinese poetry have been performed at arts festivals and exhibitions and he has made several radio and television appearances to discuss aspects of translation.

GALEN

On Diseases and Symptoms

IAN JOHNSTON

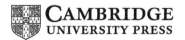

CAMBRIDGE
UNIVERSITY PRESS

University Printing House, Cambridge CB2 8BS, United Kingdom

Cambridge University Press is part of the University of Cambridge.

It furthers the University's mission by disseminating knowledge in the pursuit of education, learning and research at the highest international levels of excellence.

www.cambridge.org
Information on this title: www.cambridge.org/9780521865883

First published 2006

A catalogue record for this publication is available from the British Library

Library of Congress Cataloguing in Publication data
Johnston, Ian, 1939–
Galen on diseases and symptoms / Ian Johnston.
p. cm.
Contains 4 of Galen's treatises, three previously untranslated.
Includes bibliographical references and index.
ISBN-13: 978-0-521-86588-3 (hardback)
ISBN-10: 0-521-86588-3 (hardback)
1. Galen. 2. Medicine, Greek and Roman. 3. Medicine–Terminology–Early works to 1800. I. Galen. Selections English 2006. II. Title.
R126.J64 2006
610.938–dc22 2006023480

ISBN 978-0-521-86588-3 Hardback

Contents

List of tables   *page* vii
Acknowledgements   viii
List of abbreviations   x

PART I   INTRODUCTION

I.1   General introduction   3

I.2   Galen's life and works   7

I.3   Galen's philosophical and medical antecedents   11

I.4   Definitions and terminology   21
    I.4a   Definitions   21
    I.4b   Causal terms   31
    I.4c   General terms   37
    I.4d   Diseases and symptoms   50
    I.4e   Conclusions   63

I.5   The classification of diseases and symptoms   65
    I.5a   Introduction   65
    I.5b   Diseases (*De morborum differentiis*)   69
    I.5c   Symptoms (*De symptomatum differentiis*)   72
    I.5d   Conclusions   75

I.6   Causation in diseases and symptoms   81
    I.6a   Introduction   81
    I.6b   Theories of disease causation prior to Galen 84
    I.6c   Galen on causation   102
    I.6d   Conclusions   120

Contents

PART II TRANSLATION

II.0 Introduction   129

II.1 *On the Differentiae of Diseases*   131

II.2 *On the Causes of Diseases*   157

II.3 *On the Differentiae of Symptoms*   180

II.4 *On the Causes of Symptoms I*   203

II.5 *On the Causes of Symptoms II*   236

II.6 *On the Causes of Symptoms III*   265

PART III CONCLUSION

III.1 Conclusions   305

Bibliography   312
Index   329

Tables

1. Galen's life in summary   *page* 8
2. Other authors referred to in the four treatises   12
3. Views on disease causation in the *Anonymus londinensis*   91
4. Causes of mono-*dyscrasias*.   114
5. Causes of organic diseases   115

Acknowledgements

This work started out as a PhD thesis at the University of New England, a thesis which itself began as a translation and analysis of Galen's *De elementis secundum Hippocratem.* Redirection to the four treatises of the present work followed the appearance of De Lacy's fine CMG edition of that work. I was fortunate in many ways to have made substantial progress in the first translation before making the switch in that the four treatises are certainly best understood against the background of Galen's concepts of structure. I am, therefore, grateful to De Lacy, although I didn't necessarily recognize this at the time. More obviously, I am extremely grateful to all the members of the excellent Classics and Ancient History Department at New England where I have, intermittently, pursued my studies of Greek and Latin for more than twenty years, initially *pari passu* with a busy medical practice. My thanks go particularly to my thesis supervisors, initially Peter Toohey and John Vallance. It was Peter who, along with the others, was instrumental in my learning Classical Greek from the beginning and for setting me on the path towards this most rewarding and enjoyable work. John Vallance, a constant throughout the vicissitudes, was mainly responsible for the direction of the thesis, for the change of direction when this was needed, and was of great assistance with the further work needed to prepare the book in its present form. His help has been continuous and invaluable in all areas, and his detailed knowledge of the field absolutely critical. When Peter Toohey went to Canada, Greg Horsley took over as co-supervisor, and his contribution can only inadequately be described as substantial despite the material being outside his own areas of interest. His help has been important in many facets but especially through his detailed, painstaking and time-consuming criticism of the translations, undoubtedly the single most important piece of assistance, and through his similarly detailed criticism of the introductory sections. The assistance of Vivian Nutton has been invaluable. Not only has he helped and encouraged me from the start, both by correspondence and by direct discussion during my several trips to the UK in search of material, but he has been particularly influential in directing me towards a concentration on the medical rather than the philological aspects – 'play to your strength'. I am very grateful for this in that it has, I think, resulted in the work being of maximum possible interest to me and hopefully, as a result, better in itself. I am very grateful also to Geoffrey Lloyd, predominantly for his advice on difficult areas of the texts and in a more general way for discussion during his stimulating visits to Sydney over the last few years. Needless to say, I am also particularly indebted (as, indeed, we all are) to both Vivian Nutton and Geoffrey Lloyd for the substantial body of valuable and stimulating written work they have produced over the years. I would also like to thank Sandra Rothwell and the staff of the Dixson Library at the University of New England for their very considerable assistance, made the more valuable as it was made the more difficult by the remoteness of my present abode. Finally, I would like to thank Susan Collis who has repeatedly read through the material, often in early and almost unreadable form, and offered countless helpful criticisms and suggestions.

Abbreviations

CMG   Corpus Medicorum Graecorum.

D-K   *Die Fragmente der Vorsokratiker*, H. Diels, W. Kranz, Weidmann, Zurich, 1992 reprint.

DNP   *Der Neue Pauly: Enzyklopädie der Antike*, H. Cancik, H. Schneider, eds., Verlag J. B. Metzler, Stuttgart, 1996–.

H   Helmreich's edition of Galen's *De usu partium* (H following volume and page numbers).

K   Kühn's edition of Galen's *Opera Omnia* (K following volume and page numbers).

LSJ   *A Greek–English Lexicon*, H. G. Liddell, R. Scott, H. S. Jones, Oxford University Press, Oxford, 1990 reprint.

OCD   *The Oxford Classical Dictionary*, 3rd edn., ed. S. Hornblower, A. Spawforth, Oxford University Press, Oxford, 1996.

SVF   *Stoicorum Veterum Fragmenta*, Joannes ab Arnim, Teubner, Stuttgart, 1968 reprint.

TLG   *Thesaurus Linguae Graecae.*

PART I

Introduction

General introduction

Galen remains indisputably one of the major figures in the history of medicine, both occidental and oriental. Whilst his name may not evoke the undiluted reverence accorded to Hippocrates, he is a much more identifiable historical figure with a very substantial surviving body of work accepted as being from his own hand. In terms of influence, particularly in Western Europe, his position in medicine is somewhat akin to that of Aristotle in philosophy, characterized as it is by a dominance extending to the mid-point of the second post-Christian millennium. Unlike both Hippocrates and Aristotle, however, he has always had his share of detractors, in part a consequence of his combative and self-aggrandizing style of writing, in part because of his perceived arrogance, in part because during his lifetime he was a weighty participant in a continuing debate between conflicting schools on the theoretical bases of medicine, and in part subsequently because of the supposed stultifying effect of his ideas, seen by some as hindering further developments in medicine.

The merits of these and other criticisms are debatable. What is incontrovertible is that his writings were not only extensive in amount, but also wide-ranging in scope, embracing all aspects of theoretical and practical medicine and many areas of philosophy as well. Changing concepts of physiology and pathology may have vitiated many of his concepts and practices, but in their more theoretical aspects, his medical writings, and arguably his philosophical writings too, remain relevant. Nevertheless, only a relatively small part of his corpus has been translated into any of the modern European languages. Thus those who wish to experience the full scope of his writing must turn to the nineteenth-century edition compiled under the editorship of Karl Gottlob Kühn, which provides the Greek text and a Latin translation for most of his surviving works.[1]

---

[1] Originally published between 1821 and 1833 but reprinted by Georg Olms in 1965 and again in 1997 – see Nutton (1976). The *Corpus Medicorum Graecorum* is gradually replacing the oft-criticized Kühn

The central purpose of the present work is to provide translations of the four related treatises, *De morborum differentiis*, *De causis morborum*, *De symptomatum differentiis* and *De symptomatum causis*, the last comprising three books. These translations are the first into a modern language of these six books apart from a recent translation of *De causis morborum* in a collection of tracts related to food and diet.[2] Each translation is preceded by a short synopsis of the translated treatise. Among the secondary purposes may be mentioned the following:

(i) The attempt to examine Galen's ideas on definition, classification and causation of disease.

(ii) An analysis of his concept of the composition and structure of the body in relation to his ideas about pathology.

(iii) A consideration of Galen's place in the theoretical debate referred to, particularly with regard to causation, which defined the rival schools before and during his own time.

(iv) An evaluation of the relevance of his ideas to modern thinking on the classification and causation of diseases and symptoms.

The four treatises under examination, thought to have been written during the very prolific period after his return to Rome in AD 169,[3] form a bridge between his more theoretical and his obviously practical medical writings – between, for example, *De elementis secundum Hippocratem* and *De methodo medendi*. Galen himself, who listed them among his works of anatomical science,[4] saw them as following both Hippocrates and Aristotle in intent as well as in methodology. Thus, he wrote in the opening book of *De methodo medendi*:

Furthermore, concerning the *differentiae* of diseases, how many there are and of what kind, and likewise concerning symptoms, and in addition concerning the causes related to each, Hippocrates appears to be the first of all those we know to have made a beginning correctly, whilst after him Aristotle showed the way to the greatest degree.[5]

In this regard the books are identified as an essential prerequisite for an understanding of this, his major practical medical text of somewhat uncertain date of composition,[6] in which he also writes:

---

edition. A number of works attributed to Galen have been recovered from Latin and Arabic texts. A relatively up-to-date list is provided in López Férez (1991), pp. 309–29. See also Nutton, ed. (2002).

[2] Grant (2000), pp. 46–61.   [3] Nutton (1988), and Singer (1997), introduction, p. li.

[4] See Galen's *De libris propriis* XIX.30K.   [5] *De methodo medendi* X.15K.

[6] See Hankinson's (1991) translation of books 1 and 2 of *De methodo medendi* (introduction, pp. xxxiii–xxxiv) for a discussion of the date of composition. See also Ilberg (1889–97).

... it is then necessary for one who desires to establish the truth in every way to get away from a further concern with names, to pass to the actual substance of the matters and to reflect on and seek this – however many diseases and symptoms there are altogether and, in addition, the *proegoumenic*[7] causes of these. Therefore, we did this in other treatises, of which there is one concerning the number of diseases, which has set out the *differentiae* of diseases, and another about the *differentiae* of symptoms. And in this way we tried to discover the causes of these, each individually, those of all diseases and those of all the symptoms, so that there remains nothing further, but everything is ready and prepared for the matter now lying before us. Accordingly, I do not advise knowing the things said in what follows before being conversant with these [works], for in this way someone would misunderstand many theories and would not himself be helped, taking issue with what has been stated correctly.[8]

As evidence of the relevance and importance of these books, they remained part of the Galenic canon (*Summaria Alexandria*), both for Arabic medical teaching and for that in medieval Europe.[9]

What Galen sets out to do in these four treatises is, first, to establish certain definitions and to clarify the terminology involved in them. Secondly, he attempts to formulate a classification of diseases and symptoms. Thirdly, he endeavours to provide a detailed, and largely practical, account of causation in respect to both diseases and symptoms. These several aims, and the extent to which they are achieved, will be considered in detail in what follows. In summary, the definitions of central importance are those of health, disease, symptom and affection, whilst the terms of particular concern are those involved in these definitions. In providing a classification, and in examining causation, Galen recognizes the two competing theories of basic and bodily structure of the time. The first, a continuum theory based on the idea of four primary elements or qualities and involving humours, is the theory he himself espouses. The second, an atomic theory based on the idea of all matter as consisting of particles and void, is considered mainly with emphasis on Asclepiades' version of this,[10] and is the theory Galen opposes. What is striking in the books being considered here is the relatively even-handed way in which Galen treats these two groups of theories compared to his dismissive, indeed often vituperative, *ad hominem* arguments common elsewhere.[11]

---

[7] Galen's use of causal terminology is considered in chapters I.4 and I.6 below.
[8] *De methodo medendi* X.85–6K.   [9] See Iskander (1976), pp. 236–8; Nutton (1995), p. 87.
[10] For a detailed recent account of Asclepiades' theories and the largely Galenic sources of our knowledge of these see Vallance (1990).
[11] For example, his attacks on Thessalus, which are a prominent feature of Book I of *De methodo medendi*, and those on Erasistratus in *De causis procatarcticis*.

In part I, following these general introductory remarks, brief consideration is given to Galen's life and works, his important antecedents both medical and philosophical, and issues of terminology, disease classification and disease causation. With regard to the translations in part II, some general remarks may be apposite here. A particular aim has been to remain close to the original, avoiding paraphrase and glossing. It is to be hoped that this has been achieved without too great a cost in terms of the fluency of the English. Where, however, there has been an apparently unresolvable conflict between accuracy and readability, the latter has regrettably borne the sacrifice. Comments on the basis of the translations, and the use and availability of other manuscripts, are to be found in the introduction to the translations (chapter II.o), but this is, in effect, a translation from the oft-criticized Kühn text. The present work is, then, intended as a translation of these texts and an analysis of the ideas contained therein. It is not intended as a philological study. The focus is on accuracy of translation from the text as it is, and on the nature and relevance of the ideas expressed in relation to theories of medicine both then and now.

Before proceeding, I would like to foreshadow briefly some of the conclusions drawn from the translations and analyses. Firstly, the treatises studied are predominantly practical in intent and content. Whilst Galen does provide theoretical discussion of definitions and of causation, and, to a lesser extent, of classification, his considerations are obviously preliminary to the main purpose of the treatises, and particularly in the case of causation are somewhat peripheral to his presentation. On the matter of definitions, he does succeed in providing workable definitions of health, disease, symptom and affection although difficulties undoubtedly remain, both in the terms used in the definitions and in the overlap between them. The second problem, at least, Galen clearly recognizes. His classes of diseases and symptoms are comprehensive, perhaps even exhaustive, but are open to criticism on several grounds, as will be discussed. Causation is an issue of considerable concern to Galen. Both in these and in other works he does attempt to grapple with problems of mechanism and terminology. In the treatises here examined, there is, however, a failure to effect a systematic connection between the theoretical and the practical, and a failure also to achieve a consistent use of causal terminology. Nevertheless, the theoretical issues he raises do not depend on now outmoded concepts of anatomy, physiology and pathology. One timeless lesson, then, which might be learned from these treatises is that Galen's emphasis on the importance of the link between medicine and philosophy bears an enduring relevance.

Galen's life and works

The details of Galen's life, many of which are known from his own works, are now well established and documented,[1] and so will be considered only very briefly here. Although some aspects such as the dates of his birth and death and specific details of his training and travels remain to some degree points of contention, recent studies, especially those of Nutton, have brought considerable clarity. The matters of particular relevance for the present study are firstly, the nature of his early training and how this influenced the way he saw the role of disciplines other than medicine in the training of a doctor, and secondly, to give an outline of the range of his works so as to place the translated treatises in the overall context of his *oeuvre*. A brief biographical summary is provided in Table 1.[2]

Galen's early education, under the close and participatory supervision of his father, concentrated on mathematical and philosophical subjects, notably geometry and logic. This undoubtedly had a lasting influence on his methodological approach to medical problems and their exposition. Further, his philosophical training was eclectic and this again had a later reflection in his strong views on the importance of philosophy in medical training, not to mention his own approach to medical issues. Lack of philosophical training was a criticism he frequently levelled against his opponents.

After the redirection of his education into medicine as a result of his father's dreams,[3] he travelled widely. During this itinerant period he appears

---

[1] Among these may be mentioned the books by Sarton (1954) and Moraux (1985), the articles collected in Nutton (1988) and the relevant chapters in Nutton (2004). Earlier studies include the series of articles by Walsh (1934–9), Ackermann's *Historia literaria Claudii Galeni* in Kühn, vol. I, and the series of articles by Ilberg (1889–97).

[2] There is some variation in the dates given by different authors although all recognize the periods listed. See, for example, the chronological tables in Singer, C. (1956), pp. xiii–xv, Moraux (1985), pp. 33–4 and Singer, P. (1997), pp. l–lii.

[3] See *De ordine librorum suorum ad Eugenianum*, XIX.59K – 'Then, persuaded by clear dreams, he made me, in my seventeenth year, train in medicine at the same time as philosophy.'

Table 1 *Galen's life in summary*

AD 129/30	Born at Pergamum. Son of an erudite father (the well-to-do architect Nicias) and a termagant mother.
130–43	Early education under father's supervision. Concentration on mathematics, geometry and logic.
143–7	Formal study of philosophy under several teachers from different schools – Platonic, Peripatetic, Stoic, Epicurean.
147–9	Beginning of medical education following his father's dreams. At Pergamum under several teachers.
149–57	Travels widely in pursuit of medical training, spending time in Smyrna, Corinth and Alexandria. Teachers include Pelops, Albinus, and possibly Numisianus.
157–61	Returns to Pergamum to begin practice of medicine. Appointed as doctor to school of gladiators. First anatomical discoveries (e.g. recurrent laryngeal nerve).
162–6	First stay in Rome. Continues anatomical studies, in part under the patronage of Boethius.
167	Returns to Pergamum for reasons which are unclear – possibilities include plague in Rome, enemies in Rome and business in Pergamum.
168–?	Summoned back to Rome by Marcus Aurelius. Remains there for much of the rest of his life. His major writings are from this period.
200–16	No details. Probably died in 215 or 216. Place and manner of death unknown.

to have given particular attention to anatomy and pharmacology. It is likely he also continued his philosophical studies. In AD 157 he began medical practice in Pergamum, but shortly afterwards went to Rome where he spent the major part of the rest of his life. Details of his brief return to Pergamum remain unclear but are of no immediate relevance to the present study.

Turning to his works, the most striking feature is their sheer volume, although their breadth of scope and extent of influence are also noteworthy. Indeed, in terms of volume no ancient author of any genre surpasses, or even matches, Galen for output, although, of course, much ancient writing has been lost and, of course also, quantity alone is no true yardstick of merit. Walsh estimates his prodigious output as amounting to approximately $2\frac{1}{2}$ million words surviving and perhaps half as many again lost, particularly at the time of the fire in the vicinity of Rome's Temple of Peace in AD 192.[4] Nutton, more recently, has spoken of 434 titles of works, over

---

[4] See Walsh (1934), p. 1 and Sarton (1954), p. 23 regarding the fire. Galen himself refers to the fire in *De libris propriis* XIX.19K.

350 of which are thought to be authentic, ranging in length from 30 to 500 pages, equating with a remarkable daily output of two to three pages over 50 years.[5] A major portion of his extant writings are included in K. G. Kühn's nineteenth-century edition of his *Opera Omnia* which contains a total of 122 titles in 20 volumes (volumes 17 and 18 are divided into parts A and B, volume 20 is an index only), of which perhaps 16 are spurious. The genuine works range in length from 3–4 pages only, e.g. *De causis respirationis* and *De veneriis* to those in excess of 1,000 pages, e.g. *De usu partium* and *De methodo medendi*.[6] In the initial chapter in Kühn there are listed 100 genuine works, 44 'libri manifeste spurii', 19 fragments and 18 commentaries on works by Hippocrates.[7] A number of other works, not included in Kühn, are gradually coming to light, some in Greek but the majority from Syriac and Arabic sources. López-Férez in 1991 listed 23 such works as well as 26 additional spurious works.[8] From Galen's own account in *De libris propriis*, counting as single treatises those works described as multi-volume, one obtains a number of 187 works, although also it is not always clear what constitutes a separate work.[9] This is an extraordinary output by any measure.

The four treatises here translated have received relatively little modern attention, a neglect which seems unwarranted in the light of Galen's own evaluation of them as a bridge between the frankly philosophical and the practical medical works noted earlier, as well as their inclusion in the Alexandrian Canon. In fact, by the time of the establishment of the Alexandrian medical curriculum in the sixth and seventh centuries, Galen's surviving works had become a major component of medical teaching in conjunction with those of Hippocrates and Aristotle, just as his insistence on the necessary connection between medicine and philosophy had become an article of faith. Iskander, in reviewing the early Alexandrian curriculum, notes that Galen's books were divided into seven grades, amongst which the books here translated on the classes and causes of diseases and symptoms constituted the third grade.[10] With reference to these books, Ibn Ridwan, an important figure in Arabic medicine at the start of the second millennium,[11] is quoted as saying:

---

[5] Nutton (1995), p. 60.

[6] The references to these works in the Kühn edition are as follows: *De causis respirationis* IV.465–9K, *De veneriis* V.911–14K, *De usu partium libri I–XI* III.1–939K and *libri XII–XVII* IV.1–366K, *De methodo medendi* X.1–1021K.

[7] See Kühn, vol. 1, *Historia literaria Claudii Galeni*, pp. lxvii–clxxxvi.

[8] López-Férez (1991), pp. 326–9.   [9] *De libris propriis* XIX.8–48K.   [10] Iskander (1976).

[11] Iskander, in the article referred to in n. 10, mentions the article by Schacht and Meyerhof (1937) as a valuable source of information about him.

A third grade had one book only, on diseases and symptoms, in six treatises. Galen wrote separate treatises, but the Alexandrians assemble them in one book. It provides information on the diagnosis of diseases, their causes and symptoms. In Galen's opinion, its [treatises] bear richly upon medicine and treat of reasoning which is the major principle of this book. If studied properly and well understood, this book will disclose all the minor and major mysteries of the art of medicine.[12]

These books then remained an integral part of the medical curriculum into the second millennium. Moreover, during the great upsurge of interest in Galen's works in the original Greek, and the abundance of Latin translations and commentaries that were produced in the fifteenth and sixteenth centuries,[13] they received attention from several renowned scholars of the period, including Leoniceno and Linacre. Details of manuscripts and commentaries will be given at the start of part II.

In summary, from this brief review of Galen's life and works, there are several points of undoubted relevance to the treatises of the present study. The first is the significant role occupied by the formal disciplines of geometry and logic, and of philosophy more generally, in his early education. This must have been influential in his approach to the topics of definition, classification and causation. The second is his continuing commitment to philosophy, which would certainly have been a stimulus to him to establish a secure theoretical foundation for his practice of medicine. Thirdly, there is his continued practice itself, which inevitably reflected back on his theoretical constructions, something quite apparent in the treatises being considered, making them an interesting conjunction of the theoretical and the practical. Fourthly, in terms of the fate of the books in question, there is the matter of their continuing importance in the small kernel of Galen's works which became the basis for medical education over many centuries. Yet Galen's work, his theories and practices, did not emerge *e nihilo*, so, important as his writings unquestionably are, it is also important to examine, albeit briefly, their antecedents and to place them in their proper medical and philosophical contexts. This is the purpose of the following chapter.

---

[12] From Ibn Ridwan's *Useful Book on the Quality of Medical Education*, translation after Iskander (1976), p. 250.

[13] Durling (1961) provides a detailed list of editions and translations from this time.

CHAPTER I.3

Galen's philosophical and medical antecedents

As should be readily apparent from the brief outline of Galen's life given above, he was well versed in philosophy and this is clearly reflected in his writings. That he had a detailed knowledge of earlier medical writings and an active engagement with contemporary medical theories and practices goes without saying. The extent to which other philosophers and doctors, both predecessors and contemporaries, are mentioned in his many works is very variable as, indeed, is the treatment they are accorded. Those referred to in the translated treatises in the present work are listed in Table 2. It is noteworthy that in these works references to, and remarks about, different individuals are altogether temperate in tone, in striking contrast with those in some of his other works, for example *De methodo medendi*.

Considering philosophers first, Plato is undoubtedly the one that Galen most obviously and overtly respected. As De Lacy writes:

Plato is repeatedly praised. He is first among philosophers, as Hippocrates is the best of all physicians. Like Hippocrates, he is 'divine'. He is a member of the 'chorus' that is closest to God, whose members are devoted to the pursuit of the highest arts and sciences and are honoured equally with the gods.[1]

The matters on which Plato is of particular relevance to Galen include: the basic structure of the body, relying on ideas of elements, qualities and humours as propounded in the *Timaeus*;[2] the recognition of design in nature, involving the concept of the 'Demiurge';[3] the tripartite division of the soul, including consideration of the physical correlates of the psychic;[4] and, of special relevance to the present study, Plato's ideas on causation in general and in medicine in particular, as expounded primarily in the *Timaeus* and the *Phaedo*.[5] On a somewhat more minor (but nonetheless important) issue, Galen's agreement and identification with Plato on the

---

[1] De Lacy (1973), pp. 32–3.   [2] *Timaeus* 48b ff.   [3] *Timaeus* 28a ff.
[4] *Timaeus* 69c–71a, *Phaedrus* 253 ff.   [5] *Timaeus* 82a, *Phaedo* 97–100.

Table 2 *Other authors referred to in the four treatises*

Author	Diff. Morb.	Caus. Morb.	Diff. Sympt.	Caus. Sympt. I	Caus. Sympt. II	Caus. Sympt. III
Hippocrates		III.2 Cold diseases (*Aph*)		II.3 ref. to *De plac. Hipp. et Plat.* II.1 Visual illusions VI.1 Pleasure and pain VI.3 On terms VI.6 Tetanus (*Aph.*)	II.2 Abn. respiration (*Acut.*) II.3 On spasm (*Aph.*) V.1 Origin of pain (*Loc. hom.*) V.6 Genesis or rigors (*Aph.*) V.9 Fever and rigor (*Aph.*) VII.2 Melancholia etc. (*Aph.*)	VII.1 Diarrhoea after loss of a limb (*On joints*) VIII.3 Kidney and bladder conditions (*Aph.*) VIII.3 Failure of digestion (*Prog.*)
Plato			I.3 On affections IV.4 On naming	II.3 Ref. to *De Plac. Hipp. et Plat.* VI.1 Pleasure and pain VI.3 On terms VIII.3 Sleep		
Aristotle						IV.2 Changing characteristics
Athenaeus					III.1 Causes of fever IV.2 Cough	
Praxagoras and Philotimus				VI.5 Additional humours VII.7 Additional humours		
Thucydides			III.4 The plague		VII.1 The plague	
Asclepiades	II.4 *Anarmoi*					
Epicurus	II.4 Atoms					
Diocles of Carystus			VI.4 Sweating			
Herophilus					II.2 Optic nerve	

need to give primary attention to matters themselves rather than to terminology, something which is stressed in the translated treatises, is revealed in the following statement from the *De anatomicis administrationibus*: 'But if you are at least persuaded by Plato and myself you will always think little of names, whereas you will be attentive primarily and particularly to the knowledge of matters . . .'[6]

Aristotle, on the other hand, is not given the unqualified reverence which Plato receives. For example, De Lacy has drawn attention to two passages which clearly display a less than reverent attitude towards him on Galen's part. In the first, Aristotle is linked with Praxagoras as a target of criticism for their jointly held and major misconception of the function of the heart – 'they were either blind themselves or were addressing a blind audience'. In the second, where his views are criticized in *De semine*, he is twice addressed patronizingly as 'dearest Aristotle'.[7] Nevertheless, it could be argued that an analysis of Galen's works would support the view that Aristotle's influence was the most significant, at least in matters other than the purely medical.

Thus, in Galen's teleological views, which especially inform one of his major works, *De usu partium*, it is Aristotle's immanent teleology rather than the Platonic 'Demiurge' which is most discernible. In his methodology, Galen is clearly and profoundly influenced by Aristotle, particularly by the works of the *Organon*. In his conception of the structure of the body he is, as has been noted, a staunch supporter of the theory of elements and qualities which, whilst not attributable to Aristotle, was held and developed by him. Further, in his formulations of structural levels, which are of considerable importance to the classifications advanced in the books of the present study, Galen follows Aristotelian concepts, especially the idea of *homoiomeres*. In his consideration of causation, he is also clearly influenced by Aristotle, both in the assumption of the validity of the search for causal explanations and in the specific ideas. This is an issue which merits, and will receive, further and more detailed discussion. In his attention to taxonomy, Galen is obviously following Aristotelian principles. Moreover, he was unquestionably influenced by the psychology of *De anima*, as indeed were almost all who came after Aristotle and grappled with the same subject matter. Finally, the empirical component of his studies and

---

[6] *De anatomicis administrationibus* II.581K. According to De Lacy the reference to Plato is either '. . . *Statesman* 261E' or '. . . the conclusion of the *Cratylus*'. Singer, C. (1956), in his translation of *De anatomicis administrationibus*, also mentions *Republic* 533e and *Sophist* 244.

[7] See De Lacy (1973), p. 33. The two passages referred to are to be found in *De placitis Hippocratis et Platonis* V.187–8K and *De semine* IV.530, 553K respectively. As regards the latter, De Lacy remarks that the phrase 'dearest Aristotle' '. . . expresses a certain exasperation at the obtuseness of the person criticised'.

the use of observation of biological phenomena as the basis for theoretical formulation reveals the Aristotelian imprint.

A further predecessor who should be mentioned, both for himself and as an important representative of the Stoic school, is Chrysippus. Galen's attitude to him is somewhat ambivalent. For example, at one point in *De methodo medendi* Chrysippus is linked with Hippocrates, Plato and Aristotle in espousing what Galen himself accepts as the correct explanation of matter:

> For Hippocrates first put forward the hot, cold, dry and moist, whilst Aristotle demonstrated [these] after him. And the followers of Chrysippus took these up as already given and did not dispute [them], but said that all things are mixed from these, and that these affect and act on each other and that nature is systematic. They accept all the other doctrines of Hippocrates about nature, apart from there being some small difference between them and Aristotle.[8]

By contrast, in several passages in *De placitis Hippocratis et Platonis*, Chrysippus is roundly criticized.[9]

In summary, there are two areas where Galen is clearly in accord with Stoic thinking: (i) in his concept of the structure of matter in general (i.e. a continuum concept) and of the body in particular; and (ii) in his approach to causation and causal explanation as will be discussed further in chapter I.6. More uncertain is the degree of accord on the nature and role of *pneuma*. Whilst both Galen and the Stoics attribute considerable importance to *pneuma* in their formulations of physiology and pathology, Singer remarks that Galen '. . . is at pains to distance [his theory of *pneuma*] from that of the Stoics, who endowed *pneuma* with religious, arguably pantheistic, significance'.[10] Issues on which there is frank opposition include the structure and workings of the soul, and the importance of the heart in development and in neurological function. As these matters are only of peripheral relevance to the present subject, they are not considered further here.

Finally with regard to philosophers, Galen's position is quite clear in the case of Epicurus, taken by him as the philosophical representative of atomist theories which he unequivocally opposes. Important predecessors, such as Democritus and Leucippus, and successors, such as Lucretius, are considered only briefly or not at all. On the other hand, Asclepiades, the major member of the medical wing of atomism, is frequently referred to and mostly unfavourably (see below).

---

[8] *De methodo medendi* X.16K.   [9] See De Lacy (1973), p. 33.
[10] Singer, P. (1997), introduction, p. xii.

In terms of doctors, Galen's greatest debt, explicitly and repeatedly acknowledged, was to Hippocrates, at least to the Hippocrates whom Galen takes to be the author of certain of the works he most admires in the Hippocratic Corpus. Thus, Lloyd speaks of: '. . . the importance of the almost unbounded admiration he [Galen] always expressed, throughout his life, for Hippocrates, his "guide in all that is good"'.[11]

Three principles of primary importance to Galen were taken from Hippocrates. First, there was the humoral theory of the composition of the body, as expressed in the latter's *Nature of Man*, with its stated opposition to the existing claims of a single basic substance, characteristic of much of Presocratic philosophy. Second, there was the view, whether implicit or explicit, that each individual disease had a causal explanation which should be sought and, if identified, would be of relevance to treatment. Third, and related to the second, there was the allopathic principle underlying treatment. Of more general importance were Hippocrates' perceived emphasis on ethics and his methodology, both of which prefigure Galen's own belief in the essential nexus between medicine and philosophy. Again to quote Lloyd, Hippocrates '. . . could be used as a perfect demonstration of how, in methodology, in natural philosophy, even in moral philosophy, the best doctor is also a philosopher'.[12] It could be said, then, that properly understood and interpreted – that is, according to Galen himself – Hippocrates provided the foundation stone for all that Galen embraced in the theory and practice of medicine. In areas of doubt, any uncertainties of authorship within the Corpus could be used to Galen's advantage in dismissing aspects with which he disagreed.

Other early medical writers whose works are no longer extant but who are worthy of mention in the present context are as follows: Alcmaeon of Croton, at least on the flimsy doxographical evidence available, was the originator of the balance/imbalance concept of health and disease, so fundamental in the present treatises. Philistion of Locri, on the basis of the *Anonymus londinensis*, may be said to have held similar views to Galen on disease causation. Diocles of Carystus appears to have articulated views on the four elements or qualities, on *pneuma* and innate heat, and on digestion, which are similar to Galen's, and so may have influenced him. Finally, Praxagoras, while he attracted Galen's criticism for his cardiocentric view of the *hegemonikon* and his idea that *pneuma* was conveyed by the arteries, is quoted favourably in the present treatises in relation to his view of the expanded number of humours.

---

[11] Lloyd (1993), p. 125.   [12] Lloyd (1993), p. 140.

Galen was obviously indebted to the two great Alexandrian doctors of the third century BC, Herophilus and Erasistratus, not only for their actual anatomical discoveries, but also for the importance which they gave to anatomy in the teaching and practice of medicine. In other aspects, such as basic physiology and pathology as well as causation, he seems to be close to what we know of Herophilus, but quite at odds with some of the ideas of Erasistratus. In particular, this relates to basic structure (i.e. particles versus continuum) and to causation, as will be considered in chapter I.6.

Lastly, there is Asclepiades, who has been described by Frede as 'a pivotal figure' in the Rationalist/Empiricist debate[13] but is undoubtedly also pivotal in a wider sense. Asclepiades has a particular relevance for Galen, and a particular relevance also for the books under consideration in which his theories are given significant recognition in Galen's discussion of disease classification and causation. In essence, Asclepiades represented the culminating articulation of atomistic theories as applied to medicine up to the first century BC. Atomism was a theory that could trace its heritage back through the somewhat disparate strands of Strato of Lampsacus, Heraclides of Pontus and Epicurus to its origin with Democritus. As with a number of the significant figures already mentioned, his writings have not been preserved, although the recent collection by Vallance provides a detailed account of his views and of his intellectual progenitors.[14] Unfortunately, much of the information derives from Galen himself who, being implacably opposed to Asclepiades' key concepts, cannot be taken as an impartial source. Galen's inclusion of Asclepiadian theories and their Methodist developments in the treatises dealt with here is, however, strikingly free of polemic, as noted earlier.

Asclepiades based his physiology and pathology on the concept of fragile corpuscles (*anarmoi onkoi*) which travelled through ducts not anatomically definable (*poroi*) distributed throughout the body. Diseases occurred when this process was interfered with, in particular when there was impaction (*emphraxis*), as will be discussed further in chapter I.6. Considerable uncertainty remains about the precise nature of the structures involved, although there is agreement on the broad outlines of the theory, which formed the basis for the principles of the Methodic sect (see below). Therefore, although he was clearly a supporter of the principle of causal explanation, Asclepiades' structural concepts were so at odds with those of Galen that the nature of the causes invoked was inevitably different. Asclepiades also

---

[13] See Walzer and Frede (1985), introduction, p. xxix.   [14] Vallance (1990).

differed importantly from Galen in his rejection of teleology and in his support for Erasistratus' idea that the arteries contained *pneuma*.

In considering very briefly those philosophers and doctors who were Galen's contemporaries or near-contemporaries, the 'schools' of the period provide a convenient framework, particularly in relation to causation. Indeed, Hankinson writes: '. . . it is not much of an exaggeration to say that the differences between the principal medical tendencies of the Roman Empire, Dogmatic (Rationalist), Empiricist and Methodist, are to be located precisely in their attitudes to cause and explanation'.[15] Galen himself was, and indeed still is, clearly identified as a Dogmatist, although he was aware of the pitfalls of the Dogmatic approach and of the failure of the Dogmatists themselves to fully understand or adhere to their own principles:

On the other hand, for those who make reason [*logos*] the principle of discovery and order, who propose that this is the one road leading to the goal, there is the necessity to begin from something primary, agreed upon by all men, and in this way then proceed to the rest. They do not in fact do this, but rather the majority take up disputed starting points, not demonstrating them, and proceed to the rest in the same way, laying down the law rather than demonstrating.[16]

The criteria to be met for inclusion among the medical Dogmatists are possibly nowhere more clearly stated than by Celsus: 'Therefore there are those who, professing to a rational medicine, put forward these things as necessary: a knowledge of hidden causes involving diseases; then of evident [causes]; after these of natural actions and last of interior parts.'[17] On these grounds, Galen would certainly qualify as a fully-fledged Dogmatist. Specifically, on the issue of causation he is committed to the quest for 'hidden causes'. Furthermore, on classification, an exhaustive analysis of causes is itself the foundation for the construction of a classificatory system. There is, however, no doubt that Galen recognizes the importance of empirical knowledge, although he characterizes this as possibly 'unsystematic and irrational'.[18] He also recognizes the importance of 'evident causes'. These issues and related terminology are discussed at length in chapters I.4 and I.6.

Galen, then, was opposed in general terms to the Empirics. In characterizing the Empirical school, one may take Hankinson's observation: 'The most striking feature of the Empiricists' position, however, was their consistent refusal to let their theorising take them beyond the realm of immediate

---

[15] Hankinson (1995), p. 78.   [16] *De methodo medendi* X.32K.
[17] Celsus, *De medicina* I, *Proemium* 13.   [18] *De methodo medendi* X.32K.

experience and into the arcana of things by nature obscure . . .'[19] There is
also this more complete description offered by Frede:

What the Empiricists clearly wanted to reject were formal inferences, either deduc-
tive or inductive, in particular inferences by means of which people were supposed
to get a grasp on the theoretical truths which underlie what they could observe,
and more emphatically those inferences which were supposed to lead to theoretical
truths concerning theoretical entities, like the atoms, which can only be grasped
by reason.[20]

Certainly there is agreement on what the Empiricists took as the basis for
practice: *peira, teresis, historia* and *metabasis*, terms which may be equated
with direct experience, observation, historical information about the patient
in question or other patients, and reasoning by analogy, respectively. On
the specific issue of causation, as was recognized by Celsus, the Empiric
accepts evident causes as relevant, but regards the search for hidden causes
as fruitless and unnecessary.[21] Nonetheless, as alluded to above, Galen har-
boured an unquestionable sympathy for medical Empiricism, whilst the
foundational methods of experience, observation, history and analogy have
a continuing relevance to all medical practice.

By contrast, Methodism was relatively evanescent in both theory and
practice and was the school to which Galen was implacably opposed. Based
on the somewhat quirky development of atomism as applied to medicine,
it was attributable to Asclepiades. To characterize Methodism briefly, in
summary it relied on no authority (even the otherwise revered Hippocrates
was an object of criticism), and was based on a theory which involved
'theoretical entities' and could be said to accept 'hidden causes'. The foundational theory was, however, in large part seen as irrelevant to practice.
Medicine was reduced, in effect, to the simple recognition of phenomeno-
logically evident bodily states which, in terms of abnormality, were limited
to only two basic states, constriction and dilatation. A third, intermediary
state was also accepted, this being a mixture of these two primary states.
It was, however, further elaborated by a number of later doctors amongst
whom Themison (first century BC) and Thessalus (first century AD) were
prominent. In their hands it became a medical theory with far-reaching
consequences for both diagnosis and treatment.

Methodism was, as Sextus Empiricus observed, more complete in its
scepticism[22] or empiricism than medical Empiricism itself in that it did
not depend on cumulative experience and so had no recourse to past history,

[19] Hankinson (1995), p. 78.   [20] Walzer and Frede (1985), introduction, p. xxiii.
[21] Celsus, *De medicina* I, *Proemium* 27.   [22] Sextus Empiricus, *Outlines of Pyrrhonism* I.241.

either of the particular patient or of others, no reliance on reasoning by analogy, and did not involve memory other than the recollection required to recognize the particular state. On the issue of causation it did not, despite its theoretical substructure, make use in any way of causal analysis. Also, as Celsus observed, 'the Methodic recognized no cause whatever, the knowledge of which has any bearing on treatment'.[23] It is of some interest to note that although Galen reserved some of his most virulent criticism for the Methodist, Thessalus, this attitude did not extend to another prominent Methodist, Galen's near-contemporary, Soranus.

Less is known about the Pneumatic school than about the others. There is agreement that its founder was Athenaeus of Attaleia, although his dates are unclear and no writings survive, as is the case with other known members of the school, Archigenes of Apamea and Agathinus of Sparta.[24] Some writings do remain, of Aretaeus of Cappadocia, who was, in fact, a contemporary of Galen. In adding the role of *pneuma* to that of the four elements or qualities in their considerations of the genesis of health and disease, the Pneumatics display definite links to earlier philosophical thought, particularly to Diogenes of Apollonia and to Stoic physics, as described above. Galen himself incorporated *pneuma* into his physiological and pathological formulations and was, it might be said, sympathetic towards the Pneumatics as a group. Certainly, in terms of causation they might be seen as espousing the same basic principles, although differing in specifics, as would be expected. In classification, however, there would clearly be differences. The subjects of Galen's own relation to the Pneumatics, and the extent to which they were defined as a school, would undoubtedly bear further study.

To summarize, it may be said that Galen clearly identifies his allegiances. In medicine, his primary authority, revered almost beyond criticism, is Hippocrates. In philosophy, a similar position is held by Plato, although Aristotle is also accorded great respect and importance. In terms of basic concepts, he inherited and developed the physiological system based on the idea of the four elements (fire, air, water and earth) and their related four qualities (hot, cold, wet and dry).[25] Whilst this theory essentially originated with Empedocles, its physiological and medical implications were first substantially developed by Hippocrates. Conversely, Galen remained totally opposed to atomistic concepts, most notably associated with Democritus in philosophy and Asclepiades in medicine. Likewise, his pathology was based principally on ideas of imbalance of the four qualities and their

---

[23] Celsus, *De medicina* I, *Proemium* 54.   [24] See Wellmann (1895) and Kudlien (1962).
[25] For discussion of the latter see particularly Lloyd (1964).

related four humours (yellow bile, blood, phlegm and black bile),[26] ideas
dating back in broad outline to Alcmaeon, but again first clearly formulated by Hippocrates. In both physiology and pathology, however, the role
of *pneuma* and concepts of *dunamis* ('capacity') and *energeia* ('function'),
the former traceable to Diogenes of Apollonia and the latter particularly to
Aristotle, are both of considerable importance.

In methodology generally, Galen's debt was to Plato and Aristotle,
although here the latter must be recognized as more important than the
former even if this greater debt is not explicitly acknowledged. As will be
described later, in this area both Stoic and Sceptic influences can be discerned. In matters of practical anatomy his acknowledged debt is to the
great Alexandrians of the third century BC, of whom Herophilus is clearly
favoured, not so much for the nature of his anatomical work as for his
avoidance of the unacceptable theorizing which Galen objects to in Erasistratus. On the question of schools, Galen is most directly linked with the
Rationalists or Dogmatists, a position certainly defensible on the grounds
of his avowed allegiances. Nonetheless, he is, perhaps, more accurately characterized as a small-e eclectic, a categorization entirely in keeping with the
nature of his education and training in both philosophy and medicine.

Certainly, by the breadth of his learning and the corresponding scope of
his writing, by his acceptance of various strands of thought, some traceable
back six centuries, and by his aggressive eclecticism, it may be, as Manuli
has suggested, that Galen alone did much to still controversy on the central
issues debated by the schools.[27] To what extent our present viewpoint is
clouded by the capricious preservation of one author's works rather than
another's, and by ignorance of other significant social and intellectual forces
then operative, is difficult now to judge at such a distant remove, and
must remain an open question. The fact remains, however, that Galen
was undoubtedly a major force in medical thinking in his own time and
a dominant influence for many centuries after his death. In the following
chapter I shall examine what is, if not the cornerstone, at least a substantial
component of the theoretical foundation of his medical practice – that is,
the interwoven subjects of definition, classification and causation in disease.

---

[26] For the interconnection see, for example, Nutton, in Conrad et al. (1995), p. 25.
[27] See Manuli (1993) for discussion of this point.

Definitions and terminology

This chapter is divided into four sections. In the first of these, four groups of key terms, foundational for Galen's analysis of the classification and causation of diseases and symptoms, are considered. These are (i) ὑγίεια, νόσος, and νόσημα; (ii) πάθος, πάθημα, σύμπτωμα and ἐπιγέννημα; (iii) διάθεσις, ἕξις and κατασκευή; (iv) δύναμις, ἐνέργεια and ἔργον. In the second section, terms specifically related to causation (αἰτία, αἴτιον, πρόφασις and the various qualifying terms) are discussed, with particular focus on Galen's usage in the four treatises under examination. The third section comprises a miscellany of other terms important in the translated treatises. In the fourth and final section a glossary of medical terms used in the treatises is provided. The aim in all four sections is to clarify Galen's own usage. Although in the four treatises being considered and elsewhere,[1] Galen is disparaging about those who he considers waste their time and energies on fruitless terminological debate, it is nonetheless clear that definitions are critical to Galen's enterprise in these four treatises, as the space he devotes to the discussion of such matters indicates. In *De methodo medendi* he also explicitly acknowledges their importance thus: 'And it is shown in those [writings] that the origins of every demonstration are those things appearing to perception and intelligence and that in all things enquired into it is necessary to change the term (ὄνομα) into a definition (λόγος).'[2]

I.4A DEFINITIONS

ὑγίεια **(health).** Although there may be issues as to whether 'health' actually 'exists' and is not simply the absence of disease,[3] Galen is confident that the term signifies a definite 'thing' and so can be defined: 'And in each of

---

[1] See, for example, *De differentiis symptomatum* I.4 (VII.45–6K).

[2] *De methodo medendi* X.39K. This is taken to be a reference to Galen's lost work *On Demonstration*. 'Definition' is here the translation of λόγος following Hankinson (1991), p. 21.

[3] See Guthrie (1975), vol. 4, p. 350 (particularly n. 1).

those [so] signified there is the one same thing in all. So it is too in disease and health. Just as from the saying of "man" one thing is signified, so it is from the saying of "health". Moreover, the language that each of us speaks to others makes it clear that where there is not a homonym in these, what is signified is one thing.'[4] His outright rejection of attempts to define health in terms of the absence of disease is made quite explicit in his attack (in *De methodo medendi*) on Olympicus for presuming to do this.[5] The definitions of health and disease may be terminologically parallel but the two states are seen as independently existing.

At the outset of *De morborum differentiis*, Galen establishes his definition of 'health'. In fact, he offers alternative definitions, one functional or physiological and one structural or anatomical. In the first case, the functions of the body are in accord with nature (κατὰ φύσιν). In the second case, the constitution (κατασκευή) 'of the organs by which we function' is in accord with nature.[6] In both cases there are problems with what exactly is meant by 'in accord with nature'. Galen himself does not grapple with this particular issue in detail, but proceeds to find such accord in 'balance' or 'being in balance' (σύμμετρος – see below). This is a concept which reaches back to Alcmaeon and which is fundamental to continuum theories of structure, positing multiple elements, qualities or humours. Galen, however, accepts that it may also apply to other structural theories, specifically here the πόροι and ἄναρμοι ὄγκοι of Asclepiades. Galen's own preference, unequivocally stated both here and elsewhere, is for a continuum theory which he invokes in support of his identification of 'degrees of health'.[7] Thus, structurally health is a balance of the elements, qualities or humours throughout the body (εὐκρασία) allowing all parts, of whatever complexity, to function 'in accord with nature'. This concept is clearly stated in the pseudo-Galenic *Definitiones medicae* as follows: 'Health is a εὐκρασία in accord with nature of the primary humours in us, or function of the physical capacities that is unhindered. Health is an εὐκρασία of the four primary elements (στοιχείων) from which the body is composed.'[8]

This definition is to all intents and purposes identical with that given in *De methodo medendi*, where Galen also makes the important point that health and disease are two sides of the same coin and must, therefore, be defined in similar terms. He castigates the Methodists for their perceived failure to observe this requirement, and is particularly severe on Thessalus,

---

[4] *De methodo medendi* X.130K.   [5] See *De methodo medendi* X.54 ff. K.
[6] *De morborum differentiis* VI.836–7K.   [7] See his argument in *De morborum differentiis* VI.839K.
[8] *Definitiones medicae* XIX.382K. The definition continues in an attempt to clarify some of the terms used in the definition given.

'the author of their dementia'.⁹ In the four treatises under consideration, Galen essentially recognizes only two states, health and disease, although he accepts that there are degrees of each. This he makes clear in the opening sections of *De morborum differentiis* (particularly II.4) and also in *De sanitate tuenda* V (IV.13–29K). Whether there is some third 'intermediate' state between health and disease is not examined in these works, there being only one mention, in passing, of 'healthy, diseased or neither' without further elaboration of the 'neither'.¹⁰ In the *Ars medica*, however, there is extended discussion of medicine as 'knowledge of those who are healthy, those who are sick and those who are neither', with specific consideration of the last term.¹¹

νόσος/νόσημα (disease). First, it should be said that Galen appears to use these two terms interchangeably, at least in the books under consideration. This is in contrast, for example, to the *Anonymus londinensis*, where νόσος is defined as an 'enduring constitution' (κατασκευή) involving the whole body and νόσημα as an 'enduring constitution' involving a part. The same work further differentiates both words into a general and special sense.¹² For Galen, the situation seems clear: disease is one specific thing just as health is, and the former may be defined as the reverse of the latter. At the start of *De morborum differentiis* he offers complementary structural and functional definitions of disease as he did for health: disease is '. . . either some constitution contrary to nature or a cause of damaged function'. Just as health, then, is a 'balance' so disease is an 'imbalance'.¹³ In returning to definitions at the start of *De symptomatum differentiis*, he combines the structural and functional: 'Now disease is spoken of as being any constitution contrary to nature by which function is harmed primarily.'¹⁴ It is, then, essential to know what a disease is and to know also the basic nature of each disease – 'For in what way basically would you be able to find the means of treatments if you did not know the "substance" (τὴν οὐσίαν) of each of the diseases?'¹⁵ So, in summary, disease is an 'imbalance', just as health is a 'balance', the paired terms referring to whatever is taken to be the fundamental composition of the body – there is balance or otherwise in

---

⁹ See *De methodo medendi* X.41 and 50–1K. The final phrase is Hankinson's translation (1991), p. 26.
¹⁰ *De symptomatum differentiis* I.2 (VII.43K).
¹¹ *Ars medica* I.307–13K. See particularly von Staden's analysis of this passage and its possible Herophilean influences – von Staden (1989), pp. 103–8. The issue of authenticity of this work must also be borne in mind as discussed for example by Garcia-Ballester (1993) in his article on the 'six non-natural things' (οὐ κατὰ φύσιν). See also Kollesch (1988).
¹² *Anonymus londinensis* III.32–45.   ¹³ *De morborum differentiis* VI.837–8K.
¹⁴ *De symptomatum differentiis* VII.43K.   ¹⁵ *De facultatibus naturalibus* II.9 (II.127K).

the size of the πόροι or in the κρᾶσις of the four qualities (heat, cold, dryness, moisture). Further, both 'balance' and 'imbalance' themselves admit of differences of degree. This definition of disease, coupled with a concept of bodily structure based on a limited number of elements, qualities or humours allows a reductive analysis in terms of the permutations of changes in these elements, qualities or humours. Galen is, however, forced to recognize other, purely structural/morphological categories in his classification, as will be discussed in the next chapter (I.5). One final point of interest in relation to the definition of disease is brought out in *De methodo medendi* where he attempts to deal with the apparent difficulty of someone who might claim 'never to have seen a disease-in-itself'.[16] This bears on the issue of the ontological status of 'disease', also to be considered at greater length in the following section (I.5).

πάθος/πάθημα (affection). First, as with νόσος/νόσημα, Galen appears to make no distinction between πάθος and πάθημα in his detailed consideration of terms at the outset of *De symptomatum differentiis*. Indeed, in *De methodo medendi* he makes a specific point about the equivalence of the members of each pair: 'There is no difference in saying νόσος or νόσημα, just as there is no difference in saying πάθος or πάθημα.' He also notes here that the ancients applied the latter to the former.[17] In his definition of πάθος, Urmson has the following: 'The internal accusative of *paskhein*. It is what happens to anything that undergoes, suffers, or experiences anything.'[18] Galen's usage is essentially in accord with this, which leads him into certain difficulties in differentiating this term from others (see below). In his own definitions of the term, both in *De symptomatum differentiis* and in *De methodo medendi*, he appeals to the authority of Plato. In the latter he has:

Thus the ancients also called all movements which were in [the category] 'according to nature', at least those that were not active, affections (πάθη), just as they called the active ones functions (ἐνέργειαι). In this way too, Plato called the actual changes of the senses affections. By the moderns, and I do not know how the notion arose, the term is applied only to the movement contrary to nature. Specifically, then, affection (πάθος) was said by the ancients in the case of every external movement,

---

[16] *De methodo medendi* X.151–3K.

[17] See *De symptomatum differentiis* I.3–6 (VII.43–7K) and *De methodo medendi* X.91K.

[18] Urmson (1990), p. 126. He refers to Aristotle's *Metaphysics* (V.21, 1022b15–21): 'We call an affection (1) a quality in respect of which a thing can be altered, e.g. white and black, sweet and bitter, heaviness and lightness, and all others of the kind; (2) the already actualized (ἐνέργειαι) alterations; (3) especially, injurious alterations and movements, and, above all, painful injuries; (4) experiences pleasant or painful [which] when on a large scale are called affections.' Translation after Ross in Barnes (1984), vol. 2, p. 1615.

whereas those who misuse [the term] also call those things already arisen from an affection and are not still in motion, affections rather than conditions. A condition is not more long-lasting nor more difficult to undo than a state (ἕξις), just as a weakness is not. (X.89K)

In *De symptomatum differentiis* Galen writes: 'What is called an affection (πάθος) or an affection (πάθημα) differs from both [i.e. health and disease], just as Plato himself also made the distinction when he said that should anything at all be affected, some affection (πάθος) must be spoken of' (VII.44K). Galen's problem in these books, alluded to above, is to effect a distinction between πάθος and the other related terms. The fact is that a precise distinction is not possible. There may be a relatively clear differentiation from νόσος/νόσημα in that the latter is enduring (and therefore a διάθεσις) as well as being contrary to nature, and also from ἐνέργεια in that the latter is active as opposed to passive. Demarcation from both διάθεσις (to which Galen links πάθος/πάθημα through the verb διάκειμαι) and from σύμπτωμα is less clear. This is one of the problems Galen attempts to deal with in the initial sections of *De symptomatum differentiis*. In summary, the distinction between an affection and a condition is most clearly made on the ground that the former is still in progress whilst the latter is an established change. The distinction between an affection and a symptom hinges on what is in accord with nature and what is contrary to nature. Nonetheless, it is evident from a consideration of all the definitions in this subsection that these distinctions are not hard and fast, something of which Galen himself is obviously cognizant. It must also be borne in mind that the term πάθος has a specific usage in relation to the soul (psychology).[19]

σύμπτωμα/ἐπιγέννημα (**symptom/epiphenomenon**). At the outset of *De symptomatum differentiis* Galen writes: 'Every condition (διάθεσις), then, of the body which departs from that which accords with nature is either a disease, a cause of disease or a symptom, which some doctors call an ἐπιγέννημα (epiphenomenon) (VII.42K). This is his consistent position both in this work and in the *De methodo medendi*. In the latter, for example, he provides the following definition:

Apart from this there is another fourth class of condition (διάθεσις) which is present in bodies which are both in accord with and contrary to nature, but which neither aids nor damages functions. For example, it may happen that the colour of the whole body is changed from pale to dark in those who have spent a long time in the sun, or from dark to pale in those who have spent a long time in the

---

[19] See, for example, Galen's criticism of Chrysippus' definition of πάθος in the latter's lost work *On the Affections* in *De placitis Hippocratis et Platonis* IV.1–3.

shade, or to red in those who have washed, or to white in those who are afraid. But this is neither a function nor a condition of the body causative of function, much less a cause bringing about conditions contrary to nature. It is, rather, a symptom occurring of necessity in the case of the different changes of bodies. (X.64–5K)

In the same place he goes on to stress the distinction between symptoms that damage function (to which he here adds the term ἐξαίρετον) and those which do not (for which he offers four terms: οἰκεῖα, ἴδια, συμπίπτοντα and κατά τινα τύχην). There is undoubtedly some variation in how Galen defines a symptom, as is evident from a comparison of the excerpt from *De methodo medendi* quoted above with what is said in *De symptomatum differentiis* I.9. There, amongst other things, Galen says: "The specific characteristic of a symptom is this: it is contrary to nature" (VII.51–2K). There is, then, some blurring of the distinction between symptom and disease at one end and between symptom and affection at the other.[20]

ἐπιγέννημα is a rather problematical term for which it is difficult to find a satisfactory English rendering. I have used 'epiphenomenon', although from what follows below, 'disease symptom' might be more appropriate. LSJ offers 'after-symptom' referring to the *De symptomatum differentiis*. This does not seem to me what Galen, who only uses the term twice in these books and acknowledges that it 'is not a very usual term among the Greeks', intends.[21] The clearest statement appears to be that in *De symptomatum differentiis* where it is said: 'For example, someone may not wish to call something immediately a symptom but an ἐπιγέννημα, for a symptom is anything contrary to nature that might befall an animal whereas an ἐπιγέννημα is not anything except what necessarily follows diseases alone' (VII.51K). The pseudo-Galenic *Definitiones medicae*, however, uses the term in the definition of 'symptom' – 'A symptom is an ἐπιγέννημα of an affection (πάθος)' (XIX.395K) – and does not make the specific correlation with disease. The term is also found in Diogenes Laertius in relation to pleasure, where Hicks translates it as 'by-product' in keeping with the more general definition.[22]

---

[20] Hankinson (1991) offers the following analysis of 'symptom': 'This is a type of disposition (his rendering of *diathesis*), that is of a body or part of a body constituted in a certain way, but one which has no causal bearing on any of the *energeiai*. It will be apparent from this that a *sumptōma* differs from its contemporary homophone, either in its general or its medically exact usage (although in many cases it reasonably approximates to the former, as Galen's examples suggest). None the less, as there is no obvious modern English rendering for *sumptōma*, I have preferred simply to transliterate it with this interpretative *caveat*' (p. 152).

[21] *De symptomatum differentiis* VII.42–3K.

[22] Diogenes Laertius (Zeno) VII.86. Translation by Hicks, vol. 2 (1931).

διάθεσις/ἕξις/κατασκευή (**condition/state/constitution**). διάθεσις is a problematic term, not least because of its continuing use in medicine in a varying sense right up to the present time and also because, like δύναμις, it had in Greek writings a much wider range of use than in medicine alone. This semantic range is explicitly recognized by Galen in the opening sections of *De symptomatum differentiis* which are devoted to clarification of terminology.[23] The variation of usage of διάθεσις over time is considered in detail by Ackernecht.[24] On the specific medical use relevant to Galen, von Staden has written: 'Διάθεσις for a bodily state, condition or disposition subject to fairly quick and abrupt change had become a *terminus technicus* of medicine and biology by the time of Herophilus.'[25] Whilst any one of the three possible glosses offered by von Staden would suffice, I have chosen 'condition'. Certainly Galen's employment of the term falls within this description. He is, in fact, quite clear in his usage as the following several examples illustrate. Thus, in *De symptomatum differentiis* as noted above, he writes: 'For each thing that exists is in some sense in a condition, whether it be healthy, diseased or neither. Now the term "condition" is derived in some way from "to be in a certain condition" (διακεῖσθαι), having been brought to this usage not only by the ancient philosophers but also by other Greeks.'[26] The following statement from the *De locis affectis* brings out the temporal distinction between 'condition' (διάθεσις) and 'affection' (πάθος): 'For sometimes an affection arises from a certain cause but in some way is not yet a stable condition if the cause is separated. Sometimes it has already come about or is still coming about. Often when the cause is gone the coming about ceases and it is already a stable condition" (VIII.25K). Thirdly, from a practical point of view, '. . . there is nothing else to be cured by doctors apart from the condition of bodies'.[27] It is clear, then, that 'condition' is a critical term in Galen's definitions of health and disease, but like the other terms and phrases ('function', 'in accord with nature' and 'contrary to nature'), it has an irreducible imprecision – which is, after all, only a reflection of how things actually are.

The second term in this group, ἕξις,[28] is one which Galen uses very infrequently in these books. The distinction between ἕξις and both διάθεσις and κατασκευή appears to depend on the greater stability and duration of the first. LSJ offers 'system' as a medical meaning with reference to Mnesitheus

---

[23] See *De symptomatum differentiis* VII.43K.
[24] Ackerknecht (1982).   [25] von Staden (1989), p. 114.
[26] *De symptomatum differentiis* VII.43K.   [27] *De methodo medendi* X.63K.
[28] See Lee (1997) for a detailed consideration of this term, albeit with particular reference to its misunderstanding in New Testament lexicography.

amongst others, but this does not seem entirely appropriate here. Aristotle, who deliberates at some length on the distinction between ἕξις and διάθεσις, makes the following observation: 'A state differs from a condition by the latter being easily changed whereas the former is longer-lasting and more difficult to change. States are also conditions but conditions are not necessarily states. For those who are in states are also in a certain condition in some way on account of these, but those who are in a certain condition are not always also in a state.'[29]

I have rendered κατασκευή as 'constitution' to make the distinction from διάθεσις, although 'condition' would probably serve for both. Certainly Galen appears to accept the two as interchangeable when he writes in the *De methodo medendi* (following a further statement of his basic definitions of health and disease in terms of functions): 'If health is some condition (διάθεσις) or constitution (κατασκευή) in accord with nature, so disease will necessarily be some condition or constitution contrary to nature' (X.52K). Another statement from the same work which also helps in understanding Galen's usage of the term is as follows:

Just as we need to have the whole part for the sake of function, in the same way, I think, we also desire its constitution to be in accord with nature for the sake of function. For as was said earlier, constitution has the ground of cause with respect to function. Those things that of necessity follow the constitutions from which we function when we are healthy are called 'accidentals', but are called symptoms when we are diseased. And these are the four classes of all things involving the body, when we are either in accord with nature or contrary to nature: functions, constitutions, the things that precede these and the things that follow them.[30]

Again, either term would seem to be satisfactory here.

δύναμις/ἐνέργεια/ἔργον (**capacity/function/action**). δύναμις is not a term defined in the four treatises being considered. It is, however, a term of considerable importance in these works, as it is in a number of philosophical and medical works prior to Galen.[31] It is variously translated as 'capacity', 'faculty', 'potentiality' and 'potency'. The term is considered in detail by Aristotle in *Metaphysics* V.12. It is defined in the first of the three

---

[29] *Categories* VIII, 9a8–13. Ackrill, in his translation, uses 'state' (see Barnes (1984), vol. 1, p. 14), whilst Cooke and Tredennick (1938) use 'habit' (p. 65). In the present context the former seems the better.

[30] *De methodo medendi* X.70K. Hankinson (1991) in his translation uses 'condition' here for κατασκευή.

[31] It is not my intention here to embark on a detailed analysis of this complex term. It is found in the fragment from Alcmaeon discussed below and in the Hippocratic Corpus – see, for example, Miller (1952) and Miller (1960). Its use in Plato has been considered in detail by Souilhe (1919). Aristotle's usage is of particular relevance to Galen, especially in conjunction with ἐνέργεια; see Lloyd (1968), pp. 63–5 for an informative summary. Galen himself has a treatise ΠΕΡΙ ΔΥΝΑΜΕωΝ ΦΥΣΙΚωΝ (*De facultatibus naturalibus*) II.1–214K.

meanings given there as follows: 'Capacity, then, is the source, in general, of a change or movement in another thing or in the same thing *qua* other, and also the source of a thing's being moved by another thing or by itself *qua* other.'[32] Phillips says of Galen's use of δύναμις in *De facultatibus naturalibus*, that 'The notion of δύναμις in this book is very pervasive and mostly verbal, being a development in medicine, not of δύναμις as known in *Ancient Medicine*, but of the Aristotelian δύναμις as potentiality contrasted with ἐνέργεια, activity or actuality, also Aristotelian.'[33] Galen himself, in the work in question, has the following statement linking the three terms above: 'That is to say, I shall call the action (ἔργον) what has been already brought about and 'filled up' by the function (ἐνέργεια) of these, for example the blood, flesh and nerve. I term the active movement the function and the capacity (δύναμις) the cause of this.'[34] He also writes, in *Quod animi mores,* that

Many of the wise are openly in confusion on this matter, having an incorrect understanding of 'capacity' (δύναμις). They seem to me to wrongly conceive of 'capacity' as something which dwells in substances, as we do in houses, not being aware that the effective cause of each thing that comes about is conceived of in relation to something else, and there is some name of this cause as of such a thing which is separate and *per se.* But in it, in relation to what is brought about from it, the 'capacity' is of what is brought about, and because of this we say that substance has as many capacities as it has functions (ἐνέργειαι). (IV.769K)

I have chosen to translate ἐνέργεια consistently as 'function' in accord with one of the definitions given in LSJ as 'physiological function'. The reference is to *De sanitate tuenda*, where Galen writes:

Certainly one must not, therefore, determine those who are healthy and those who are diseased simply by strength or weakness of functions, but one must attribute 'in accord with nature' (κατὰ φύσιν) to those who are healthy in contrast to 'contrary to nature' (παρὰ φύσιν) to those who are diseased, that is for the former to be a healthy condition (διάθεσις) in accord with nature effecting functions, and for the latter to be a diseased condition (διάθεσις) contrary to nature harming function. (VI.21K)

This statement is clearly relevant also to the definitions of health and disease, and to that of διάθεσις. Several translators render ἐνέργεια as 'activity' whilst I have distinguished it from ἔργον by using 'action' for the latter. But Galen himself makes the specific point that the two terms are essentially interchangeable when he writes in *De methodo medendi*, in relation to the

---

[32] *Metaphysics* 1019a18–21, translation after Ross in Barnes (1984), vol. 2, p. 1609.
[33] Phillips (1987), p. 176.   [34] *De facultatibus naturalibus* I.2. See Brock (1916), pp. 12–13.

eye: 'For it is agreed then, in this case, by all men, not only by doctors but also by those they meet, that it is its [the eye's] action [ἔργον] to see. And whether I say 'action' (ἔργον) or 'function' (ἐνέργεια) certainly makes no difference now in this case' (X.43K).

A similar indifference is displayed by Linacre in his sixteenth-century Latin translation where, within the space of two sentences, he uses *actio* and *functio* interchangeably for ἐνέργεια. Galen himself does not define the term in the four treatises under consideration but does do so as follows in *De methodo medendi*:

Vision is the function of the eyes, speech of the tongue, walking of the legs. Again, the function is this active movement and the movement of these things is a change of what there was before. The active movement is that which is from the thing itself, whereas the passive at any rate is from something external. For example, flying is the function of what flies and walking of what walks. (X.45–6)

ἔργον, then, becomes the 'action' carried out by the 'function', although Galen's own remarks on the equivalence of ἐνέργεια and ἔργον quoted above should be borne in mind. Nevertheless, my own understanding of the use of the three terms is essentially identical to that of Brock in his introduction to *De facultatibus naturalibus*.[35]

In attempting to summarize Galen's usage of these key terms it might be said that the body as a whole, or each one of its identifiably separate parts (μόρια), are at all times in a certain condition (διάθεσις) or have a certain constitution (κατασκευή), which amounts to the same thing. In a condition of health, the body and its parts have the capacity (δύναμις) to carry out a series of different functions (ἐνέργειαι), the results (ἔργα) of which maintain the status quo in accord with nature (κατὰ φύσιν). For example, in the case of digestion, the body (or at least its relevant parts), when in a normal condition, has the capacity to digest food (the exact mechanism need not be specified). If this capacity is unhindered in its function, the result is digested food. However, factors both external and internal, acting jointly or in isolation (i.e. αἴτια), can act on this system (ἕξις) to produce changes in its condition. These changes may be accommodated within the range of normal (κατὰ φύσιν), in which case they are affections (πάθος, πάθημα) or they may be abnormal (contrary to nature – παρὰ φύσιν), in

---

[35] See Brock (1916), introduction, pp. xxix–xxxi. There he writes: 'Any of the operations of the living part may be looked on in three ways, either (a) as a δύναμις, faculty, potentiality; (b) as an ἐνέργεια, which is the δύναμις in operation; or (c) as an ἔργον, the product or effect of the ἐνέργεια.' He then continues his analysis by means of a comparison with some concepts advanced by Bergson in his then very influential work, *L'Évolution créatrice* – see n. 1, pp. xxx–xxxi.

which case they are either diseases (νόσος, νόσημα) if they involve damage (βλάβη) to function, or symptoms (σύμπτωμα) if they do not. It must, however, be recognized that within this scheme there is, first, an irreducible vagueness in the key definitional terms (διάθεσις, κατασκευή, κατὰ φύσιν, παρὰ φύσιν), a range of causal terms (see below), and an inevitable overlap in the resulting altered states (affections, symptoms, diseases).

I.4B   CAUSAL TERMS

These terms may be considered under two headings: primary, nominal terms of which there are, in essence, two – αἰτία/αἴτιον and πρόφασις – and qualifying terms which are relatively numerous. Some of the latter Galen makes use of and some he does not. These will be listed and briefly considered below after initial discussion of the primary terms.

Primary causal terms

αἰτία/αἴτιον **(cause).** The root meaning of both words is 'responsibility/guilt/blame'. When 'cause' is intended, at least broadly, it must still be determined whether it is meant in the sense of an 'agent' or more as 'explanation'. This is especially relevant in Aristotle's writings which are themselves of considerable significance in early discussions of causation. This is a problem recognized long ago, for example by Schopenhauer, but recently brought to attention again by Vlastos in particular.[36] A further issue is whether a distinction is to be made between the two forms themselves, αἰτία and αἴτιον. Several modern writers have addressed this question, notably Frede, who refers to Stobaeus' account of Chrysippus' distinction as follows: 'But an αἰτία, he [i.e. Chrysippus] says, is an account of the αἴτιον or the account about the αἴτιον as αἴτιον.'[37] How far this distinction, which might be characterized as that between non-propositional cause and propositional explanation, is preserved in the various accounts of causation is an issue not addressed here. What does seem incontrovertible is that in the four treatises being dealt with here, as in others of his works, Galen generally does not make this distinction. Thus, in *Synopsis librorum suorum de pulsibus*, having listed *synektic, proegoumenic* and *prokatarktic* causes, he writes: 'It is quite clear that it does not matter whether one says

[36] See Schopenhauer's *On the Fourfold Root of the Principle of Sufficient Reason* (1847), translated by Payne (1974), pp. 9–13, Vlastos (1969) and Hocutt (1974). See also section I.4c below.
[37] Frede (1980), p. 134.

"causes" in the feminine or "causes" in the neuter' (IX.458K). Galen does provide a clear definition of 'cause' in *De symptomatum differentiis* I.6:

That which from its own nature contributes some part of the genesis by its occurrence is called its cause. There are a number [of causes] according to class: the material, the useful, the objective, the instrumental and that from which there is origin of movement. Each of these contributes some joint action to what happens, whereas those which contribute nothing, yet are not separate from those that do, hold the relation of those not without.[38]

There is the following definition of αἴτιον in the pseudo-Galenic *Definitiones medicae*: 'A cause is what does something in the body but is itself "asomatic". The cause, as the philosophers say, is the effector of something or by which something happens. Cause is threefold: there is the *prokatarktic*, the *proegoumenic* and the *synektic*' (XIX.392K). The Latin version in Kühn has here *evidens*, *antecedens* and *continens* respectively. This last differentiation suggests Stoic influence and may also owe a debt to Athenaeus, but overall the definition does correspond closely to Galen's usage in the four treatises, although there may be some question about 'asomatic'.

In summary, I have taken Galen to be using 'cause' (αἰτία/αἴτιον) in the modern sense in relation to disease. His employment of the qualifying terms enumerated below is variable and inconsistent, depending in part on his subject matter and in part on his polemical purpose.

πρόφασις (cause). This is a word of considerable interest, particularly in early historical texts, and has been the subject of at least three specific studies.[39] Unlike αἰτία/αἴτιον, there are doubts about its derivation and also about the significance of the prefix. Like αἰτία/αἴτιον, the basic meaning is not 'cause' but rather 'pretext' or 'excuse'. Pearson draws attention to Pindar's description of πρόφασις as 'the daughter of afterthought'. For present purposes the issue is, how, and how frequently, Galen uses it. Is it simply an alternative word for 'cause' carrying no additional or different connotation, or is something more implied? LSJ gives its medical use as 'external exciting cause', whilst Hankinson suggests it is, '. . . simply the ostensible reason or surface cause for something, as contrasted with its full cause or complete reason (generally denoted in the Hippocratic corpus by the term αἴτιον)'.[40] It is, in fact, not a widely used term in Galen. In the four treatises under examination, it is used twice in *De causis morborum* and five times in *De symptomatum causis*. Galen makes no attempt to define it as he does with the other causal terms, and it is not defined in the pseudo-Galenic *Definitiones medicae*. In answer to the question posed above, it seems to be used simply as another word for 'cause'. This is how I have translated πρόφασις — without embellishment — as indeed De Lacy does in *De placitis Hippocratis et Platonis* V.2.4 and V.2.9. The term also appears, for example, in *De facultatibus naturalibus* II (II.121K) where Galen speaks of the cause of disproportionate heat producing *dyscrasia*, and also in *De methodo medendi* (X.805K) where in using the word in relation again to disturbances of heat, he feels obliged to add 'external'.

Qualifying causal terms

In the four treatises under consideration, Galen draws attention to three distinct groups of qualifying causal terms as set out below. In addition, he uses the two terms πρόδηλα and ποιητικόν once only in each case and without further elaboration.

προηγούμενος/προκαταρκτικός/συνεκτικός (*proegoumenic/prokatarktic/synektic*). Although these terms may have Stoic origins, it is Athenaeus' classification on which Galen's use of them is based, as he makes clear in the following passage from *De causis contentivis*:

As for Athenaeus the Attaleian, he founded the medical school known as that of the Animists. It suits his doctrine to speak of a cohesive cause (*coniunctam causam*) in illness since he bases himself upon the Stoics and was a pupil and disciple of Posidonius. But it does not suit the theories of those other doctors who hold different views to look for a cohesive cause in every illness nor the try to find it in the *homoiomeres* in their narural state and they cannot say, as Athenaeus did, that there are three types of primary cause that are ultimate in their class: first that of the cohesive causes (*coniunctarum*), then that of the prior causes (*antecedentium*) while the third type is compossed of the matter of the immediate causes (*procatarcticarum*). This latter term is applied to externals *whose function it is to produce some change in the body, whatever this change may be.*[41]

---

[40] Hankinson (1998), p. 58.

[41] *De causis contentivis* II.1–3; see Lyons (1969), p. 55. The Latin terms in parentheses are from Kalbfleisch's text included in the same volume (p. 134). The author's italics in the final sentence indicate an area of difference between Arabic and Latin texts.

Galen himself offers a succinct definition of *proegoumenic* and *prokatarktic* causes in *De causis morborum* II.5 where he writes: 'They then call either conditions pertaining to the animal itself, or movements contrary to nature, *proegoumenic* (internal antecedent) causes of diseases and those things that befall [the animal] from without and greatly change or alter the body, initiating or *prokatarktic* (external antecedent) causes' (VII.10K). The same statement is also made in *De methodo medendi* X.65–6K. Each of these two is used only twice more in the four treatises. In *De morborum differentiis* VII.4 (VI.861K) *proegoumenic* is used with specific reference to the constriction of the nasal channels which might follow a blow. It is the nasal distortion which is the *proegoumenic* cause of disease, being a deviation from the form which accords with nature. Subsequently, in *De symptomatum differentiis* I.8 (VII.54K), he makes the point that *proegoumenic* causes of diseases which exist in the body of the animal may be subsumed under the heading of symptoms. In the first of the two further references to *prokatarktic* causes (II.2, VII.54K), Galen stresses that these are not symptoms (in distinction from *proegoumenic* causes). In the second reference the distinction is made from the following pair of causal terms (*per se* and *per accidens*) as follows:

It is appropriate presumably to consider in all such cases what is primary and *per se*, and not through another intermediary, the cause of the final result, not what is called *prokatarchontic* or *prokatarktic*, which Hippocrates saw fit to remind us of many times in other places and in saying: 'It is sometimes the case in *tetanos* without a wound (*helkos*), in a well-conditioned young man during the middle of summer, that a pouring on of copious cold brings about a restoration of heat, and heat relieves these things.'[42]

Du Bois, in his sixteenth-century Latin commentary on these treatises, offers the following definitions of *proegoumenic* and *prokatarktic* causes: (i) 'προηγούμενος – that is preceding or internal, is an affection or movement outside nature occurring in the animal itself'; (ii) 'προκαταρκτικός – that is, evident and external, which approaching externally, forcefully alters and changes bodies'.[43]

The third of these three terms (συνεκτικός) is somewhat more problematic. If we accept that this is a Stoic term, and closely linked to Stoic concepts of bodily structure, especially involving *pneuma*, it is questionable how far it is relevant to Galen's account of disease causation. This will be considered further in chapter I.6 below. It should be noted, however, that it appears only three times in the four treatises, all in *De symptomatum causis* and all related to specific examples as follows:

[42] *De symptomatum causis* VI.6.   [43] Du Bois (1539), p. 4.

For, as one might say, the *synektic* cause of its genesis is tension of the choroid membrane, just as conversely relaxation is of constriction. And since it is stretched in a twofold way when it is affected by virtue of itself, either being dried as an *homoiomeric* [part], or made moist as an organic [part], its dryness is difficult to cure but its moistness is not. (VII.93K)

Therefore, the *synechic* cause, or *synektic*, or *prosechic*, or however someone might wish to term it, is some such condition in the nerve as to impede the capacity being sent down to it from the *arche*. So then, it is impeded if the nerve has some channel, just as is clearly seen with respect to those in the eyes due to obstruction or compression. If it does not have [a channel], it is due to contraction, cooling or compression. (VII.109K)

Especially in these, heat is a *synektic* cause of not being hungry inasmuch as it loosens solid bodies by relaxing them and makes them weaker in terms of attraction, whilst moist bodies are stretched still more by dissolving. (VII.132K)

Three points that might be made about *synektic* causes are: first, that they are internal causes; second, that it is probable that they must be synchronous with their presumed effects; and third, that they might be taken as the final internal mechanism responsible for the effect.

καθ' ἑαυτό/κατὰ συμβεβηκός. These are somewhat problematical terms which I have translated throughout as *per se* and *per accidens* respectively although Urmson for one takes exception to this rendering.[44] The terms are attributable to Aristotle, particularly in the *Physics* (192b22 and 211a18–25). In the latter place he writes: 'There is that which is moved by an action *per se* and that *per accidens*. Of the latter there is that which admits of being moved *per se*, like the parts of the body or the nail in a ship, and that which does not admit of [being moved] but is always [moved] *per accidens*, like whiteness or wisdom, for these have only changed place insofar as they are in that which changes.'[45] Galen is at some pains to clarify these terms, equating them with 'primary' and 'secondary' respectively although he does not, in fact, use them extensively. The basic definition follows his Aristotelian listing in *De symptomatum differentiis* and makes his use, at least, quite clear:

... it is often possible when causes succeed one another, for a certain series to occur, as when many small stones are placed next to each other and someone moves the first one, this [moves] the second, and that the third, and so on in order, each [moving] the one adjacent to it. In all such things, unless one distinguishes that which is said to act *per se* from that which acts *per accidens*, many very absurd

---

[44] Urmson (1990), pp. 85–6.
[45] See also Aristotle, *Metaphysics* (1020a16 and 1052a18) as well as Theophrastus, *De sensu* (22.2).

errors will occur in the arguments. Moreover, *per se* signifies the same as 'primary', even if some Atticizers avoid the term, whereas *per accidens* specifies the same as 'secondary'. Therefore, the one applying a finger to the first stone moves this 'primarily', whereas [he moves] the one following it *per accidens* or 'secondarily', and in the same way then also all the others. In this way too the first stone moves the second *per se*, whilst [it moves] the third and others in turn *per accidens*. (VII.48K)

Shortly after, in specific relation to disease, he states:

... it is possible that some other condition precedes the disease itself that is contrary to nature yet not, in fact, harmful to function by reason of itself, but through the mediate disease. We shall not call such a condition a disease but a cause antecedent to a disease, and here we shall give careful consideration to those who assert that that condition is a cause of damage to function. For not *per se* and primarily, but *per accidens* and secondarily, shall we say function is hindered and harmed by this, whereas primarily and by reason of itself by the actual disease. (VII.49–50K)

ἡ ὕλη, ἡ χρεία, ὁ σκοπός, τὸ ὄργανον, τὸ ὅθεν ἡ ἀρχὴ τῆς κινήσεως. In *De symptomatum differentiis*, following a general definition of cause, Galen gives this 'Aristotelian' list of causes:

That which from its own nature contributes some part of the genesis [of something] by its occurrence is called its cause. There are a number [of causes] according to class: *the material, the useful, the objective, the instrumental and that from which there is the origin of movement*. Each of these contributes some joint action to what happens, whereas those which contribute nothing, yet are not separate from those that do, hold the relation of 'those not without'. (VII.47–8K)[46]

Having offered this classification, Galen makes no further use of the terms in these treatises.

In summarizing Galen's use of causal terms in the four treatises, the following points may be enumerated.

1. He predominantly uses αἰτία or αἴτιον to denote cause and makes it clear that he regards the two terms as interchangeable.
2. Occasionally he uses πρόφασις, apparently with the general sense of 'cause', but does not elaborate on his use of this term. There is, however, no evidence, either in the four treatises examined or in other texts, that it has some more specific or restricted meaning.
3. He does define 'cause' in *De symptomatum differentiis* and there speaks of a fivefold classification similar to Aristotle's four causes and his own

---

[46] For a discussion of Galen's use of Aristotle's analysis of causation see chapter I.6 below and also Hankinson (1998), pp. 379–85.

discussion of these in *De usu partium* VI. He does not, however, use this classification in his description of the causes of diseases or symptoms.

4. He makes a point of clarifying the usage of the two terms προ-ηγούμενος and προκαταρκτικός with the definitions of each given at VII.10K and quoted above, but barely mentions these terms again.

5. προηγούμενος is used on two further occasions. The first describes it as a cause '. . . which exists in the actual body of the animal' and as 'subsumed under the notion of the class "symptom"' (VII.53K). The second is a specific example – the physical distortion of the nose due to a blow which interferes with the respiratory channel so causing a disease (VI.861K).

6. προκαταρκτικός is also used on two further occasions, the first stating that such causes are not symptoms (VII.54K) and the second that they act through an intermediary (VII.125K).

7. συνεκτικός is used three times in specific examples: tension in the choroid membrane as a cause of pupillary dilatation; a condition of nerves which impedes the flow of capacity from the *arche*; heat as a cause of loss of appetite by relaxing bodies. All are, then, internal, structural and coexisting with the effect.

8. He does also at times use the terms καθ' ἑαυτό and κατὰ συμβεβηκός in the sense of primary and secondary, the latter being a type of cause mediated through something else.

9. Of other possible terms, he uses ποιητικόν once in the general sense of 'effecting' (VII.212K) and πρόδηλα once to describe a list of causes of rupture of blood vessels, all traumatic and all external (VII.232K).

10. In the four treatises he addresses the issue of disease and symptom causation from a very practical standpoint, making very little, indeed no significant use of qualifying terminology to clarify causal mechanisms.

I.4C GENERAL TERMS

αἴσθησις (**sense perception**). The pseudo-Galenic *Definitiones medicae* has the following:

Sense perception (αἴσθησις) is an affection of the soul through the body convey-ing information of movement. How do αἴσθησις, αἰσθητήριον, αἰσθητόν and αἰσθητικόν differ? They differ [as follows]: αἴσθησις is the capacity functioning; αἰσθητήριον is the organ entrusted with a certain αἴσθησις; αἰσθητόν is what falls on the sense; αἰσθητικόν is the thing actually sensing. For example, αἴσθησις is sight, taste, smell or the remaining senses hearing and touch; αἰσθητήριον is the eye, nose or tongue, and the sensing organs being presented; αἰσθητόν is wood, stone and pillar and all things falling on those sensing; αἰσθητικόν is Theon or Dion or whatever other animals sense. (XIX.378–9K)

These definitions make the distinction between several aspects or components of the sensory process and are of particular relevance in *De symptomatum causis* I. The concept of process implied is that there is a functioning capacity responsible for sensation which acts primarily in the actual organ of sensation in response to the presentation of the sensed object to the perceiver. Whilst the usage of the first three terms is clear and might correspond to 'sense perception', 'sense organ' and 'sensibilia' respectively, the last is less clear where the definition appears to be somewhat at odds with usage in *De symptomatum causis* I. Specific issues of terminology in relation to sensory function will be given in the footnotes to the translations where applicable. An extended analysis of Galen's concepts is provided by Siegel.[47]

ἀλλοίωσις/ὁμοίωσις **(alteration/assimilation).** Galen is quite clear in his use of these two terms which, in general, may be taken as 'change/alteration' and 'the making like [of something]' respectively. In their application to digestion, common in Galen, I have rendered them 'alteration' and 'assimilation' respectively. In relation to ἀλλοίωσις Galen follows the Aristotelian use (see *Physics* 226a26–8) in regarding the alteration or change as a form of movement (κίνησις).[48] In *De locis affectis* Galen writes: 'Movement is twofold according to class; alteration (change – ἀλλοίωσις) and spatial movement (φορά)' (VIII.32K). In a more extended definition he writes, in *De facultatibus naturalibus*:

. . . and at any rate it is not only those things changed with respect to colour or flavour that we say are moved, but also with what becomes hot from being cold or cold from being hot, we say that they are moved too, just like with something becoming dry from being moist or moist from being dry. The common term we apply to all these things is 'alteration' (ἀλλοίωσις). (II.3K)

A little later in the same passage he makes reference to Aristotle's writing (*On the Complete Alteration of Substance*) and to Chrysippus' work on the same topic (II.4K). With particular reference to digestion, and a comparison of the mechanisms of the stomach and intestines, there is detailed discussion in *De facultatibus naturalibus* II.164–6K. The second term, ὁμοίωσις, is less frequently used and is largely specific for digestion in Galen's works. Both terms are used adjectivally (as ἀλλοιωτικός and ὁμοιωτικός) and may be applied to δύναμις (see *De facultatibus naturalibus* II.143K).

[47] Siegel (1970).   [48] See also Theophrastus, *De causis plantarum* IV.5.5.

ἄμετρος/σύμμετρος (**imbalance/balance**). These two terms are essential components of Galen's definitions of health and disease where they are translated as above. In other contexts, 'disproportion' and 'proportion' may be more appropriate. In the initial definitions in *De morborum differentiis* (II.1) the former has been used. Galen at first leaves open the question as to what health and disease are a balance and imbalance of respectively, but then identifies two possibilities: 'pores' (see πόρος) and 'qualities' (see εὐκρασία/δυσκρασία). He makes the following somewhat more expanded statement in *De sanitate tuenda*:

Health surely is a balance (συμμετρία) according to all the schools. According to us it is [a balance] of moisture, dryness, heat and coldness, but according to others of 'masses' (ὄγκος) and 'pores' (πόρος) and to others again of 'indivisibles' (ἄτομος), or of *anarmoi* (ἄναρμος), or of 'things without parts' (ἀμερής), or of *homoiomeres* (ὁμοιομερής), or of whatever, in fact, [there is] of primary elements (στοιχεῖον). But according to all [schools] at least, we function through a balance of these things in the parts. So if, then, we function differently, the difference is the balance in relation to each of the elements, which was health. (VI.15K)

The paired terms are used by Plato also in relation to health and disease (as well as virtue and vice), although not as definitions (*Timaeus* 87d). ἄμετρος is a term also used in other disciplines such as mathematics (Aristotle, *On Indivisible Lines* 968b6), writing (Aristotle, *Poetics* 1451b1) and ethics (Plato, *Laws* 690c).

ἀνάδοσις/διάδοσις (**distribution**). I have taken these two terms together to indicate the whole process of distribution of food following the preparatory processes which take place in the stomach: the former (ἀνάδοσις) to indicate distribution to the tissues, and the latter (διάδοσις) distribution into the tissues. In this I am influenced by May in her translation of *De usu partium*, although she simply leaves the terms in their transliterated form.[49] In his translation of the *De facultatibus naturalibus*, Brock appends this note to I.2: 'In Greek *anadosis*. This process includes two stages: (i) transmission of food from alimentary canal to liver (rather more than our "absorption"); (ii) further transmission from liver to tissues. *Anadosis* is lit. a yielding-up, a "delivery"; it may sometimes be rendered "dispersal". "Distribution" (*diadosis*) is a further stage.'[50] For Galen's use of ἀνάδοσις

---

[49] See May (1968), vol. 1, pp. 226–8 for ἀνάδοσις and vol. 2, p. 465 for διάδοσις. In her note 5, p. 465 she writes: '*Diadosis* (διάδοσις) means for Galen the assumption by the tissues of the nutriment delivered to them by the veins.' But also, referring to *De facultatibus naturalibus* I.2 and II.6 (II.7K, 104K) she speaks of '. . . assumption of the nutriment . . .' taking place '. . . directly, without the benefit of veins'.

[50] Brock (1916), p. 13, n. 5 – see also p. 163, n. 4.

see, for example, *De symptomatum differentiis* IV.9 (VII.73K). He does not, in fact, use διάδοσις in the four treatises.

ἀπαθής **(impassible).** This term, of obvious derivation, has a wide range of meaning. Galen uses it in these four treatises in the metaphysical sense of 'something incapable of being acted upon' applied to elementary particles. Elsewhere, he uses it to describe tissue unaffected by a disease process (see *De atra bile* V.122K). For a more general usage see, for example, Aristotle, *Topics* 148a20 and *Metaphysics* 1019a27.

ἀπόκρισις **(separation).** I have retained the more general and fundamental meaning for this word (see, for example, Anaxagoras, *Fragment* 4, SVF, vol. II, p. 34). This is in preference to the more specific medical meanings of 'excretion' and 'secretion' listed as such in LSJ. In referring to the capacity so named, my translation is, then, the 'separative capacity'. Brock (1916) speaks of the *eliminative faculty*, even in relation to the pregnant uterus (see *De facultatibus naturalibus* II.148–9K). The more basic and general term 'separation' seems to fit better with the range of processes to which it is applied by Galen. Guthrie, in his discussion of the philosophical use, takes the term to be the same as ἔκκρισις.[51] (See also ἔκκρισις below.)

ἀρρωστία **(weakness).** This term is widely used by Galen, not only in the nominal but also in the adjectival and adverbial forms, in a general sense to describe 'weakness'. In the four treatises it is particularly used in those on symptoms in relation to function – see, for example, *De symptomatum differentiis* IV where Galen speaks of 'weakness of function' in relation to the stomach, for which he also uses the more specific term 'debility' (ἀτονία). The term is similarly used in *De facultatibus naturalibus* (II.152–3K), and in relation to muscles in *De usu partium* I.XIX (III.67–73K). Other biological/medical examples of the terms are to be found in Hippocrates, *Ancient Medicine* VI and Aristotle, *History of Animals* 634b14.

βλάβη **(damage, harm).** This is a recurring term in these four treatises insofar as it figures in the basic definition of disease as well as more generally in relation to function (ἐνέργεια), itself a term of particular importance. Like many of the terms considered here, it has a much wider application than to medicine or biology alone. Galen, however, is relatively specific in his usage, at least in these treatises. A typical example of his usage from outside these treatises is the following passage from *De methodo medendi*:

---

[51] See Guthrie (1962), vol. 1, p. 89.

Heat is the name of a simple thing. And, further, damage to function is a simple thing. However, such an amount of heat as already to damage function is no longer similarly simple. If, moreover, it involves the whole body, it is then far less a simple thing. So that men do not commonly speak thus, it being in their nature to practise brevity, but term such heat 'fever', for it is easier to say that Dion is febrile than that he has such an amount of heat in the whole body as to damage many functions. (X.150–1K)

διάπλασις (**conformation**). This term is of particular relevance in classification, being one of the kinds in the genus of diseases of organic bodies. It may refer to congenital and acquired abnormalities of form exemplified not only by visible disturbances of outward form but also by changes in internal cavities and channels, and by alterations in the roughness or smoothness of their surfaces – see *De morborum differentiis* VII.1–4 (VI.856–62K). Hankinson, in his translation of Books I–II of *De methodo medendi*, renders διάπλασις as 'configuration'.[52] In *De usu partium* it is listed with 'position', 'size' and 'contexture' as a 'contingent attribute'.[53]

διαφορά (*differentia*). Although a common term meaning 'difference' generally, διαφορά, which is a recurring term in all four treatises, and particularly the first and third where it appears in the titles, has for the most part in these works the meaning it carries in logic and taxonomy. This usage is particularly attributable to Aristotle – see, for example, *Metaphysics* 1057. It also occurs repeatedly in the first and second books of *De methodo medendi* in a similar context – see, for example, Book I, X.20–9K and Book II, X.83–6K. Nevertheless, in the titles of these two treatises it is usually translated as 'differences'. Even Hankinson, in his translation of Books I and II of *De methodo medendi*, gives the titles as *The Differences of Diseases* and *The Differences of Symptoms* despite using '*differential differentiae*' throughout the text and giving a detailed analysis of its specific usage (pp. 99–103). Other renderings in the titles include 'distinctions' (Singer) and 'differential diagnosis' (Siegel). Galen himself provides an analysis of the term in *De differentiis pulsuum* (VIII.628–30K). One further point is whether the use in the titles is singular (perhaps 'differentiation') or plural, as I have taken it to be. Certainly there is use of the singular by Galen in referring to the works in some instances in other texts. Latin versions generally use the

---

[52] See Hankinson (1991), p. 63 where he has, 'Of the complete organs, one type of disease is concerned with configuration . . .' (X.125K).
[53] These are May's (1968) terms for θέσις, μέγεθος and πλοκή. She also uses 'conformation' for διάπλασις — see May (1968), p. 80 (I.19H, III.26K). A similar group of attributes including conformation is also discussed in *De usu partium* VI.7 (I.316H).

plural in the titles, even where the singular is indicated by the article in the text.

ἔκκρισις (**separation**). As with ἀπόκρισις above, I have retained what I take to be the basic meaning of this term – 'separation'. Urmson refers to the use by Simplicius to describe Anaxagoras' concept of the 'separating out' of the *homoiomeres* from the original confusion as also discussed in relation to ἀπόκρισις above.[54] It is a term widely used by Galen, but particularly in the treatises on symptoms, in *De locis affectis* (where Siegel translates as 'excretion'), in *De usu partium* (where May uses 'elimination' or 'evacuation'), and in *De alimentorum facultatibus*. Aristotle in his biological works uses the term with reference to menstrual fluid and semen amongst other things (see, for example, *Parts of Animals* 689a16, *Generation of Animals* 727a2 and *History of Animals* 583a2), where 'excretion' would not be appropriate and 'elimination' or 'evacuation' also not entirely satisfactory. The brief entry in the pseudo-Galenic *Definitiones medicae* – 'ἔκκρισις is the passage out of superfluities present in bodies' (XIX.363K) – is in accord with Galen's usage in the four treatises.

ἐλλιπής/πλημμελής (**deficient/defective**). The basic meaning of these two words might be taken as 'wanting' or 'defective' in the former and 'out of tune', 'faulty' or 'erring' in the latter. They are the two terms which Galen uses in the treatises on symptoms to describe disturbances of function, which are the bases of his classification of symptoms. In this context, I have taken the first to indicate reduced normal function and the second to indicate abnormal function. Interestingly, the two terms are only used together in the two works (*De symptomatum differentiis* and *De symptomatum causis*), six times adjectivally and twice adverbially. In several instances they are used in association with στέρησις (privation) and μοχθηρός (distress/distressing) – see below.

ἔμφραξις (**obstruction**). LSJ gives 'stoppage' as the meaning of this term, but in a medical text 'obstruction' seems more appropriate. Galen makes considerable use of the term in all four treatises. It is used in relation to sweat in the pseudo-Aristotelian *Problems* (870b19). With respect to Galen's usage, the important point is that it is in relation to both the 'theoretical' πόροι of Asclepiades and the Methodics and macroscopic channels such as the bowel – see *De morborum differentiis* V.1 and VII.2 respectively.

[54] Urmson (1990), p. 51.

ἐπίκτητος **(acquired).** The transition from the basic meaning of 'gained in addition' to 'acquired' in relation to characteristics is unremarkable. The sense of Galen's use is well exemplified by Aristotle's use in *Generation of Animals* 721b30, where the distinction is made between 'congenital' (τὰ σύμφυτα) and 'acquired' (τὰ ἐπίκτητα): 'And these opinions are plausibly supported by such evidence as that children are born with a likeness to their parents, not only in congenital but also in acquired characteristics . . .'[55]

εὐκρασία/δυσκρασία **(*eucrasia/dyscrasia*).** These two terms are fundamental to the definitions of health and disease, describing a normal and abnormal 'mixing' of the components of the body (elements/qualities/humours) respectively. They are typically rendered 'good temperament' and 'bad temperament' but I have chosen rather to transliterate them both. The definition from the pseudo-Galenic *Definitiones medicae*, already given on p. 22 above, is repeated here: 'Health is a εὐκρασία in accord with nature of the primary humours in us, or function of the physical capacities that is unhindered. Health is a εὐκρασία of the four primary elements (στοιχείων) from which the body is composed' (XIX.382K).

εὐρύτης/στέγνωσις **(dilatation/constriction).** These are the two terms which Galen uses to refer to contrasting abnormal states of the 'theoretical' πόροι, as in the *De morborum differentiis* in relation to the primary division of diseases in simple bodies (IV.1, VI.842K). Health, on the basis of Methodic pathology as interpreted by Galen, is a balance in the calibre of the πόροι, whilst disease is an imbalance due to deviation in either direction. As above, I have used 'dilatation' and 'constriction' respectively in translation.

λύσις συνεχείας **(dissolution of continuity).** This is an important term in that it designates one of Galen's three major genera of diseases: (i) *dyscrasias*; (ii) disorders of morphology; (iii) dissolutions of continuity. With regard to the term itself, two points should be made. The first is that Galen believes it to be a class of diseases not previously named (*De causis morborum* XI.1); and the second that there is variation in terminology. Thus Galen also uses διαίρεσις or διαφθορά instead of λύσις, and ἕνωσις instead of συνεχεία. De Lacy gives a list of different works in which the components of the term differ in the course of a general consideration of Galen's concept of 'continuity' (συνεχεία).[56] In the same article he also examines previous usage of similar terminology, particularly by Hippocrates, Diogenes

---

[55] Translation after Platt in Barnes (1984), p. 1121.
[56] See De Lacy (1979), and particularly p. 356 for the list.

of Apollonia, Aristotle and Diocles of Carystus, as well as considering the wider application of the terms. In addition, Kollesch and Nickel have two entries under the title *De dissolutione continua* in their recent 'Bibliographia galeniana'.[57] With respect specifically to the four treatises, Galen himself foreshadows the use of the term in *De morborum differentiis* IV.5 before introducing it in section XI.1 of the same work as λύσις ἑνώσεως. He again discusses it in *De causis morborum* XI.1 where he speaks of three terms: λύσις ἑνώσεως, διαφθορά ἑνώσεως and λύσις συνεχείας. In Galen's classification, the main distinguishing feature of this genus is that it is applicable to both *homoiomeric* and organic structures, unlike the other two classes. Whilst it is clear what kinds of diseases Galen is including in this class – fractures in bones, avulsions in sinewy or ligamentous structures, ulcers in flesh – the lines of demarcation are not altogether clear in that the first two could conceivably be considered under disorders of morphology whilst Galen himself notes that the last can be due to a *dyscrasia*.

μάνωσις **(rarefaction)**. This term, defined in LSJ as 'making loose or porous, rarefaction' is taken to be the converse of πύκνωσις. It is a term rarely used by Galen: five times in *De causis morborum* in opposition to στέγνωσις and four times in *De methodo medendi* in opposition to πύκνωσις. In the former, I have rendered it 'rarefaction' consistently although in some of the instances 'dilatation', which I have used for εὐρύτης (vide supra), might be preferable. In the latter, Hankinson uses 'looseness' in relation to the Asclepiadian πόροι.[58] In their translation of Theophrastus' *De causis plantarum* (IV.14.2), where the term is used in opposition to πύκνωσις, Einarson and Link use 'open texture'.[59]

μοχθηρός **(abnormal)**. This is a common term, widely used by Galen. In the four treatises it is extensively used in *De symptomatum causis* (52 instances according to the TLG). I include it here because I have employed a somewhat unusual translation as 'abnormal', quite remote from the usual moral overtones.[60] It is also common in *De locis affectis*, particularly in association with χυμός. Siegel speaks of 'noxious humours' but 'abnormal' might also be preferable there.[61] In his translation of *De placitis Hippocratis et Platonis* (another text in which the word is commonly used) De Lacy renders it as 'faulty' in relation to movements (κίνησις) and actions (ἐνέργεια).[62]

[57] Kollesch and Nickel (1993), p. 1394.
[58] *De methodo medendi* X.95K – see Hankinson (1991), p. 48.
[59] Einarson and Link (1990), vol. 2, p. 347.
[60] See, for example, Hankinson's use of 'wicked' in *De methodo medendi* X.10K – Hankinson (1991), p. 7.
[61] For example, *De locis affectis* VIII.2K, Siegel (1976), p. 16.   [62] De Lacy (1978), vol. 2, p. 256.

ὁμοιομέρεια/ὁμοιομερής (*homoiomere/homoiomeric*). Both the noun and adjective have been directly transliterated in the translation. The LSJ entries are limited to single meanings – 'having like parts' and 'having parts like each other and the whole' – for noun and adjective respectively, meanings obviously in accord with derivation and certainly applicable to Galen's usage. A common English translation is 'uniform'. There is some suggestion of the attribution of the terms to Anaxagoras – indeed, Galen refers to this in *De placitis Hippocratis et Platonis* V.3.18 (De Lacy, vol. 1, p. 308). Usage is, however, particularly associated with Aristotle, both in relation to inanimate things (*Meteorologica* X–XIII, 388a10–390b20) and animate things (*Parts of Animals* II, 648a6–655b27). There are several places where Galen clearly defines what he means by *homoiomeres*. Thus, in *De elementiis secundum Hippocratem,* he describes them as '. . . the primary parts with respect to perception', and lists arteries, veins, nerves, ligaments, membranes and flesh as *homoiomeres* in humans (I.493K). In *De placitis Hippocratis et Platonis* the list differs slightly, including cartilage, bones, nerves, membranes, ligaments and all other such things (VIII.4.7–15, De Lacy, vol. 2, p. 500). Here he also provides the following definition, having considered the term's biological application to stem particularly from Aristotle: 'Therefore, bodies in one outline (προσγραφή) are often called *homoiomeres* because all their parts are similar to each other and to the whole, and they are also often called simple or primary.' In *De morborum differentiis* Galen lists arteries, veins, nerves, bones, cartilage, ligaments, membranes and flesh as *homoiomeric* structures and clearly states that these are the components of organic bodies (see below), and are themselves formed from the primary elements (III.1, VI.841K). In *De methodo medendi* he writes: 'A part is *homoiomeric*, as the name itself also clearly shows, which is divisible into similar parts throughout, like the vitreous and the crystalloid and the specific substance of the membranes in the eye' (X.48K). Galen has a specific work on the subject, *De partium homoeomerium differentia libelli*, not included in Kühn because not surviving in Greek.[63]

ὄργανον/ὀργανικός (**organ/organic**). The basic meanings of these terms are 'instrument' and 'instrumental'. In application to the structures of the body, they then come to mean what carries out a function, or is the instrument by which a function is carried out. May, in her translation of *De usu partium*, retains 'instrument' as the translation.[64] Galen offers the following clear definition of 'organ' in *De methodo medendi*:

---

[63] Strohmaier (1970), CMG, Suppl. O, III (Arabic and Latin).
[64] See May (1968), vol. 1, pp. 67–8.

I term an organ a part of an animal which carries out a complete function, like the eye with respect to vision, the tongue to speech and the legs to walking. In this way too artery, vein and nerve are organs and also parts of the animal. And according to this usage of terms at least as defined, not only by us but also by the Greeks of old, the eye will be termed a 'constituent part' (μόριον), a 'part' (μέρος) and an 'organ.' (X.47K)

There is, then, overlap between *homoiomere* and organ, as is brought out in the almost immediately following discussion of the eye in the same work: 'For the organ is the eye whilst the function is vision. One of its parts is both *homoiomeric* and the primary organ of vision – the crystalline humour – as is shown in the works on these' (X.48K). As to the combination of *homoiomeres* to form organs, there is the following from *De elementiis secundum Hippocratem*: 'For each of the *homoiomeres* arises from these humours, whilst when these [*homoiomeres*] come together with each other they form a primary and most simple organ which arises through nature for the sake of a single function. And when these in turn come together with each other they create another and greater organ . . ." (I.481K). These accounts are closely akin to Aristotle's descriptions in *Parts of Animals* II.[65]

περίττωμα **(superfluity).** I have translated this term as 'superfluity' throughout in the interests of consistency, although there are clearly times when 'excretion' or 'excrement' would be appropriate. Peck, in the introduction to his translation of Aristotle's *Parts of Animals*, writes: 'This term I have translated throughout "residue", as being more literal and at the same time less misleading than "excrement". "Surplus" would have been even better if the word had been a little more manageable.'[66] De Lacy uses both 'residue' and 'waste' in his translation of *De placitis Hippocratis et Platonis*.[67] Galen, in the four treatises, uses the term in relation to a variety of bodily processes. 'Superfluity' seems to capture the essential meaning as, indeed, Peck's 'surplus' would.

πόρος **(pore/channel).** This is another word with a wide range of meaning, applying to both inanimate and animate things. In relation to the latter,

---

[65] A description of the biological usage and the distinction between 'uniform' and 'non-uniform' parts in Aristotle's biology may be found in Peck's (1965) introduction to the *History of Animals*, pp. lxii–lxiv. Aristotle's own detailed description in relation to biology is found in *Parts of Animals* II (646a6–655b27), and in relation to inanimate structures in *Meteorologica* X–XII (388a10–390b20). Hankinson's (1991) discussion of Galen's usage in *De methodo medendi* is also helpful (pp. 139–40). Finally, the discussion of μόριον by Peck and Forster (1937) in their introduction to Aristotle's *Parts of Animals* is informative, especially in relation to Galen's use of the terms involved in his disease classification (pp. 28–30).

[66] Peck and Forster (1937), pp. 32–3.   [67] For example, De Lacy (1978), vol. 3, p. 387.

the following passage from Vallance's work on Asclepiades, referring not only to πόροι but also to ἀγγεῖον, ὀχετός and ὁδός, gives a clear idea of Galen's usage:

Such words are often, though not always, used to refer to visible passages which can be discovered anatomically. Aristotle uses πόρος (usually qualified in some way) of blood vessels and the urethra; the term has a history, perhaps going back to Alcmaeon, of being applied to various sensory tracts – in particular the optic 'nerve'. Galen uses the word in a variety of ways, some of which look remarkably close to those he attributes to Asclepiades. But most often Galen's pores are visible passages: the urethra (or ureter), for instance, the 'bile-ducts', the windpipe, the 'spermatic ducts', the ethmoid passages, the 'optic passage', and the 'acoustic passage'. Galen is always keen to set himself up as someone who does not believe what he cannot see by experiment and observation, and he frequently qualifies πόρος with αἰσθητός.[68]

In the treatises translated here, the distinction between 'Asclepiadian' and macroscopic πόροι (in such structures as listed above) is signalled by the use of 'pores' for the former and 'channels' for the latter, although perhaps 'lumina' would be a more appropriate rendering in a medical text. The term was also used, as it is now, for the pores of the skin through which, according to ancient physiology, 'superfluities are transmitted' – see Galen's *De sanitate tuenda* (VI.218–19K) for this usage in conjunction with both στέγνωσις and ἔμφραξις.

στέρησις **(privation).** I have used 'privation' consistently for this term although simple 'loss' or 'absence' might be preferable. In Aristotle's definition in *Metaphysics* V.22 (1022b22–1023a8), considering the broad application of the term, translators commonly use 'privation'.[69] Galen's usage in the four treatises is particularly in relation to 'function' (ἐνέργεια) where he speaks of the tripartite classification of disturbed function – loss or privation (i.e. complete absence – στέρησις), deficiency or reduction (ἐλλιπής), and defect or abnormality (πλημμελής, μοχθηρός).

στοιχεῖον **(element).** Galen uses this term both in the specific sense of primary structural component of matter, the sense broadly that has endured in modern science, and in the more general sense of a fundamental component of any composite entity or system. The two uses are found close together, for example, in *De morborum differentiis* (VI.840K for the former and VI.836K for the latter). Knowledge of what the primary elements in the first sense are, is of critical importance to medical practice in Galen's view. As he writes elsewhere in *De morborum differentiis*: 'From this it is

[68] Vallance (1990), pp. 50–1. [69] For example, Ross in Barnes (1984), vol. 2, p. 1615.

also obvious that none of the primary diseases, such as are specific to the *homoiomeres* themelves, will be able to be treated rationally without due consideration being given to the primary elements' (VI.854K). He is quite clear, both in these works and in others (see particularly *De elementis secundum Hippocratem*) as to what he considers these primary elements to be – hot, cold, moist and dry. The pseudo-Galenic *Definitiones medicae* has the following definition:

An element is that from which, as primary and most simple, all things arise and to which, as most simple and least, all things are resolved. So Athenaeus the Athenian says in the third book. The elements of medicine are, as certain of the ancients understood, heat, cold, moisture and dryness, from which appearing primary, simplest and least, man is put together, and to which as seeming extreme, most simple and least, he suffers (takes) resolution. (XIX.356K)

θερμόν, τὸ ἔμφυτον (**innate heat**). Whilst this is a concept of fundamental importance in Galen's thinking, it does not feature to a major extent in his analysis of diseases and symptoms in the four treatises. The main discussion of 'innate heat' is in relation to cold *dyscrasias* in *De causis morborum* (III.2–5). It is, however, considered in his specific work on abnormal movements (*De tremore, palpitatione, convulsione et rigore*), movements which are themselves given detailed consideration in Book II of *De symptomatum causis*. In the former, there is the following clear statement of how Galen understands 'innate heat':

We do not posit masses and pores as elements of the body, nor do we declare that heat comes from motion or friction or some other cause; rather, we suppose the whole body breathing and flowing together, the heat not acquired nor subsequent to the generation of the animal, but itself first and original and innate. This is nothing other than the nature and soul of life, so that you would not be wrong thinking heat to be a self-moving and constantly moving substance. (VII.616K)[70]

A good summarizing discussion on Galen's view of 'innate heat' is given by May and a broader consideration by Siegel.[71]

φύσις (κατὰ φύσιν, οὐ κατὰ φύσιν, παρὰ φύσιν) (**nature, accord with nature, non-accord with nature, contrary to nature**). 'Nature' is itself an important and complex term. Galen's usage of the word is undoubtedly influenced by Hippocratic and Aristotelian considerations which won't be entered into here.[72] The main relevance in the four treatises is the usage in

---

[70] Sider and McVaugh (1979), p. 199.
[71] See May (1968), vol. 1, pp. 50–2, Siegel (1968), pp. 164–8 and also Solmsen (1957).
[72] For discussion of this matter see, for example, Miller (1952) re the former, and Lloyd (1968), chapter 4, pp. 68–93, and Ross (1995), pp. 69–71 re the latter.

the terms κατά and παρά φύσιν, key elements in his definitions of 'health' and 'disease' respectively. A third, and possibly intermediary, state οὐ κατά φύσιν (or οὐ φύσει), which is found particularly in the *Ars medica* and is discussed in English as (the six) 'non-naturals',[73] is not mentioned in this manner in the four treatises. Returning to the two principal definitions, clearly an understanding of φύσις itself is essential to a proper understanding of the definitions. Galen does not, however, address this issue in these texts. In general, the terms are translated as 'in accord with' and 'contrary to' nature, respectively. This assumes an understanding of what 'nature' means in this context. The pseudo-Galenic *Definitiones medicae* has the following which relates the terms to health and disease:

Health is that which is in accord with nature. Disease is that which is contrary to nature. What is 'natural' (φύσει) but neither 'in accord with nature' nor already 'contrary to nature', is like someone very thin, or dry, or thick-set, or fat, or sharp-nosed, or grey, or snub-nosed, or grey-eyed. Those who are thus are not in a condition 'in accord with nature' for they have gone beyond 'balance' but neither are they 'contrary to nature' for they are not hindered with respect to functions. Such a thing that is 'non-natural' (οὐ φύσει) is neither 'contrary to nature', nor 'in accord with nature', nor 'natural'. Examples are those having *leuke*, leprous warts, warts and the like. For these are not 'in accord with nature' as they are outside what accords with nature, but nor are they 'contrary to nature' for they do not hinder the functions that accord with nature. They are not, however, 'natural' in that they do not occur from the beginning, nor are they from the initial genesis. They remain, therefore, 'non-natural'. What is 'non-natural' by definition is close to what accords with nature and what is contrary to nature. (XIX.384–5K)

χρεία (use). This is a term only infrequently used in the four treatises, although it is obviously important to Galen as evidenced by its use in the title of one of his major works, *De usu partium*. Certainly, in the four treatises χρεία does not feature in the major definitions – ἐνέργεια is the key term. May, in the introduction to her translation of *De usu partium*, has the following to say about the distinction between χρεία and ἐνέργεια which I think summarizes Galen's position admirably: 'The Greek χρεία of the title, which I have chosen in most cases to translate "usefulness", does not mean function, as one might naturally suppose. Function is more nearly ἐνέργεια or "action", in Galen's terms. χρεία means for him rather the suitability of a part for performing its action, the special characteristics of its structure that enable it to function as it does.'[74]

---

73 For example, Niebyl (1979), Bylebyl (1979), Garcia-Ballester (1993).
74 May (1968), vol. 1, p. 9.

χυμός **(humour).** Apart from the occasional use in the general sense of 'juice' or 'flavour', this term is used to indicate the four basic humours of the body. The pseudo-Galenic *Definitiones medicae* has the following explanation:

χυμός in Hippocrates is invariably applied to the humours in the body of which our structure is – that is, of blood, phlegm, and the two biles, yellow and black. In Plato and Aristotle the gustatory quality which each of these has in us is also termed humour. These are the qualities of sharpness, dryness, harshness, acridness, saltiness, sweetness and bitterness. So Mnesitheus meant in his pathology. (XIX.457–458K)

1.4D   DISEASES AND SYMPTOMS

This is intended as a more or less exhaustive list of the diseases and symptoms mentioned by Galen in the four treatises. Those that he identifies clearly as symptoms are marked *. A double * is used to indicate the rendering[s] given in the translation. The reference to the text in each case is to the most significant description but other references are given where appropriate. The three modern works referred to are Grmek (1991), Mettler (1947) and Siegel (1976 – unless otherwise stated).

*ἀγρυπνία **(insomnia**, wakefulness).** Linked with κῶμα as a symptom of the sensory component of the soul (VII.58K). According to Galen both are, '. . . due to involvement of the "primary sense" itself which is . . . common to all sensations'.

ἀθέρωμα **(tumour full of gruel-like matter).** Listed with diseases in which 'excess' causes disturbed function (VI.863K). See also VII.22K.

αἱμορροΐς **(haemorrhoids).** As in present usage. See Mettler, p. 806 for early descriptions, and VII.82K.

αἱμωδία **(a sensation of having the teeth set on edge, haemodia**).** Identified as a symptom of the tactile capacity and brought on especially by acidic and sour foods – see VII.108K. There is a more detailed description in *De locis affectis* (86–110K) where Siegel, in his translation of this work, equates it with gingivitis.

ἀκροχόρδων **(wart** – pedunculated).** Listed among examples of diseases in which 'excess' causes disturbed function (VI.863K).

ἀλφός **(alphos).** LSJ gives 'dull-white leprosy, esp. on the face'. This is not leprosy in the present sense of the word, but probably a loss of skin pigmentation, i.e. a skin disease. It is classified by Galen (VI.849K) among the *dyscrasias* of *homoiomeric* bodies due to a substance flowing in from without.

ἀλωπεκία (**bald patches on the head, a disease like mange in foxes in which hair falls out,** *alopecia***). For the first description see the pseudo-Aristotelian *Problems* 893b38. Attributed by Galen to a nutritional failing – see VII.63K. For Celsus' description see Mettler, p. 665.

*ἀμβλυωπία (**dim-sightedness**). One of the three symptoms of disturbed vision indicating deficient function – see παρόρασις, τυφλότης (VII.56K). For causes see VII.99K.

*ἀναισθησία (**lack of sensation,** *anaesthesia***). Included among *dyscrasias* of cold but as a symptom rather than a disease (VI.851K). LSJ also gives 'unconsciousness, insensibility, mental obtuseness, stupor' but Galen's usage in these treatises appears to correspond quite closely to modern usage.

ἀνὰ σάρκα (*anasarca*). One of the forms of dropsy; also called *leukophlegmasia* or *hyposarca* – see Mettler, p. 339. For Galen's definition see *De locis affectis* V.7 (VIII.353K).

ἄνθραξ (**carbuncle, pustule***). Linked with φλεγμονή, ἐρυσίπελας and ἕρπης as diseases that give rise to another disease i.e. fever (VI.860K).

*ἄνοια (**amentia**). A complete failure of mental function – see VII.60K. See also Siegel, pp. 274–5 for related terms and a list of causes. Mettler, in her table on p. 524, takes it to indicate underactivity of the rational component of the *hegemonikon* specifically.

*ἀντίας (**tonsillitis**). Attributed in *De sympt. caus.* III to a flux from the head affecting '. . . the glands situated opposite each other on both sides in the boundary of the mouth' (VII.270K).

ἀνωμαλία (**irregularity, indisposition, malaise***). A sense of unease indicating the early stages of a *dyscrasia* – see *De morborum temporibus* VII.435K.

*ἀπεψία (*apepsia*). Complete failure of digestion. Part of the symptom range, *apepsia, bradypepsia, dyspepsia* (VII.66K).

ἀποπληξία (**apoplexy***, **paralysis**). Listed as a primary *dyscrasia* of cold (VI.850K). See Mettler, pp. 490 ff. for a discussion of this and related terms.

ἀπόσπασμα (**avulsion****, **tearing away of bone, severing**). An example of dissolution of continuity (VI.872K).

ἀπόστημα (**abscess**). Listed with diseases in which an 'excess' causes disturbance of function (VI.863K). Also a disease which may interfere with the patency of a cavity or channel (VII.31K).

ἀρθρῖτις (**gout, of or in the joints**). Listed as a disease in which altered form impairs function (VI.856K).

ἀσκίτες (*ascites*). One of the forms of dropsy and a term still in use – see *anasarca* above. Attributed to serous superfluities by Galen (VII.224K).

ἀτονία (**slackness, enervation, debility****). Galen appears to use this term in a general way to describe a mild *dyscrasia* without visible manifestations. He goes to some length to define it in VI.853–4K.

ἀτροφία (**atrophy**). Taken to be a non-specific loss of substance – see VI.869 where Galen makes a somewhat unclear distinction between atrophy and *phthisis*.

ἀχώρ (*achor*). A skin condition affecting the scalp (VII.22K). For Paul's description see Mettler, p. 666.

*βαρυηκοΐα (**hardness of hearing**). One of the three symptoms of disturbed auditory function – see παράκουσις, κωφότης (VII.56K). For causes see VII.102K.

*βήξ (**cough**). Grouped with the disordered movements at the start of *De sympt. caus.* II (VII.147K).

βλαισός (**bent, distorted, splay-footed, knock-kneed****). Listed as an example of a disease in which an abnormality of form impairs function.

βλάστημα (**outgrowth****, **excrescence**). Used in a general way. A potential cause of obstruction of a channel.

*βορβορυγμός (*borborygmus*). A symptom detected by hearing – like ἦχος and τρυσμός – see VII.79K.

βουβών (**swollen glands**). Listed among causes of hot diseases (VII.5K).

βούλιμος (*bulimia***, **ravenous hunger**). see VII.136K. For a detailed description see Siegel, pp. 253–5.

*βραδυπεψία (*bradypepsia*, **slowness of digestion**). Indicates reduction or slowness of normal digestion (VII.66K).

γαγγλίον (*ganglion***, **encysted tumour on a tendon or aponeurosis**). Probably similar to present usage. Attributed by Galen to 'fluxion' and included as a disease in the class of change of form (VII.22, 35K).

γάγγραινα (**gangrene**). Attributed by Galen to inflowing material and linked with *herpes, erysipelas* etc – see VII.21–2K.

*γονόρροια (**spermatorrhoea**). A disordered movement; a form of spasm (*spasmos*) or a weakness of the retentive capacity – see VII.150K.

*δῆξις (**gnawing**). Considered as a symptom of a disturbance of the retentive capacity (VII.68K).

*διαβήτης (*diabetes*). See VII.81K for three types. See also Mettler, p. 347 for a detailed description of the term's usage in ancient times including a translation of part of Aretaeus' *On the Causes and Symptoms of Chronic Diseases.*

διαπυΐσκομαι (**to suppurate throughout**). Linked with σκιρόομαι (to become indurated), φλεγμαίνω (to be heated, inflamed), σφακελίζω (to be gangrened, mortify), and οἰδίσκω (to swell, enlarge) as processes causing distortion or obstruction of channels within bodies (VI.858K).

δυσεντερία (**dysentery**). Classified in detail in VII.246–7.

*δυσθυμία (**despair, depression****, **ill-temper**). Attributed to the action of black bile on the rational part of the soul (VII.203K).

*δυσουρία (**difficult micturition**). Used as a general term for disturbance of micturition (VII.59K).

δυσπεψία (*dyspepsia***, **disordered digestion**). An abnormal rather than a reduced or absent digestion – see *apepsia, bradypepsia.* A more general use than at present – see VII.53, 62, 66K.

ἐγκανθίς (**tumour in the inner angle of the eye**). A disease in which increase in size causes disturbed function (VI.870K).

ἔγκαυσις/ἔκκαυσις (**sun-stroke, heat-stroke****). Listed among the hot *dyscrasias.* I have taken the two terms to be interchangeable although LSJ has 'sun-stroke' for the former and 'heat-stroke' for the latter.

εἰλεός (**intestinal obstruction****, *ileus* **). A general term for types of failure of the retentive capacity in the gastro-intestinal tract (VII.69K). See also VII.220K where *ileus* is used.

ἐλεφαντίασις (*elephantiasis*). This is not elephantiasis in the present sense but possibly leprosy – see Grmek, pp. 168–76. Galen classifies it among the *dyscrasias* of *homoiomeric* bodies due to a substance flowing in from without (VI.849K).

ἐλέφας (*elephantiasis*). Taken as interchangeable with ἐλεφαντίασις.

ἕλκος (**wound, sore, ulcer****). See VI.853K with regard to the stomach and VII.37K as an example of 'dissolution of continuity'.

*ἐμπνευμάτωσις (**flatulence**). A possible symptom in disturbed digestion (VII.269K).

ἐμπροσθοτονία/ἐμπροσθότονος (**tetanic procurvation, drawn forward and stiffened, *emprosthotonos*****). Listed as a primary *dyscrasia* of cold (VI.850K). For a detailed description of this and related terms see Mettler, pp. 349–56.

ἐντεροπλοκήλη (**intestinal hernia**). Listed as a disease due to disturbed combination of parts (VI.870K).

ἐξάρθρησις/ἐξάρθρημα (**dislocation**). Grouped with παράρθρησις (subluxation) among diseases in which changes in (relative) position disturb function (VI.870K). For a more complete description see VII.36K.

ἐπιληψία (**epilepsy**, epileptic fit, stoppage**). Listed as a primary *dyscrasia* of cold (VI.850K). See *De locis affectis* III.11 for Galen's identification of three types of epilepsy (VIII.193K ff.).

ἐπιπλοκήλη (**hernia of omentum**). Listed as an example of an organ disease due to abnormal position (VI.870K, VII.36K).

*ἐρεθισμός (**irritation**). Linked with insomnia as due to excessive dryness or heat (VII.144K).

ἕρπης (*herpes***, **shingles**). See ἄνθραξ above. Grmek argues that the ancient descriptions may be of chickenpox – see pp. 335–6. See also Mettler, p. 666.

*ἐρυγή (**belching**). Grouped with the disordered movements at the start of *De sympt. caus.* II (VII.147K).

ἐρυσίπελας (*erysipelas*). This probably does include what is currently termed erysipelas, a β-haemolytic Streptococcus pyogenes skin infection, but has, in Galen's time, a wider application. Grmek writes: '. . . the term erysipelas in Greek medical parlance designates various diseases that "redden the skin" and also diffuse, purulent inflammations of internal organs, but in its commonest sense it designates a group of skin diseases with hot, painful, reddish swelling, now thought to be streptococcic dermatitis' (p. 129). In Galen's classification it is *dyscrasia* of *homoiomeric* bodies due to an inflowing substance (VI.849K).

*ἡσυχία (**stillness, inertia****, **quiescence****). Included as a symptom – see the 'three quiescences' (VII.153K).

ἴκτερος (**jaundice**). Described as a symptom relating to improper separation of superfluities (VII.63K).

*ἰσχουρία (**retention of urine**). As an injury of a physical function see VII.150K.

*καρδιαλγία (**heartburn**). Used as an example of pain at a particular site (VII.58K). Described at VII.135–6K as '. . . a sensory symptom of the opening of the stomach distressed due to mordant humours'.

*καρηβαρία (**heaviness in the head****, **headache**). Mentioned as a possible symptom in disturbed digestion (VII.269K).

καρκινός (**an eating sore or ulcer, cancer****). Used in relation to a superficial abnormality in VI.874K and attributed to black bile (VI.875K).

*κάρος (**heavy sleep, torpor, unconsciousness****). Probably best taken as applying to a reversible loss of conciousness, possibly including deep sleep. Mentioned as a consequence of both head trauma and trephining – see *De locis affectis* VIII.231–3K.

κάταγμα (**fracture**). An example of a disease due to 'dissolution of continuity' (VI.872K).

*κατάληψις (**catalepsy**). This term does not have the specific meaning it has acquired in relatively recent times. It is, to a significant degree, interchangeable with κατόχος/κατοχή although neither of these terms is used in the translated treatises. See Mettler chapter 8, pp. 487–600 for use of the terms over the centuries and also pseudo-Galen *Definitiones Medicae* XIX.414K.

*κατάπτωσις (**collapse****; **also used for epileptic seizures**). Linked with *leipopsychia* in relation to gastric disturbances (VII.136K).

*κάταρρος (**running from the head, catarrh****). Grouped with *coryza* as a symptom pertaining to the nose (VII.107K).

56   Galen

καῦσος **(a bilious remittent fever)**. See VII.183K.

*κεφαλαλγία **(headache)**. Used as an example of pain at a particular site (VII.58K). For the distinction from κεφαλαία see Siegel, p. 245.

κίττα **('longing' of pregnant women, craving for strange food, *kitta* **, *pica* **)**. Described in VII.132–4K where it is attributed to the presence of abnormal qualities (e.g. bad humours) in the covering of the stomach. The term is still used in its Latin form of *pica*.

*κλονώδης **(shaking)**. An abnormal movement representing a symptom due to malfunction of the motor component of the soul (VII.58K).

*κλύδων **(splashing in the stomach or chest)**. A symptom of disturbed functioning of the retentive capacity (VII.67K).

*κνῆσις **(itch)**. Discussed at VII.196K ff. where it is attributed to the presence of superfluities.

κόπος **(fatigue)**. It is not altogether clear whether this is a disease or a symptom. For description and tripartite classification see VII.178–80K.

κορύζα **(*coryza***, cold)**. See κάταρρος above.

*κῶμα **(lethargic state, coma**)**. Siegel takes this term to be essentially synonymous with κάρος – see his analysis of the three terms κῶμα, κάρος, λήθαργος on pp. 295–8. In one instance termed a disease.

*κωφότης **(deafness)**. One of the three symptoms of disturbed auditory function (VII.56K).

λειεντερία **(passing one's food undigested, *leientery* **)**. Complete failure of the retentive capacity in relation to food (VII.67K).

λειόπους **(flat-footed)**. Linked with βλαισός and ῥαιβός as a disorder of form impairing function (VI.856K). See also *In Hipp. de art. libr. comm.* XVIIIA.613K.

*λειποψυχία **(swooning)**. Taken as having the same meaning as λειπο-θυμία – see VII.136K and re causes, VII.194K. See also *De meth. med. ad Glauc.* XI.48, 56K and Mettler, p. 510.

λέπρα **(leprosy which makes the skin scaly, *lepra* **)**. This is not leprosy in the modern sense but a skin disease characterized by eruptions and loss of skin pigmentation. It is often linked with *alphos* and *leuke* – see Grmek pp. 163–6. Galen classifies it among the *dyscrasias* of *homoiomeres* due to an inflowing substance.

λεύκη **(a skin disease, so called from its colour, *leuke***).** Initial mention in these treatises is on VI.863K in conjunction with *alphoi* and *leprai* as well as other conditions exemplifying 'excess' as something that may damage function.

λευκοφλεγμασία **(*leukophlegmasia*).** A form of dropsy – see ἀνὰ σάρκα.

*λήθαργος **(lethargy).** May also be taken as 'drowsiness' or 'forgetfulness'. See *De meth. med.* X.929–31K, Mettler, pp. 497 ff. (in particular pp. 502–3) and Siegel, p. 255. In one instance it is called a disease.

*λήθη **(forgetfulness, amnesia**).** Failure of function of one component of the rational soul (memory) and related to cooling. See VII.200–2K.

*λύγξ, λυγμός **(hiccup).** Defined by Galen as a type of spasm of the stomach associated with deficient functioning of the retentive capacity (VII.68–9K).

μανία **(madness, *mania***).** Contrasted with *phrenitis* in VII.202K. Possibly a subclass of delirium (*paraphrosune*).

μελικηρίς **(cyst** or wen resembling a honeycomb).** Listed as an example of 'excess' causing disturbance of function (VI.863K).

*μωρία **(folly, dullness**).** Both this and the following term are classified by Galen as symptoms of impaired function of the rational component of the soul (VII.60K).

*μώρωσις **(dullness, sluggishness, dementia**).** Clearly defined in *De loc. aff.* III (VIII.160K) as a joint disturbance of memory and reasoning. Attributed to a cold *diathesis*.

*ναρκή **(numbness**, deadness).** Listed among the *dyscrasias* of cold but considered a symptom rather than a disease (VI.851K). Defined as '. . . a combination of disturbed sensation and disturbed movement involving the whole body or the limbs and due to cooling or compression' (VII.108–9K).

οἴδημα **(swelling**, oedema, tumour).** I have taken this to be a general term for swelling rather than specifically indicating fluid accumulation. Galen classifies it as a *dyscrasia* of *homoiomeric* bodies due to inflowing material (VI.849K).

ὀπισθοτονία /ὀπισθότονος **(tetanic recurvation; a disease in which the body is drawn backward and stiffens, *opisthotonos***).** Listed among the primary *dyscrasias* of cold (VI.850K). Still in use to describe a generalized spasm in extension in neurological disease.

*ὀστοκόπος (*ostokopos*). A form of fatigue in which there is a sensation of one's bones giving way (VII.179K).

ὀφθαλμία (*ophthalmia*). An inflammatory disease of the eye with discharge – possibly severe conjunctivitis (see Mettler, pp. 1006–19, particularly p. 1016).

ὀφίασις (**a bald patch** on the head, of serpentine or winding form**). Attributed to nutritional failure and linked with *leuke* and *alopecia* – VII.63K.

*παρακοπή (**delirium**). Mentioned only as a sympathetic affection in relation to disturbances of the stomach (VII.128K).

*παράκουσις (**defect of hearing, false hearing****). One of the three symptoms of disordered auditory function (VII.56K). At VII.108K where Galen returns to disturbances of hearing, he gives three terms all of which appear to indicate 'false hearing' or auditory illusion. The other two are παρακοή and παράκουσμα.

παράλυσις (**disabling of the nerves, paralysis****). As Siegel points out, Galen uses this term to indicate '. . . a simultaneous loss of both motor and sensory activity, using paraplegia to indicate involving arm and leg of the same side' (pp. 237–8). In *De sympt. caus.* Galen makes the point that paralysis and numbness (*narke*) are of the same class, differing only in magnitude.

*παράνοια (**derangement**, madness**). Taken as a non-specific term for mental disturbance – see VII.202, 270K.

παράρθρησις (**subluxation**). See ἐξάρθρησις (dislocation) above.

*παραφροσύνη (**madness**, delirium****). Siegel differentiates this term from *phrenitis* by calling the former 'delirium without fever' and the latter 'delirium with fever' – see pp. 264–72.

παρίσθμιον (**fauces, tonsils****). Used in *De sympt. caus.* III for adenitis in conjunction with ἀντίας indicating tonsillitis.

*παρόρασις (**false vision**, illusion**). One of the three symptoms of disturbed vision, i.e. defective vision – see ἀμβλυωπία, τυφλότης (VII.56K). See also VII.99K.

περιπνευμονία (**inflammation of the lungs**). Siegel suggests this might equate with lobar pneumonia – see his discussion (1968), pp. 325–6 and VII.174K. See also Grmek, p. 131.

πῆξις **(coagulation, freezing)**. Classified as a primary *dyscrasia* of cold (VI.850K). See also Hippocrates, *Airs, Waters, Places* 8.

πλευρῖτις **(pleurisy)**. See references for περιπνευμονία above.

πνίξ **(choking**, suffocation)**. A sympathetic affection occurring in certain uterine disturbances – see VII.128K.

πληθώρα **(over-abundance of blood or humours, fullness of habit, *plethora* **)**. For the causes of *plethora* see VII.16–17K.

*πνευμάτωσις **(inflation)**. A symptom of impaired function of the retentive capacity (VII.67K).

πριαπισμός **(priapism)**. Term still in use. Listed here as disease in which an abnormality of size interferes with function (VI.869K). See also VII.266K.

πρόσπταισμα **(whitlow)**. Mentioned as a cause of sympathetic *leipopsychia* (VII.136K).

*πταρμός **(sneezing)**. Grouped with the disordered movements at the start of *De sympt. caus.* II (VII.147K).

πτερύγιον **(*pterygium*)**. Term still in use in ophthalmology as 'pterygium' (VI.862K), this being the use which Galen employs. In Greek the term has a number of other meanings, both medical and non-medical.

πύον **(discharge from a sore, pus**)**. A disease in which 'excess' causes disturbance of function (VI.863K).

πυρετός/πυρετώδης **(fever/feverish**, inflamed)**. A primary *dyscrasia* due to excess of heat (VI.850K). In this initial statement the term appears to be interchangeable with τυφώδης. Given detailed consideration among the 'hot' diseases in VII.4–10K. The interrelationships with *rigor* and the types of fever (tertian, quartan, bilious remittent) are considered in VII.182K ff.

πῶρος **(chalkstone formed in the joints**, stone in the bladder)**. Taken in the former sense as an example of a disorder of form – VI.857K.

ῥαιβός **(crooked, bent, bandy-legged**)**. An example of a disease where form is altered impairing function – see βλαισός and VI.856K.

ῥῆγμα **(breakage, fracture)**. Linked with κάταγμα and σπάσγα as diseases due to dissolution of continuity (VI.872K).

ῥῖγος **(shivering fit as in ague, *rigor***)**. Described by Galen as an '... irregular shaking and agitation of the whole body' (VII.145K).

ῥύας (**discharge****). A disease of the eye causing a continual watery discharge. This is the sense used by Galen at VI.870K, where it is included among diseases due to an increase in size of a part. The term can also mean urinary fistula.

σατυρίασις (*satyriasis*). A potentially severe, even fatal disease. There are detailed descriptions by Aretaeus, Paul of Aegina and Caelius Aurelianus given by Mettler, pp. 518, 610–11.

σκίρρος (**hardened swelling or tumour, induration****). Initially included among diseases of *homoiomeric* bodies due to an inflowing substance (VI.849K).

*σκορδινισμός (**stretching**). Grouped with the disordered movements at the start of *De sympt. caus.* II (VII.147K).

σπάσμα (**sprain or rupture of muscle fibres**). Listed with κάταγμα (fracture) and ῥῆγμα (breakage) as a disease due to dissolution of continuity (VII.39–40K).

σπασμός/σπασμώδης (**convulsion/ive, spasm/odic**). Listed with *apoplexy, epilepsy,* and τρομώδης as a primary *dyscrasia* of cold (VI.850K). Translated as 'spasm' or 'convulsion' according to context. Siegel (p. 245) writes: 'The Greek term *spasmos* meant both a continued contraction by a tetanic stimulus and an alternating violent contraction and relaxation of skeletal muscle. Both types of movement are also symptoms of epilepsy. *Spasmos* (convulsion), however, appeared to Galen as exaggeration of normal motion intensified by heat, cold or dryness of the spinal nerves.'

στεάτωμα (**sebaceous tumour**). An example of a disease in which 'excess' causes disturbance of function (VI.863K). Possibly corresponding to the common sebaceous cyst.

*στραβισμός (**squinting**). A disordered movement of the eyes (VII.150K).

*στραγγουρία (**strangury**). See VII.251 and *De locis affectis* VIII.402K.

*συγκοπή (**sudden loss of strength,** *syncope* **). A term with broader connotations than in modern usage – see VII.127K and *De meth. med.* X.850K for a list of causes, and Siegel, pp. 251–3 for detailed consideration.

σφακελίζω (**to suffer from** σφάκελος, **to be gangrened, mortify**). Given as a cause of distortion or obstruction of channels in bodies – see VI.858K and διαπυΐσκομαι above.

τεινεσμός (**a vain endeavour to evacuate**). Linked with δυσεντερία and λειεντερία – see for example VII.170K.

τερηδών (**caries**). See VII.37–9 for a detailed consideration of this term and its distinction from τρῆμα (perforation) below.

τέτανος (**convulsive tension, *tetanos*****). Listed as a primary *dyscrasia* of cold (VI.850K). See Aretaeus' distinction between this term and the terms *opisthotonos* and *emprothotonos* translated by Mettler, pp. 349–50.

τρῆμα (**perforation**). See τερηδών above.

*τριγμός (**rasping**). Grouped with the disordered movements at the start of *De sympt. caus.* II (VII.147K).

τρόμος/τρομώδης (**tremor/trembling****, quaking, quivering**). See σπασμός above (VI.850K). Generally translated as 'tremor'. Also classed as a symptom indicating disturbance of the motor component of the *psyche* – see VII.51, 58K.

*τρυσμός (**gurgling**). Said to be synonymous with τριγμός but Galen appears to use it to indicate a sound (VII.79, 170K), whilst the latter is an abnormal movement – see above.

*τυφλότης (**blindness**). One of the three symptoms of disturbed visual function – see ἀμβλυωπία, παρόρασις (VII.58K).

τυφώδης (**of persons in fever, delirious**). As for πυρετώδης above (VI.850K).

ὕδερος (**dropsy**). Related to maldistribution of nutritive materials – see VII.62K.

*ὑπόσφαγμα (**hyphaema**). Taken to be equivalent to the current term *hyphaema* – a suffusion of blood into the anterior chamber of the eye (VII.99K). May also be or include subconjunctival haemorrhage.

ὑπόχυμα (**cataract**). Taken as identical to the cataracts that occur in the eye – see particularly VII.89K, VII.95K.

φαγέδαινα (**cancerous sore**). Listed as a disease due to an abnormal influx of humour (VII.22K).

φθίσις (**consumption, wasting****, atrophy, emaciation, *phthisis*****; also constriction of the pupil of the eye**). Used by Galen (along with ἀτροφία) as an example of a disease in which alteration in magnitude affects function – see VI.869K, VII.63K.

φθόη (**consumption****, *phthoe*). Given as an example of a disease in which the form of the whole body is changed (VII.29–30K).

φλεγμονή (**inflammation**). Initially defined as a *dyscrasia* of *homoiomeric* bodies due to an inflowing substance (VI.849K).

φρενῖτις (**inflammation of the brain**, *phrenitis***). Termed by Siegel 'delirium with fever' – see his discussion, pp. 270–2, and also Mettler, pp. 490 ff. For Galen's account see VII.143–4K and also VII.202K.

*φρίκη (**shaking**). Grouped with the disordered movements at the start of *De sympt. caus.* II (VII.147K).

φύγεθλον (φύγεθρον) (**swelling of the glands, especially of the groin or armpit**). Included in the *dyscrasias* of *homoiomeric* bodies due to inflowing material (VI.849K).

φῦμα (**tumour****, **tubercle**). Grmek writes: '. . . the word *phuma* corresponds primarily to our terms "abscess" and "tubercle", but also functions as the name for certain forms of cancer and hydatid cyst' (p. 188). Galen includes it in his class of *dyscrasias* of *homoiomeres* due to a substance flowing in (VI.849K).

χαλάζιον (*chalazion*). A small cyst growing on the eyelid, a term now used for a tarsal cyst. Like cataract and pterygium, a term which has essentially retained its original meaning, all three being used by Galen as ophthalmological examples of 'excess' causing impaired function (VI.862–3K).

*χάσμη (**yawning**). Grouped with the disordered movements at the start of *De sympt. caus.* II (VII.147K).

χήμωσις (**chemosis**). An affection of the eyes when the cornea swells like a cockle-shell so as to impede sight – see VII.101K. Another ophthalmological term still in use.

χοιράς (**scrofulous swelling**** **in the glands, particularly of the neck**). Listed among the *dyscrasias* of *homoiomeric* bodies due to an inflowing substance (VI.849K).

χόλερα (*cholera*). For Celsus' description as a condition with simultaneous diarrhoea and vomiting (which appears to coincide with Galen's use – VII.218K) see Mettler, p. 340.

ψώρα (**itch, mange, scurvy,** *psora***). Listed among the *dyscrasias* of *homoiomeric* bodies due to an inflowing substance (VII.849–50K).

*ὠταλγία (**earache**). Used as an example of pain at a particular site (VII.58K).

1.4E CONCLUSIONS

This section on definitions and terms has three aims. The first is to provide support for the view that the whole edifice of Galen's enterprise in these four treatises rests on a foundation of definitions. Galen himself undoubtedly recognizes this despite his often dismissive attitude, both in these works and elsewhere, towards those who allow themselves to be diverted from a proper attention to practical matters into what he would see as the sterile areas of theoretical dispute. The critical definitions are those of health, disease and symptom. One cannot classify, nor even give a proper account of the causes of diseases and symptoms without first defining what these terms mean, that is what their extension is. To do this a definition of health is also necessary. It is probably also necessary to define related terms such as affection, syndrome and cause of disease, not to mention the terms contained in the primary definitions – these being condition, constitution, function and in accord with/contrary to nature.

As Suppe writes: 'In the most fundamental scientific sense, to define is to delimit. Thus definitions serve to fix boundary phenomena or the range of applicability of terms or concepts.'[75] This idea is inherent in the Greek term for definition, as the following definition of definition from the pseudo-Galenic *Definitiones medicae* makes clear: 'A definition (ὁρισμός) is a concise statement (λόγος) which makes clear the nature of the underlying matter. ὁρισμός is used from a transfer (μεταφορά) of the boundaries (ὁροθεσία) in regions' (XIX.349K). Galen himself (quoting Plato) speaks of 'taking a comprehensive view of widely scattered particulars and bringing them under one form, so that a person may clarify by a definition the subject about which he may at any time choose to give instruction . . .'[76] Galen's problem is that what he is attempting to define in these treatises (the *definiendum*) does not have clear boundaries. In fact, as Suppe also points out, 'In many scientific cases, definitions function more as explications

[75] See Suppe in Newton-Smith (2000), p. 76.
[76] *De placitis Hippocratis et Platonis* IX.5.15. The quotation from Plato is from the *Phaedrus* 265d and the translation after De Lacy.

than as meaning specifications or real definitions.⁷⁷ Galen, then, should be taken as offering explications rather than definitions. Whilst quibbling over such terminological niceties might be just the kind of activity that would elicit Galen's scorn, the distinction does bring out the fundamental difficulties in establishing the precise extensions of the relevant terms. These are difficulties that have important implications for the whole project of classification and analysis of causation.

Causation itself is a further problem and one which will be considered at length in chapter I.6. Insofar as the problems relate to definition, however, the main point to be taken from section I.4b above is that whilst Galen has at least three more or less distinct approaches to draw from (Aristotelian, Stoic and 'common-sense'), his usage of terms is inconsistent and *ad hoc*, certainly not systematic. In brief: (i) He seems to make no distinction between αἰτία, αἴτιον and πρόφασις; (ii) his digression into a quasi-Aristotelian classification (*De symptomatum differentiis* I.6) is not pursued in these treatises; (iii) the two descriptive terms he is at pains to clarify (προκαταρκτικός, προηγούμενος) are not subsequently employed to any extent. In fact, he ends up by giving what is essentially an empirical and common-sense account of disease and symptom causation.

The second aim is to clarify Galen's own usage of important and recurring terms (I.4c). Inclusion in the list given is based on importance in Galen's arguments in the translated treatises rather than general importance. Therefore, the analysis of each term has a somewhat narrow focus. In respect to this list there are no general points to be made. The third purpose is to provide a list of the diseases and symptoms (I.4d) included in the treatises with particular attention again being given to Galen's use specifically, although wider issues and areas of uncertainty are at least referred to where appropriate.

⁷⁷ In Newton-Smith (2000), p. 78.

The classification of diseases and symptoms

I.5A INTRODUCTION

In the four translated treatises, two on diseases and two on symptoms, the first of each pair is devoted to definition and classification. In any nosological endeavour, classification depends on definition. Here the entities (if, in fact, they are entities)[1] to be defined (if, in fact, definition is applicable)[2] are disease and symptom. The two provisos, obviously interrelated, are intended to indicate the difficulties of Galen's taxonomic undertaking, difficulties which he himself clearly acknowledged, not least when he considered the issue of 'disease in itself'.[3] It is undeniable, however, that a satisfactory classification of, and distinction between, diseases and symptoms is of considerable value in both the theoretical and the practical aspects of medicine. Prior to these treatises there is no attempt at systematic and exhaustive classification, at least none that is extant, which invests these works with particular historical interest, not to mention their relevance to medical practice at the time. As has been noted earlier, Galen himself saw them as a necessary bridge between his theoretical writings and his manuals of practical medicine.

This is not to say there were not some prior attempts at definition and classification – there were – but what is notable is their paucity both in number and content. This is especially surprising given the attention paid to these matters in other fields, including biology generally, by such notables as Aristotle, Speusippus and Theophrastus.[4] Nonetheless, it is worthwhile to consider, at least briefly, three early ventures into classification that do

---

[1] For a modern discussion of the different approaches to characterizing disease see Cohen (1981).
[2] Suppe provides a summarized account of the nature of definitions and the distinction from explication in Newton-Smith (2000), pp. 76–8. References to more detailed considerations are given there.
[3] See *De methodo medendi* X.152K.
[4] For discussion of Aristotle's contribution in these areas see Lloyd (1968), pp. 86–90, and the articles in Part II of Gotthelf and Lennox (1987), pp. 65–198.

remain: those in the Hippocratic Corpus, that in Plato's *Timaeus*, and that given by Celsus.

With respect to the Hippocratic Corpus, Lonie has written: 'It is a strange circumstance that in all the treatises of the (Hippocratic) Collection, some of which stand under the influence of the sophists who were professionally interested in definition, there is no explicit attempt to define disease – nothing for instance, like Galen's "condition contrary to nature which impairs functioning (sc. of a particular organ or of the whole body)".'[5] There are, however, some taxonomic endeavours, albeit fragmentary and incomplete, in what may be recognized as the nosological treatises such as *Diseases* II, *Diseases* III and *Internal Affections*. The first of these, *Diseases* II, in its 75 sections deals individually with diseases and symptoms but does not differentiate between the two nor is the material arranged systematically. In *Diseases* III, 16 of the 17 chapters consider an individual disease or symptom, but again no distinction is made between the two and the list is, needless to say, incomplete. *Internal Affections*, which focuses predominantly on treatment, does order the diseases discussed to the extent that 'each of its 54 chapters deals with a specific nosological entity', as Potter writes.[6] It must be reiterated, however, that none of the Hippocratic works attempts a systematic definition and classification of diseases and symptoms.

Plato, in the *Timaeus*, does make a specific attempt to classify diseases, although as in the Hippocratic texts this is again without distinction between disease and symptom and also without prior definition. He identifies three classes of disease, the divisions being based on theories of causation and on a continuum theory of bodily structure (elements/qualities). The three classes, considered in greater detail in the following section on causation, are in summary:

1. Those due to imbalance or maldistribution of elements.
2. Those due to a disordered sequence of formation of tissues.
3. Those due to an abnormal accumulation of air (wind), phlegm or bile.

Galen is not altogether sympathetic to these attempts by Plato, writing on this section of the *Timaeus* in the *De placitis Hippocratis et Platonis*:

It particularly behoves Plato to impart this order of instruction, inasmuch, at least, as it is proper for a philosopher to use order and method in teaching more than it is for doctors. But perhaps he was unable to go over such things accurately, lacking experience, as he was not himself engaged in the tasks of a doctor.[7]

[5] Lonie (1981), pp. 328–9.   [6] Hippocrates, vol. 6 (Loeb), Potter (1988), p. 68.
[7] *De placitis Hippocratis et Platonis* VIII.6 (De Lacy, vol. 2, p. 518).

A third example of early classification of disease is to be found in Celsus' *De medicina*. Again, this is not so much a classification of diseases as an ordering of material for purposes of presentation. At the outset of Book III he writes: 'All those things which pertain to entire classes of diseases having been dealt with, I shall come to the treatments of individual diseases. The Greeks, in fact, have divided these into two kinds and have said that some of them are acute and some chronic.'[8] Although he goes on to criticize this simple bipartite division, he nonetheless accepts the time course of disease as the basis for classification. It is notable that this same division is also followed by Caelius Aurelianus in his later compendium of diseases.[9] In Book IV, in dealing with diseases of particular parts, he imposes a topographic division which is set out in summary form by Mettler who remarks that, 'What is here considered is a category of symptoms rather than particular diseases.'[10]

What might be said, then, on the basis of the texts that have survived, is that prior to Galen there were no systematic attempts to define disease or symptom (although Aristotle does give some thought to the definition of health),[11] nor to draw the distinction between health and disease or between disease, symptom and affection. Nor were there any systematic attempts to furnish an exhaustive classification of diseases or symptoms, either separately or jointly. All that could be claimed is that there were some attempts at arrangement of material on diseases and symptoms considered jointly and organized, if at all, topographically.

Galen's own attempts at classification are particularly to be found in treatises I and III of the present study – *De morborum differentiis* and *De symptomatum differentiis*. As noted at the start of this section, each work begins with discussion of the definitions essential to the classificatory exercise. The section on definitions is relatively brief in the work on diseases whereas it is rather more discursive prior to the classification of symptoms. This disparity reflects the difficulty of determining the extension of the terms 'disease' (*nosos*), 'symptom' (*symptoma*) and 'affection' (*pathos*) and the degree of demarcation which they have from one another, problems which do not so obviously exist with the terms 'health' (*hugieia*) and 'disease' (*nosos*) in the first work. Some indication of the purpose of the whole exercise, and of Galen's recognition of his predecessors and their influences on him, both with regard to the importance of taxonomy in general, and its application to medicine in particular – as well as the anatomical basis

---

[8] Celsus, *De medicina* III.1.   [9] See Drabkin (1950).
[10] Mettler (1947), pp. 339–42.   [11] For example, in the *Topics* 106b34–107a2, 110a19–21.

of his own classification – is to be found in the following passage from *De methodo medendi*:

If someone, then, wishes to know how much such people err, and how great a number of diseases they overlook, and how many more things they are ignorant of than they know, let him read the work *De morborum differentiis*. For he will learn how Hippocrates was the first of all to use the right path, and how it was necessary for those who followed him to complete it and how no one did complete it but many, in fact, destroyed the things properly discovered. Aristotle and Theophrastus, and those around them, came nearest to completing and extending the way transmitted by Hippocrates, and if the truth is to be told, they did virtually complete it in distinguishing that the diseases in *homoiomeric* bodies and in those [bodies] termed organs were not [of] the same class.

A somewhat similar view is expressed earlier in the same work: 'Moreover, regarding the differentiation of diseases, how many there are and of what sort, and likewise of symptoms, Hippocrates appears as the first of those we know to have made a proper beginning, whilst after him Aristotle led the way still further.'[12] In the absence of specific evidence to the contrary, one must assume that the reference to Aristotle and Theophrastus relates to their endeavours in other fields, as mentioned above.

In fact, issues of background, purpose and method pertaining to the classification of diseases and symptoms are given extended treatment in *De methodo medendi* I.3.3–15 (X.20–31K). Two passages of particular relevance to Galen's method from within this section are as follows:

And here too it must be stated precisely what a disease is and what a symptom and an affection (*pathos*) are, and distinguished in what way each of the aforementioned things is the same and in what way not the same and, by this means, attempt to 'cut' these things into their proper *differentiae* according to the method which the philosophers taught us.

A little earlier he has said, 'In this way then too, anyone who attempts to speak about the number of diseases, how many there are altogether, must not stay fixed in the first *differentia* but go on dividing this until he should reach the particular kinds of those things no longer able to be cut into another species.'[13]

Whilst on the subject of the *De methodo medendi*, two further passages of relevance to the present discussion are, first, that in which Galen provides the following summary of the classificatory scheme he employs in *De morborum differentiis*:

---

[12] See *De methodo medendi* X.117–18K and X.15K for these two passages.
[13] *De methodo medendi* X.27K and X.25–6K respectively.

There are then six classes of diseases in all: one specific to *homoiomeres*, which is *dyscrasia*, four specific to each of the organs, as was said just now, and in addition to these what is common to organs and *homoiomeres*, which is dissolution of continuity. The *differentiae* in relation to each of these up to the particular kinds are written about in the work on the *differentia* of diseases.[14]

Then there is the further summary statement, albeit embedded in some typical Galenic vituperation, on the Methodist position: 'But like a tyrant, he [Thessalus] "orders" that according to regimen there are only two diseases altogether, flow and stasis, not knowing that he is stating a certain *differentia* of diseases, and one known moreover to earlier doctors, as we shall show.'[15]

In the two of the four treatises of the present study devoted to classification, Galen embarks on his project – how many diseases and how many symptoms are there and of what classes and kinds are they? As Hankinson writes, 'The point is not that the successful doctor needs to know the actual number of diseases, but that he needs to know how many types there are in reality; that is, he needs to know the proper taxonomical structure of disease.'[16] In each case Galen begins with a consideration of the definitions of health, disease, symptom, affection (*pathos/pathema*) and cause. He does not, in these works, consider the term 'syndrome' which, although he does himself use it, he seems to associate with the Empiricists.[17] Having clarified the issues of definition to the best of his ability, whilst recognizing the variable but inevitable overlap between classes, he then proceeds to his classification in each case. What follows below is an analysis of the taxonomical schemes in the two books on *differentiae*, culminating in some concluding remarks on the success or otherwise of Galen's nosological endeavour, and on later attempts at the same undertaking.

1.5B DISEASES (*DE MORBORUM DIFFERENTIIS*)

In this work the key definition, that of disease, is given first in terms of a constitution (*kataskeue*) or condition (*diathesis*) damaging or interfering

---

[14] *De methodo medendi* X.126K. I take *eschaton eidos* to indicate the particular or individual diseases, following Aristotle's usage in *Metaphysics* 998b16 and 1059b26. Hankinson (1991) translates as *infimae species* (see p. 63, for example). I have left *differentia* as singular here on the basis of the genitive singular definite article. Latin versions have the plural, as in the titles.

[15] *De methodo medendi* X.20K. Similar statements can be found elsewhere, for example in *De sectis ad eos qui introducuntur* I.80K.

[16] Hankinson (1991), p. 167.

[17] In *Ad Glauconem de medendi methodo* Galen speaks of a 'plethoric syndrome' (XI.59K). Elsewhere, for example *De methodo medendi* X.100–1K and *An Outline of Empiricism* (Walzer and Frede, 1985, p. 30), he links this term explicitly with the Empiricists.

with function (*energeia*) and then more specifically in terms of being 'out of balance' (*ametros*). Galen does give recognition (*sans* vituperation) in this work to the alternative definitions proposed by Asclepiades and the Methodics, at least with regard to *homoiomeres*. His own preference for a continuum theory based on elements or qualities is, however, clearly stated and provides the basis for his own classification. In either case there is the other important preliminary step of division of bodily structure into: (i) *homoiomeres*; (ii) organs; (iii) the whole body.

Considering first *homoiomeric* structures on the basis of Asclepiadian theory, Galen speaks initially of two primary affections – a dilatation and a constriction of the 'theoretical' pores.[18] This distinction is reiterated as he begins his systematic classification in section V.1.[19] Here, however, he introduces a further twofold differentiation in each case. He divides dilatation into a generalized outward movement of all parts of the pore-containing body itself, and an expansion of the actual pores due to a 'falling away of their elements'. Constriction he divides into an inward collapse of the pore-containing body, and a destruction of the pores themselves.

The essentials of his own classification are as follows. First, there are three genera:

1. *Dyscrasias* – applicable to *homoiomeres*.
2. Abnormalities of morphology and composition – applicable to organs.
3. Dissolution of continuity – applicable to both *homoiomeres* and organs.

On the basis of the theory of elements and qualities, *dyscrasias* of *homoiomeric* bodies are brought about by a change in one or more of the four primary qualities – heat, cold, moisture and dryness. This, in turn, may occur in one of two ways. Either there is a change in the body itself, i.e. the process is entirely internal to the body, or the change results from something flowing into the affected body from without which alters the balance of qualities. One practical point is that the first may be relatively hard to detect, whilst the second is not, in that such changes are commonly associated with an obvious swelling. Galen lists *erysipelas*, inflammatory swelling, *oidema* and tumours as examples of the latter. He introduces a further distinction which is basically one of degree: '. . . *dyscrasias* of the parts which are slight and escape the notice of most are called by them "debilities" (*atoniai*)'.[20] He does not provide an exhaustive listing of diseases under the several possible headings of the four 'mono-*dyscrasias*', the

---

[18] *De morborum differentiis* IV.1 (VI.842K).
[19] *De morborum differentiis* VI.848K.   [20] *De morborum differentiis* V.6 (VI.853K).

four regular 'bi-*dyscrasias*' and the two irregular 'bi-*dyscrasias*', the last two groups not being mentioned until later.

In considering diseases of organic structures, Galen stresses the distinction in these structures between what might be called the primary part, responsible for carrying out the specific function of the organ in question, and the secondary or subsidiary parts which act in a facilitating role. The classification of the diseases of organic parts is on a different basis from that of the *homoiomeric* parts and is essentially morphological. The subdivisions are as follows:

1. Disorders of conformation – including abnormalities of overall form both congenital and acquired, changes in the number and configuration of channels and cavities, and changes in the roughness and smoothness of their surfaces.
2. Disorders of the number of parts – the basic division is into 'increase' (again divided into congenital and acquired) and 'decrease' (for which he introduces the term 'docked').
3. Disorders of the size of parts – with a basic division into 'increase' and 'decrease'.
4. Disorders of relative position – these are exemplified particularly by dislocations and hernias.

The final genus is that of dissolution of continuity which applies to both *homoiomeric* and organic structures. In his initial consideration of this disease class, Galen is satisfied solely with the provision of some obvious examples such as bone fractures, avulsions of arteries and ligaments, and ulcers. These are, of course, principally of traumatic origin. There are two problems with this class. The first and more important is whether it is justifiable to regard it as a discrete class. The second is the numerical problem of Galen's description of it as 'a fifth class'. On this putative class, Hankinson writes as follows: 'Finally there is one type of affection, breakdown of cohesion, which can happen to either organic or *homoiomerous* parts (presumably in virtue of the fact that both types of part have extension essentially; that this constitutes a disease depends in part on the thesis that all causing is by contact, and consequently any rupture of contact must affect the causal power of the whole).'[21] These matters will be further discussed in section I.6d below.

In the final sections (XI–XIII) Galen considers what he calls 'combined diseases', focusing mainly on those occurring in similar structures, i.e. in *homoiomeres* or in organs. In the former, combined diseases will be either a

---

[21] Hankinson (1991), p. 201.

combination of constriction and dilatation if considered from the viewpoint of Asclepiadian theory, or one of the 'bi-*dyscrasias*' if considered on the basis of a theory of elements and qualities. With regard to the latter, there is again subdivision into diseases arising from primary change in the qualities within the affected body, and those due to the inflow of some substance altering the balance of qualities. He does not here introduce the concept of anomalous or irregular 'bi-*dyscrasias*' which is deferred to the following work.[22] He also points out that dissolution of continuity, such as an ulcer, can occur in combination with a *dyscrasia* in a simple *homoiomeric* body. Combined dissolutions of continuity involving organic parts he illustrates in detail by consideration of eye disease in the case of multiple involvement of its components, e.g. cornea, pupil, choroid etc.

1.5C SYMPTOMS (*DE SYMPTOMATUM DIFFERENTIIS*)

In the case of symptoms, the taxonomic basis is somewhat different from that for diseases. Although there are what might be called subsidiary classifications, the basic criterion in this case is the nature of the disturbance of function. The treatise *De symptomatum differentiis* is divided into six sections which will be considered in sequence in the following analysis. In terms of the main classification of symptoms the key sections are II and III.

The first, long section, which occupies over a quarter of the entire book, is devoted to a reiteration of definitions and, particularly, to the clarification of terms. Although there are significant digressions, as for example the attempt at a definition of cause (I.6), the crux of this section is the endeavour to establish a clear idea of what actually constitutes a symptom. This is a singularly difficult undertaking with problems of demarcation at both 'ends' – that is, distinction from normal conditions or affections at one 'end' and from diseases and their causes at the other 'end'. Ultimately Galen recognizes that a clear line of demarcation is impossible, particularly with his focus on 'damage to function' as the central feature of his proposed definition. So, at least theoretically, diseases and their internal antecedent (*proegoumenic*) causes may be considered as symptoms according to his definitions. This is reflected in the actual terminology of diseases and symptoms.

The second section is brief. Having announced his intention to go over individual symptoms, Galen makes his first taxonomic distinction into

---

[22] See *De causis morborum* VI.2 (VII.20–21K).

1. Those symptoms that are conditions of the body itself.
2. Those symptoms that are damages of function.
3. Those symptoms that follow both.

He does not, however, really develop this differentiation. He then makes a second, and fundamental, distinction between total and partial loss of function which becomes, in effect, the basis of his classification. After some further reflections on the difficulties considered in the first section, he concludes the second section with the summarizing statement that anything contrary to nature that is not a disease or cause of disease is, by exclusion, a symptom.

In the third section, having made the further general distinction between the psychical and the physical, he proceeds to a consideration of symptoms that are psychical. His classification of psychical symptoms depends on several of the subsidiary classifications referred to earlier. The first is the threefold division of the psychical into sensory, motor and authoritative. The second is the fivefold division of the sensory into the five modalities (sight, hearing, smell, taste, touch) and the threefold division of the authoritative into imagination, reason and memory, the motor being left undivided. The third is an elaboration of the earlier subdivision of damage of function into three subclasses rather than two, the three being:

1. Privation (complete loss) of function.
2. Deficient (reduced) function.
3. Defective (abnormal) function.

Considering the five sensory modalities first, in the case of sight and hearing this threefold classification is signalled by specific terms for each, which Galen gives.[23] For the other three modalities no specific terms are available but the same division applies nonetheless. Thus, as Galen makes explicit, sensory symptoms are divided into anaesthesias and dysaesthesias with the dysaesthesias being further divided as above into 'deficient' and 'defective'. This basic distinction is indicated by several different terms, but here *amudros* and *paratuptikos* are used. Two other sensory symptoms, which do not entirely fit into the threefold division, are pain and itch, which are both taken to be aspects of touch even when involving, in the case of pain, the organs of special sense.

Motor symptoms are also included in this section and again the basic divisions apply – *akinesia* and *dyskinesia* with the latter being further divided, as with the sensory symptoms, into 'deficient' (diminished, weak) and 'defective' (abnormal). Of the latter, tremor, spasm/convulsion, palpitation and

---

[23] See *De symptomatum differentiis* VII.56K.

a variable fourth (shivering, rigor, agitation) are given special attention.[24] The final part of this section is devoted to the 'authoritative' or *hegemonical* functions which are divided, as indicated above, into imagination, reason and memory. Here the different forms of malfunction are indicated by the more usual terms of *ellipes* and *plemmeles*. One important point here is that Galen rather passes over memory, noting only that it can be involved with the other functions. Indeed, he indicates that combined disturbances of the three primary components of the 'authoritative' function are common. Also, as in the case of pain and itch in relation to sensory symptoms, there are two further symptoms which fall outside the basic threefold classification and which Galen links to what he calls '. . . the primary sense itself, which is definitely common to all the senses'.[25] These are insomnia and coma, although in this context the latter might more properly be called hypersomnia.

The physical symptoms, which are considered in detail in the long section IV, are also susceptible to the same basic division into loss of function and disturbance of function, the latter being again subdivided into deficient and defective. The division and its associated terminology is illustrated by the digestive function of the stomach, the disturbances of which fall into one of three categories: *apepsia, bradypepsia* and *dyspepsia*. In fact, Galen makes the point that recognition of physical symptoms in general is closely dependent on an understanding of the four physical capacities – attractive, retentive, alterative and separative. If the basic division (no function/disturbed function) is observed in relation to these capacities, each physical organ will have eight possible symptoms, applying no function or disturbed function to the four capacities. Thus, as Galen indicates, armed with this knowledge coupled with that of the total number of physical organs, the total number of possible symptoms of these organs could be calculated. Adjustment can be made to include the psychical symptoms, in particular the two additional 'unclassified' symptoms of insomnia and hypersomnia/coma.

The final two sections (V and VI) concern symptoms that do not directly conform to the basic classification although, as Galen stresses at the start of section V, they are consequences of disturbed function just as the others are. The groups of symptoms in these two sections comprise, first, symptoms gathered under the rubric of 'means of perception' (section V), and second, under that of 'things separated from the body' (section VI). In

[24] See also the work, *De tremore, palpitatione, convulsione et rigore* (VII.584–642K).
[25] *De symptomatum differentiis* III.2 (VII.58K).

the first case, the means of perception can refer either to the doctor or to the patient, so Galen deals with abnormal colours, noises, tastes, smells and what is palpable. In the second case, the materials considered include blood, faeces, urine and sweat. Here, particularly, the dividing line between normal and abnormal is often hard to draw. Galen clearly recognizes this. These two groups are, in fact, something of a problem taxonomically and in relation to definitions. With respect to the latter, although an important criterion is contrariety to nature, this too may be hard to establish, whilst the other important component of definition – damage to function – is also somewhat variable.

1.5D CONCLUSIONS

Galen, then, attempts in these four treatises to provide a comprehensive classification of diseases and symptoms despite the several difficulties involved. It is an ambitious, and to a significant extent successful, undertaking. It is ambitious in that Galen has chosen a basis other than simple topography for his classification. Herein, however, lies his first major problem. Can he be said to have identified or established natural class divisions? Are there, in fact, such natural divisions as there are in other areas of successful taxonomy?

Having decided that the programme is feasible and that his definitions are sufficiently secure, he classifies diseases into what I have taken to be three major genera: (i) *dyscrasias*; (ii) disorders of organ morphology; (iii) dissolutions of continuity. Hankinson, however, in his commentary on Galen's relatively brief statement of this classification in *De methodo medendi*, speaks of 'six genera of disease' and writes as follows: 'Galen treats the eight *duskrasiai* as falling under one genus, while the four organic diseases are each *sui generis*: it is not immediately clear what if anything the theoretical import of this is, nor what the reasons behind it might be; my analysis above implicitly suggests a different way of making the cuts.'[26] Further, Galen himself speaks of dissolution of continuity as 'a fifth class', although this could be construed as the fifth after the four subclasses of the main class of disorders of morphology applicable to organs.

Barnes appears to accept the tripartite division but not without criticism, remarking of the classification, that it '. . . lacks symmetry and elegance; the initial introduction of the distempers provided a pleasantly neat theory; the addition of the four organic diseases seems *ad hoc*; and "loss of continuity"

---

[26] Hankinson (1991), p. 202.

is appended without any attempt to integrate it into a unified theory. But Galen is not interested in elegant symmetry: his concern is for truth.'[27] Is this criticism justified? In terms of Galen's reliance on a continuum theory of structure based on qualities and humours, his identification of the mono- and regular bi-*dyscrasias*, even perhaps his later addition of the 'irregular' bi-*dyscrasias* (hot and cold, dry and moist) grouped under the single class heading of *dyscrasia*, seems theoretically acceptable. The question arises, however, whether 'theoretically acceptable' translates into 'practically applicable', in short, recognition in general and recognition specifically as to what they are without theoretical interpolation. It is one thing to postulate that a particular disease is, say, a hot and moist bi-*dyscrasia*, but another thing to say that this is a *natural* subclass or kind.

Galen's use of a morphological basis for the classification of organic diseases is less exceptionable, Barnes' comments notwithstanding, particularly as he accepts the existence of combined diseases in which *homoiomeric* parts of an organ can be affected by a *dyscrasia* at the same time as the whole organ is affected by one of the four morphological disturbances. The main problem with this morphological basis is that an obvious morphological abnormality does not necessarily constitute a disease on the basis of Galen's own definition of disease in which a critical component is disturbance of function. What, for example, is the status of a supernumerary digit, or of a pterygium that has not yet encroached on the pupil? Both are obviously *para phusin*, but neither actually compromises function.[28]

The final class, dissolution of continuity, is the most problematical. Galen's own discussion of this in *De morborum differentiis* is undeniably somewhat superficial whilst that in *De methodo medendi* is even less detailed.[29] He certainly fails to establish why this must be taken as a separate class. The impression is that he is endeavouring to include abnormalities of *homoiomeric* structures which do not fit into the class of *dyscrasias* and cannot, on the grounds of his structural division, be included in the morphological disturbances affecting organs. Otherwise, dissolution of continuity, as in bone fractures which is one of his examples, would seem to fit more comfortably into the fourth subclass of his morphological abnormalities. There is also the question of whether ulcers, another of his examples of dissolution of continuity, inevitably bring about damage to function.

---

[27] Barnes (1993).
[28] Although see his comments on supernumerary digits in *De usu partium* I.23 (I.61H). May (1968) has: '. . . a superfluity, by imposing an extra burden, hinders parts that are strong enough in themselves to function and thus causes injury. Finally, the abnormal formation of a sixth finger confirms my reasoning' (p. 109).
[29] See, for example, *De methodo medendi* X.83K, X.126K.

Turning to symptoms, the different basis of classification which he employs seems, at first sight, more promising. He does not here depend on the division into *homoiomeres* and organs with the inherent difficulties due to the presence of *homoiomeric* structures within organic structures. Instead, he makes the much more 'natural' division into psychical and physical, setting aside for the moment the issue of psycho-physical interaction (psychosomatic disease) and the further generally accepted subdivisions of these, and proceeds to classification on the grounds of disordered function. If there are three kinds of functional disturbance – loss, reduction and abnormality – and there is an identifiable finite number of discrete organs, psychical and physical, then there is the basis for a comprehensive or even exhaustive classification. This will, moreover, be a workable classification with practical relevance if these various disturbances of function are clearly recognizable. Even if, in a particular instance, there were to be problems of recognition, this would not in itself invalidate the classification.

As with diseases, however, the issue of whether function is actually damaged could present a problem. Is an abnormal taste, for example, a symptom if there is no detectable disturbance of function – or is the abnormal taste itself a disturbance of function? Also, in the case of materials separated or expelled (which Galen allocates to a separate class), there are again problems differentiating normal from abnormal. One only has to consider the difficulty in evaluating variations in the qualities and quantities of faeces, urine and menstrual flow to realize that this is so. Amongst other problems there is the question of why Galen does not here add excess to his threefold subdivision. Perhaps this is to be included under 'abnormal'. Organs with multiple functions also present difficulties, although this was a matter much less clearly understood in Galen's time. In addition, there is the question of why he felt obliged to describe the two extra classes, 'means of perception' and 'materials expelled from the body' in sections V and VI, respectively. It may be, in fact, with more detailed knowledge of functions, more sophisticated means of testing, and greater perseverance on the part of the taxonomist, that all examples of these two appended classes could be subsumed under the two major classes.

Clearly, then, there are difficulties with Galen's system of classification. The major ones may be enumerated in summary as follows:

1. Definition. It is arguable that all such attempts at classification are doomed to at least some degree of failure owing to the inevitable imprecision of the foundational definitions. As noted in the introductory remarks to this section and in the preceding chapter on definitions and terms (I.4), a strict definition of disease is impossible. Moreover, clear

demarcation between diseases, causes of disease, symptoms and affections, to use the terms Galen is at pains to define, is likewise impossible.
Apart from his recognition of this problem in the two treatises on classification under scrutiny, Galen also acknowledges its existence in a number
of other works.

2. Rationale. On what grounds does Galen choose the bases for his two
   classifications, and why are they different for diseases and symptoms? In
   particular, why is a functional basis chosen for symptoms when damage
   to function is the key element in the definition of disease? Further,
   is it permissible to have such different bases for the major classes in
   such taxonomic systems? Whatever basis is decided on, there will at
   any time be deficiencies in knowledge in the particular area chosen –
   for example, the precise nature or location of morphological change,
   the precise understanding of physiological mechanism, or the exact and
   comprehensive recognition of relevant causal factors.

3. Nomenclature. Although not discussed in the two treatises under examination, this issue is raised in *De methodo medendi* where Galen draws
   attention to the quite variable bases for the naming of diseases and symptoms. One highly desirable result of a successful classification would be
   systematization of nomenclature.

These fundamental difficulties notwithstanding, attempts at disease classification of varying degrees of complexity and comprehensiveness extend
back before Hippocrates, as Jouanna has pointed out,[30] and continue to the
present time, reflecting the inescapable human impulse towards ordering
and sorting data to make it more manageable, and the perceived usefulness
of such an enterprise. As Galen makes explicit, such attempts unquestionably derive at least part of their motivation from other taxonomic projects,
particularly those in which more exact results are possible.[31] In this respect,
it is of interest to note that Galen's identifiable antecedents, Aristotle and
Theophrastus, were instrumental in developing elaborate systems of biological classification, as mentioned above. Similarly, many centuries later,
the taxonomic work of Linnaeus and others was closely associated with
a resurgence of interest in disease classification and the publication of a
number of influential works on nosology, including one by Linnaeus himself. Of particular significance in this regard were those of François Boissier

[30] Jouanna (1999), in his general study of Hippocrates, remarks on attempts at disease classification
prior to Hippocrates, finding scattered evidence in records of Egyptian medicine and even in some
of the early Greek poets, specifically Homer and Pindar – see pp. 145–6.

[31] See the references to Aristotle and Theophrastus in the passages from *De methodo medendi* quoted
in I.5a above (X.15K, X.117–18K).

de Sauvages and William Cullen. The question arises as to what purpose such classifications actually serve, for example in diagnosis and prognosis as well as in therapy and prophylaxis. In broad terms, grouping of like with like should, at the very least, be facilitatory in the four aspects of practical medicine listed earlier. In addition, there are clearly benefits to teaching and documentation. Nevertheless, a need for flexibility must be recognized which is considerably greater in diseases and related phenomena than in many other areas of biology – a need which Galen himself recognized. It may even be that whilst classification is appropriate where there is clear divisibility into natural kinds, where the lines of division are blurred it is significantly less useful.

Finally, in attempting an evaluation of Galen's achievement in these two books on the classification of diseases and symptoms, it is of interest to look at what are deemed to be the desirable features of a system of classification in a modern work on the theory of medicine. Thus, Murphy, who describes the overall aim as '. . . for something to fall into one of a finite number of unambiguous classes', lists the following six factors – naturalness, exhaustiveness, disjointness, usefulness, illumination and simplicity – as desirable.[32]

If examined critically against these criteria, one must conclude that the Galenic system, particularly in these two treatises, has significant deficiencies. On naturalness, it could be argued that only the disease class of morphological disturbance has this characteristic. *Dyscrasia*, dependent as it is on an underlying theory, then contentious, now outmoded, cannot be a natural class. Neither, for different but equally cogent reasons, can dissolution of continuity. A classification based on types of disorder of function has more claim to naturalness but there are still difficulties, as discussed. Exhaustiveness is important for Galen and is a claim he explicitly makes for his endeavours more than once in these treatises. If exhaustiveness is taken to mean all diseases and all symptoms are covered by his two taxonomic systems, even if not individually mentioned, then perhaps his claim is justified. But such a result is achieved only at the expense of naturalness and the third criterion, disjointness. For diseases, dissolution of continuity seems to transgress this criterion, as has been argued above. For symptoms, the same may be said of the two appended classes.

On usefulness, a more confident claim might be made despite difficulties with respect to the other criteria. This is a moot point insofar as Galen and like-minded contemporaries would presumably argue, for example,

---

[32] Murphy (1997), pp. 121–31.

that identification and recognition of the class of *dyscrasias* would allow appropriate choice of allopathic therapy. If the theory is wrong, however, the therapy would be wrongly based even if empirically successful. Nevertheless, in terms of then current practice, usefulness could legitimately be claimed. Illumination could also be claimed if the explanations inherent in the taxonomic system are themselves illuminating, which they might reasonably have been taken to be at the time. Lastly, on simplicity, one must look again to the difficulty in establishing the necessary functional deficit, the addition of questionable further classes outside the basic divisions, and the use of different bases of classification for diseases and symptoms, and find Galen's systems wanting in this respect.

Despite these reservations a concluding reiteration of the ambitious nature of Galen's attempts at definition and classification and their success, at least partial, in meeting the required criteria is, however, appropriate. These treatises should, then, be recognized as ground-breaking in these areas to a significant degree and worthy of their long-enduring position within the medical curriculum. Indeed, they might justifiably be regarded as models of the marriage between the theoretical and practical which should form the foundation of the practice of medicine.

CHAPTER I.6

Causation in disease and symptoms

I.6A INTRODUCTION

The terms cause and causation are relevant to a large part of day-to-day experience yet the concepts and theories underlying them have been matters of contention since the beginning of philosophy and remain so today. Galen, in the two treatises on causation in the four works under consideration, sets out to give an account of the causes of diseases and symptoms. This should be distinguished from an attempt to give a theoretical analysis of causation in disease and its related symptomatology, although he does make a brief excursion into the latter. In other words, he is aiming to provide an exhaustive (as he sees it) list of causes of diseases and symptoms which is of practical relevance to the practising doctor in that elimination or counteraction of causative factors is of primary importance in prophylaxis and treatment, just as recognition of causative factors is critical to diagnosis. So these are practical works. But they are also works with a significant embedded theoretical component which, when taken in conjunction with his other works on causation, signal Galen's interest in the fundamental aspects of the subject. This is as it should be for a doctor who is also a philosopher.

The purpose of this chapter is, then, primarily to examine Galen's views on causes and causation in diseases and symptoms, particularly as revealed by the presently considered treatises, but also to consider his views expressed in other works in which causation has an important role.[1] Before focusing on Galen's views in detail, I shall give a brief outline of views on causation, either in general or as applied to specific disciplines such as medicine and biology, which existed prior to or contemporary with Galen, so establishing the intellectual context of his own formulations. Galen's views, both as

---

[1] These additional works are the two specifically on causation (*De causis contentivis, De causis procatarcticis*), the two on 'biological' causation (*De causis pulsuum, De causis respirationis*), the *De usu partium* and, to a lesser extent, *De methodo medendi* and *De locis affectis*.

expressed in the translated treatises and in the other works referred to, will then be considered in some detail before attempting to summarize his position and, briefly, to relate it to current thinking on causation in medicine.

Before embarking on these matters, some preliminary observations, brief and general, might be apposite. First, at least for the purposes of the present discussion, I think it is worthwhile to make an arbitrary division into 'pure' and 'applied' causation. By 'pure' causation I mean the fundamental nature of causation – whether there is an actual causal nexus, if so what it connects, and the linguistic ramifications of discussion of such issues. In short, this is the subject matter of philosophical discussions of cause and causation independent of reference to a specific system. By 'applied' causation I mean the existence of causation in, and the application of causal concepts to, specific systems or disciplines. These include, notably, sciences and quasi-sciences (the latter to include medicine), other philosophical issues, and ethics. In the present context, medicine is the dominant concern, but also of importance are biology and psychology, the last including the vexed question of mind–body interaction. The overall implication here is that the application of causal concepts may differ in different systems.

With regard to what I have called 'pure' causation, the central requirement is to give a philosophically plausible account of what, in everyday life, is taken to be a universally operative process. The essential question is whether causation involves a physical nexus, or a logical connection, or an *a priori* mental 'structure', or merely more or less constant conjunction (to the extent that these accounts are mutually exclusive). And in the event of finding an answer to this question, however provisional, there is the further issue of what the causal relation is between. Is it between events, property instances, objects, variables, facts, states of affairs, propositions, events under a description etc.,[2] and how it is to be spoken of? Undoubtedly these issues are to a significant degree peripheral to the kind of account Galen is concerned with in the treatises on causation of diseases and symptoms, but not so much so that they can be ignored or lost sight of. At the very least, section I.6 in his *De symptomatum differentiis* reveals Galen's awareness of this.

On the matter of 'applied' causation, the particular issues of importance for Galen are those mentioned above. To reiterate, and amplify slightly, these are:

---

[2] This list is taken from Humphreys in Newton-Smith (2000), p. 31.

1. The causes of diseases generally, along with what might be called related phenomena such as symptoms, syndromes and affections – the subject matter of the treatises under consideration.
2. The causes of basic biological phenomena, specifically why bodily structures are as they are, and what the causes are of such essentially invariable and regular functions as the pulse and respiration.
3. The causes of mental disturbances and diseases, which takes Galen into two problematic areas: the then still contentious field of the anatomical locus of mental functions and the now still contentious issue of psychophysical interaction.

Even the most cursory reflection on the points above makes it obvious how inextricably linked the practice of medicine is to ideas of causation even if, under ordinary circumstances, these ideas and the issues referred to are largely unexamined. Anscombe, in a recent article, poses the following question rhetorically: '. . . might it not be like this: knowledge of causes is possible without any satisfactory grasp of what is involved in causation?'[3] In the same article, laced with references to medicine, she downplays the role of causation, writing, '. . . doctors seldom even know any of the conditions under which one invariably gets a disease, let alone all the sets of conditions.' It is, however, at the root of Galen's endeavour, in these treatises and elsewhere, that these causes/conditions must be sought, the underlying assumption being that the extent to which this endeavour is successful determines the success of recognition and treatment of diseases and also the ability to formulate a satisfactory classification. It is also, I would suggest, a fundamental credo of current conventional medical practice. In what follows the primary focus will be on point 1 above, but the other two points will also be considered.

In concluding these introductory remarks, I would like briefly to presage the overall argument. As outlined in the following section, in the time before Galen there were five particularly influential individuals or schools who expressed views on (more or less) 'pure' causation, or at least, causation in general, as I have here termed it. These were Plato, Aristotle, the Atomists/Epicureans, the Stoics and the Sceptics. Each, however, could be said to have had something of a particular axe to grind – for example, the Atomists on the nature of matter and the Stoics on ethical issues – so the accounts that emerge are, to a degree, conflicting or, perhaps, non-overlapping. The medical accounts of causation, given in outline below, were heavily dependent on prior or contemporary philosophical accounts

---

[3] Anscombe, in Perry and Bratman (1993), p. 252.

and became distilled essentially into the three main 'schools' existing in Galen's time: the Empiricists, casting doubt on causation, or at least on the possibility of understanding causation and applying it fruitfully to medical practice; the Methodics, giving an idiosyncratic and severely reductionist account of disease causation which essentially took it out of play in ordinary practice; and the Dogmatics who sought to give as complete a causal account of disease as possible and to make this a basis for therapy. I shall argue for two conclusions. The first, for which I shall argue only weakly and briefly, is that in terms of causation in general (or 'pure' causation), the main strands of thinking and the areas of contention that existed before and during Galen's time remain discernible today. The second, for which I shall argue strongly and at greater length, is that Galen, by the range and force of his arguments, dominated the debate on causation in medicine to the extent that his became the defining and enduring view, not seriously challenged until his basic structural concepts were definitively overthrown. And even when this happened, the difference between Galen and the moderns was not in what the concepts of causation were and how they were applied, but in what the physical nature of the causative factors and what they acted on actually was, Thus, whilst one must be conscious of the realism/instrumentalism issue in science in general, it could be argued that Galen's brand of Dogmatism, seasoned with Empiricism (for example, a particular causal analysis is subject to empirical verification), is still what informs the attitudes towards causation in medicine today despite the very substantial advances in knowledge and understanding of specific causes.

1.6B THEORIES OF DISEASE CAUSATION PRIOR TO GALEN

There is, as noted above, a close correspondence between the ideas formulated on causation in general, and the more restricted field of causation of disease, although the correspondence is not exact. One important question specific to the latter is whether it is feasible to achieve, or even reasonable to attempt, the theoretically desirable perfection of causal analysis in a system which is complex and non-isolated. So there is not only the fundamental issue of whether a causal account is possible, but also the practical issue of whether it is desirable, necessary and relevant. On these matters, broadly speaking three positions may be identified:

1. All diseases are ultimately susceptible to a complete causal analysis and only when this is achieved will satisfactory prophylaxis, diagnosis and treatment be possible for the particular disease in question. This position

presupposes the discrete existence of individual disease 'entities' (see I.4a above).

2. Causal analysis of disease is either impossible or irrelevant and should not be pursued. The doctor recognizes what has been seen before and treats it in a way that he and others have found to work. There is no necessity to understand why. Clearly, the doctor's approach can be continuously modified on the basis of changing experience.

3. A middle way can be pursued in which theoretical constructions related to disease causation and mechanism can be established, but are not necessarily relevant to the immediate practical aspects of diagnosis and treatment.

Galen himself characterizes this range of attitudes as follows:

For some have said that no cause of anything exists; some have doubted if there is [a cause] or not, like the Empiricists; some have accepted [causes] on the basis of supposition, like Herophilus, whilst others in fact, of whom he himself [Erasistratus] was the leader, set aside the *prokatarktic* among causes as being wrongly believed in. All these have changed the signification of the term to suit the purposes of their arguments. For if they concede that since all men say there is the useful cause of those things which come about, and the effective cause which is the origin, and with these the material and the instruments, it would certainly be easily discovered that they are sophistical.[4]

It must also be remembered that in practical matters like disease, causation cannot be considered independently from the system in which it is supposedly operating. Thus, the concept of the basic structure of the body is a critical component of any causal account of diseases and symptoms. In this case there were two quite distinct prevailing theories, atomic and continuum, the latter with or without the addition of *pneuma*. Differing causal accounts will clearly be required for each major theory with appropriate modifications for variations. What follows is a summarized account of the various theories associated with individuals or sects prior to Galen.

(i) Alcmaeon

It is agreed, albeit on very flimsy evidence, that the first to advance a rational account of disease causation was Alcmaeon in the fifth century BC. The relevant fragment (from Aëtius) is as follows:

---

[4] *De causis procatarcticis* XII.162, Hankinson (1998), pp. 128–30.

[According to] Alcmaeon the essential requirement for health is the balance (*isonomia*) of the capacities, moistness, dryness, coldness, hotness, bitterness, sweetness, and the remainder, whereas what brings about disease is a preponderance (*monarchia*) in them, for a preponderance of each is destructive. And disease occurs by excess of heat or cold, and from this through excess or lack of nutriment, and in these [things] – blood, marrow or brain. Sometimes [disease] occurs to them from external causes, from the kinds of waters, from place, from fatigue, from necessity, or from things near them. Health on the other hand is a balanced mixture of qualities.[5]

There are three key aspects of this fragment: (i) the supposition of basic qualities or capacities (the latter term – *dunamis* – having a different sense from its later use) as fundamental in the composition of the body; (ii) the idea of balance of these qualities corresponding to health and imbalance to disease; (iii) the idea of both internal and external factors as being capable of disturbing balance. This is, in essence, Galen's position as elaborated on in the four treatises being considered, particularly with respect to causation.

(ii)　Hippocratic Corpus

As indicated earlier, the Hippocratic Corpus is now widely accepted as being a heterogeneous collection of works by an unknown number of different writers compiled over a period of up to two centuries.[6] The inconsistencies embedded in this composite material are clearly in evidence when the disparate views on the causation of disease contained in the Corpus are examined. In general terms, however, the various components contain some of the earliest surviving sustained attempts to provide a natural, as opposed to a supernatural, account of disease causation. Moreover, despite some notable variations, this account is generally based on a continuum concept of bodily structure involving elements and qualities. Jouanna provides a full discussion of the transition from the divine to the rational in medical explanation, showing, *inter alia*, how this corresponds to changes in the nature of the explanation of historical events, as exemplified in Herodotus and Thucydides.[7] In the present brief survey, the concept of disease causation in the Hippocratic Corpus – a topic of considerable complexity in itself – will be considered only in relation to several key works, as follows.

The *Sacred Disease* provides a useful starting point: 'Nor does this disease (i.e. epilepsy) seem to me to be any more divine that the rest, but it has

[5] D-K, Frag. B4, vol. 1, pp. 215–16.
[6] See, for example, Gomperz (1911), Lloyd (1975), Jouanna (1999), chapter 4, pp. 56–71.
[7] See Jouanna (1999), ch. 8, pp. 181–209.

a nature as other diseases do, and a cause (*prophasis*) from which each one arises.'[8] Apart from the obvious importance of the work as a whole, marking historically the transition to a rational explanation of disease, articulated clearly in the statement above, there is the detail of the attempted explanation which follows, although what this is does not immediately concern us here.[9] What is notable is the detail of the analysis of the disease mechanism and, incidental to present concerns, the recognition of the brain as the *locus affectus* of neurological disease.

In contrast, the author of *Ancient Medicine*[10] begins with a strong statement against those who seek causal factors in disease:

All those who attempt to speak or write about medicine put forward for themselves a hypothesis for their argument – heat, cold, moisture or dryness or whatever else they might wish. They narrow down the origin of the cause of diseases and death in men, making it the same in all cases, postulating one thing or two. They are clearly in error in the many and varied things they say, and are particularly worthy of censure in that these relate to what is an art, and one which all use on the most important occasions and honour particularly the good practitioners and craftsmen.[11]

Subsequently, there is a further strongly worded statement against those who base their theoretical formulations on concepts of structure.[12]

Nonetheless, the author's position against causal analysis is not intractable: 'And it seems to me necessary to know these things, i.e. which affections in a person arise from capacities, and which from forms.'[13] Is the writer taking a general anti-theoretical position, or are particular theories pertaining especially to causation being attacked? Lloyd, who has given detailed consideration to the question of who is being attacked in *Ancient Medicine*, writes: 'Among many different theories of disease which are found in the Hippocratic Corpus, there are several to which the author of *Ancient Medicine* would have objected, either because they were based on a postulate or because they laid too great an emphasis on heat, cold, moisture and dryness.'[14] Elsewhere, he identifies particularly Alcmaeon and the Hippocratic treatises *Breaths* and *Regimen* I, although he mentions also a number of other treatises including *Nature of Man*, a work which has a special relevance to Galen's own theoretical formulations.[15] Certainly, this

---

[8] *Sacred Disease* V (Jones).   [9] See *Sacred Disease* VI–X (Jones).
[10] It is not clear who this was – see, for example, *Hippocrates*, ed. Jones (1923), vol. 1, introduction pp. 3–11, particularly p. 3, and Lloyd (1975).
[11] *Ancient Medicine* I.1–11.   [12] *Ancient Medicine* XX.
[13] *Ancient Medicine* XXII.   [14] Lloyd (1963), pp. 117–18.
[15] See the two important Galenic works, *De elementis secundum Hippocratem* (I.413–508K) and *In Hippocratis De natura hominis librum commentarii* (XV.1–173K).

last work is a possible target in that here, most clearly, it is the theory of structure involving elements and qualities which is advanced in relation to disease causation thus: 'For there are in the body many things present which, whenever they are heated, cooled, dried or moistened contrary to nature by other things, bring about diseases.'[16]

External factors are also recognized as important: 'Diseases arise in some cases from ways of life and in some cases from the breathed air which, by taking in, we live.'[17] To the author, knowledge of causes is clearly of more than theoretical importance: 'Those diseases which arise suddenly and the causes of which are readily discerned, are the most securely prognosticated on.'[18] In several works, in fact, the role of environmental factors in the causation of disease is given prominence. Particularly is this so in *Airs, Waters, Places*, where a more or less systematic account is given of problems associated with specific environmental and climatic conditions together with examples of activities which have apparent adverse effects. A well-known instance is that of the unfortunate Scythians.[19] The roles of climatic factors and seasonal variations are also considered in other treatises, for example in *Humours* ('For the seasons too are apt to recur and so are disease-causing')[20] and in *Aphorisms* ('The changes of the seasons especially give rise to diseases . . .').[21]

The Hippocratic treatise *Breaths* is generally taken to be advancing a single major cause of disease. Thus Jones, in his somewhat derogatory comments about the author, remarks: 'The writer of *Breaths* would prove that air, powerful in nature generally, is also the prime factor in causing diseases. He is a rhetorical sophist who, either in earnest or perhaps merely to show his skill in supporting a *hypothesis*, adopted the fundamental tenet of a rather belated Ionian monist.'[22] There are, however, more general points being made in this work, not least the importance of causal explanation itself: 'For if someone knew the cause of a disease, he would be the kind of person to bring things of benefit to the body.'[23] Moreover, food and drink are recognized as causally important. Nonetheless, it is *phusai* that are of primary importance: 'Therefore breaths appear to be particularly troublesome throughout all diseases, whereas all other things are *sunaitia* (cooperative causes) or *metaitia* (joint causes).'[24]

---

[16] *Nature of Man* II.16–20.   [17] *Nature of Man* IX.11–13.
[18] *Nature of Man* XIII.1–3. It is notable that here and elsewhere *prophasis* is used for 'cause' – see section 1.4b above.
[19] See *Airs, Waters, Places* XVII–XXII.   [20] *Humours* XIII.26–7.
[21] *Aphorisms* III.1.   [22] *Hippocrates*, ed. Jones (1923), vol. 1, pp. 221–2.
[23] *Breaths* I.24–6. Jouanna (1999) adds here, "using opposites to combat the disease" (see p. 208).
[24] *Breaths* XV.1–3.

What can be said in summary about disease causation in the Hippocratic Corpus? First and foremost, there is the generally pervasive, and in a number of places specifically stated, view that causal explanation of individual diseases can not only be given, but is of critical importance for prophylaxis and treatment. Second, there is the assumption that causal accounts must be based on a proper understanding of the structure and composition of matter in general and of the body in particular. The treatise *Ancient Medicine* does raise a dissenting voice from within the Corpus against both these supposedly fundamental premises, but still speaks of the knowledge of causation in relation to structural variations as the basis for taking appropriate measures.[25] Among the causal factors given prominence in the Hippocratic Corpus are the four elements, four qualities or four humours, and disturbance of their proper harmony. External factors are also recognized as important, not only the more obvious ones such as trauma causing wounds or fractures, but also those related to environment and way of life. All these aspects are accorded considerable importance in Galen's own accounts of the causation of diseases and symptoms.

(iii)   Philolaus and Philistion (Anonymus londinensis)

Subsequent, and interrelated in ways not altogether clear, are the formulations on the causation of disease by Philolaus of Croton, Philistion of Locri and Plato. First, it would seem that all accepted, at least broadly, the continuum theory of bodily structure involving elements, qualities and humours. Longrigg considers that Philolaus was the only Pythagorean known to have done this.[26] Secondly, there are no surviving writings of the first two men. Unfortunately then, as is often the case, reliance must be placed on fragments and doxographical material. Galen himself lists Philistion, along with Empedocles and Pausanias, among the Italian doctors but has no mention of Philolaus.[27] The main source of information on the causal views of both Philolaus and Philistion is the *Anonymus londinensis*. In section XVIII of that work there is an account first of Philolaus' ideas on the structure of the body, and then the following statement of his views on disease causation:

He says diseases occur due to bile, blood and phlegm, these being the origin of diseases. He says that the blood is made thick when the flesh is pressed inwards, whereas it becomes thin when the vessels in the flesh are divided up. He says

---

[25] *Ancient Medicine* XXIII.   [26] Longrigg (1993), p. 114.
[27] The reference to Philistion is in *De methodo medendi* X.5K. Philolaus is spoken of several times in the pseudo-Galenic work *De historia philosophica* XIX.222–345K.

phlegm is made up from waters and bile is a liquor (serum) of the flesh. In this the man himself proposes what is paradoxical. For he says that the bile is not assigned to the liver but is, rather, a liquor (serum) of the flesh. Again, while the majority say phlegm is cold, he postulates that it is hot in nature, in that 'phlegm' is derived from 'to burn' (*phlegein*). It is in this way, by partaking of phlegm, inflamed things are inflamed. And these, he proposes, are the origins of diseases whereas excesses of heat, nourishment and cold are contributory [factors].[28]

Subsequently, in section XX of the *Anonymus londinensis* there is a similar account for Philistion, who is described in a way that suggests he had a more orthodox view of the elements, qualities and humours. His theory of disease causation is given as follows:

Philistion thinks we are compounded from kinds, that is from elements – fire, air, water and earth. And that there are capacities of each – heat of fire, cold of air, moisture of water and dryness of earth. According to him, diseases occur in many ways but to speak in outline and more generically [they are] threefold: because of the elements, because of the condition of bodies, and because of external things. It is because of the elements then, whenever the hot or the moist is in excess, or whenever the hot becomes less or weak. It is because of external things through wounds or ulcers, or through excess of heat or cold or similar things, or through the change of heat to cold or cold to heat, or through nutriment which is inappropriate or corrupted. It is because of the condition of bodies thus: whenever, he says, the whole body breathes well and the breath passes through unhindered, health occurs. For respiration occurs not only in relation to the mouth and nostrils but also in relation to the entire body. Whenever the body does not breathe well diseases arise, and in a variety of ways. For when breathing is restricted in relation to the whole body, diseases . . .[29]

The *Anonymus londinensis* also sets out the views of a number of other writers. These are listed in summary in Table 3. Broadly, they fall into two groups: (i) Those who attribute diseases to some disorder of nutrition, whether it involves disposal or distribution. (ii) Those who postulate an imbalance of the bodily components.

(iv)   Plato

We turn next to Plato's somewhat extraordinary account of the classification and causation of disease in the *Timaeus*. His theory is founded on a concept of structure based on elements, qualities and humours, augmented by his own curious and idiosyncratic concept of geometric shapes. On grounds of causation specifically, he identifies three classes of disease.[30]

---

[28] *Anonymus londinensis* XVIII.30–49.   [29] *Anonymus londinensis* XX.25–50.
[30] For a recent consideration of Plato's theory of disease see Lloyd (2004).

Table 3 *Summary of views of lesser writers on causation of disease in the* Anonymus londinensis

Name	*Anon. Lon.*	Cause(s) of diseases
Eurypion of Cnidos	IV.31	Retention of nutriment with build-up of superfluities
Herodicus of Cnidos	IV.40	Nutriment not assimilated; formation of superfluities – one acid, one bitter
Alcmanes of Abydus	VII.41	Superfluities from nutriment
Timotheus of Metapontum	VIII.11	Blocked distribution of nutriment and build-up of superfluities
Aias(?)	VIII.35	Purging from the brain via nose, ears, eyes and nostrils
Herodicus of Selymbria	IX.20	Way of life (regimen)
Ninyas the Egyptian	IX.37	Two kinds of disease: congenital (innate in bodies) and acquired (failed distribution of nutriment)
Hippon of Croton	XI.22	Drying of natural moisture, excess heat or cold.
Thrasymachus of Sardis	XI.43	Changes of blood giving phlegm, bile or pus due to excess cold or heat
Dexippus of Cos	XII.8	Superfluities of nutriment – particularly bile and phlegm
Phasilas the Coan	XII.36	Emanations from moistures or excretions themselves; balance of ?elements
Aegimius of Elis	XIII.21	Excess of superfluities or due to nutriment
Menecrates	XIX.18	Disturbed harmony of elements/humours: two hot (blood, bile), two cold (breath, phlegm)
Petron of Aegina	XX.1	Disproportion of elements/qualities; excess of superfluities

1. Those due to the basic material elements. For Plato these were earth, fire, water and air. This class he subdivided into diseases caused by excess or deficiency of one of the elements, diseases caused by transfer of one of the elements from its proper place to a foreign place, and diseases due to the existence in the body of the wrong variant of a particular element.
2. Those due to a disordered sequence of formation of the tissues which Galen would include under the heading of *homoiomeric*, themselves formed from the elements. The term *deuterai sustaseis* is used.
3. Those due to the accumulation of air (wind), phlegm or bile.

It is a matter of considerable interest why Plato provided such a detailed account of the classification and causation of diseases. With respect to content, Taylor comments: 'The doctrine he (i.e. Plato) puts forward, though not wholly clear or coherent, is what we should expect from a speculative thinker anxious to fuse Pythagoras and Alcmaeon with Empedocles. Hence it is probably deliberately based by Plato on actual syntheses of this kind attempted by fifth-century Italian or Sicilian teachers.'[31] As to motive, Taylor elsewhere writes, apropos of the second class particularly:

It is hardly conceivable that Plato, who was, as Galen rightly insists, an *idiotes*, though an intelligent one, in medical matters, should have been at the pains to elaborate such a detailed theory for himself merely to fill two or three pages of T's discourse. The whole passage smells of the medical text-book. . . . we may probably conclude with reasonable probability that in all Timaeus has to say about disease arising in the *deuterai sustaseis* he is following the authority of Philolaus, as would be natural, since Philolaus, like himself, was concerned to bring biology, for which Empedocles was the great source in Sicily and Magna Graecia, into union with Pythagoreanism.[32]

Galen provides detailed criticism of this expression of Plato's views in his *De placitis Hippocratis et Platonis*.[33]

(v) Aristotle

Aristotle is included here despite the fact that he had nothing of any significance to say, at least in his extant writings, on the causation of disease. There is one work now lost entitled *Medicine* (in two books) included in Diogenes Laertius' list.[34] Given Aristotle's own medical background, and his profound subsequent interest in biology generally, it is somewhat surprising that he did not, as Plato did, make some contribution of importance in this matter. Certainly he gave some consideration to what disease is, in particular its existence as the contrary to health, which bears on the issues discussed in the previous section.[35] Also, in the first book of the pseudo-Aristotelian *Problems* there are some more or less random questions about disease, a number of which relate to causation. Two issues of interest among these are, firstly, the role of excess in the causation of disease and, secondly, why plague is likely to affect those who come into contact with those already suffering the disease.[36] Most of the rest of the material concerns external factors, particularly climatic conditions. As discussed in section I.6a, where Aristotle most notably influenced Galen with respect to causation was in

---

[31] Taylor (1928), p. 608. Possible direct influences are identified as Philolaus and Philistion.
[32] Taylor (1928), pp. 598–9.
[33] See Books VII–VIII (V.586–719K, De Lacy, vol. 2, pp. 428–531) and Taylor (1928), pp. 608–10.
[34] For a full list of titles, including Diogenes Laertius' list, see Barnes (1984), vol. 2, pp. 2386–8.
[35] See, for example, *Metaphysics* 1032b5 and 1044b31.
[36] *Problems* I.1 (859a1–10) and I.7 (859b15–20) respectively.

the areas of biological structure and function. The application of concepts of causation aimed at teleological explanation is, at first sight, hardly appropriate to disease and death, fundamental and ineluctable aspects of biology though they might be. This is, however, a complex issue which neither Aristotle nor Galen apparently addressed and which, therefore, will not be considered further here.

(vi) Diocles of Carystus

Diocles is listed among the Rationalists in the pseudo-Galenic work *Introductio sive medicus* as follows:

Hippocrates of Cos stood first among the Rationalist sect. He was the originator of the sect and the first to set up the Rationalist sect. After him [there came] Diocles of Carystus, Praxagoras of Cos, Herophilus of Chalcedon, Erasistratus of Ceos, Mnesitheus of Athens, Asclepiades of Bithynia who was also called of Prusias, and Athenaeus of Attaleia in Pamphylia.[37]

However, the exact position of Diocles in the causation debate is somewhat uncertain, as, indeed, are other aspects of his life and work. Like Praxagoras after him, he is said to have written a work entitled *Affections, Causes, Therapies*.[38] What little can be gleaned about his ideas of disease causation on the basis of the available fragments would align him clearly with other continuum theorists in attributing diseases primarily to an imbalance in elements, qualities or humours, whilst acknowledging also the role of external agents such as climatic conditions.

In the fragments of the *Anonymous of Paris* referring to specific diseases, Diocles is usually mentioned along with Praxagoras and others in relation to his views on causation. Scrutiny of the substantial collection of fragments in van der Eijk[39] reveals a significant variety of causal explanations for a range of particular diseases. The level of explanation is itself variable insofar as the attribution of a disease to inflammation clearly requires a further level of causal explanation to account for the inflammation. In addition, there is the problem posed by the apparently direct quotation from Diocles which Galen gives in *De alimentorum facultatibus*.[40] Although this is ostensibly about the effects caused by different kinds of ingested material, there is the possibility that the argument becomes more generalized. Thus, Vallance

---

[37] *Introductio sive medicus* XIV.683K. For other fragments stating the same see van der Eijk (2000), pp. 12–27.

[38] Galen is said to have written about Praxagoras' theory – see for example van der Eijk (2000), vol. 2, p. 53.

[39] van der Eijk (2000), vol. 1, pp. 142–241.   [40] *De alimentorum facultatibus* VI.454–7K.

writes that '. . . he seems to be arguing for more flexibility in the assignment of pathological effects to given causes'.[41] The evidence of this fragment notwithstanding, there seems to be insufficient in the collected fragments generally to necessitate revision of the view that Diocles' basic concept of disease causation depended on alterations in elements, qualities or humours coupled with external factors.

(vii)   Praxagoras

Like that of Diocles, Praxagoras' contribution to the development of ideas on disease causation has to be pieced together from relatively few scattered fragments, a number of which are from Galenic or pseudo-Galenic works where he is mentioned in conjunction with other doctors. He, too, is said to have written a work on causation of disease.[42] On the basis of what information there is, it is reasonable to accept that his concepts of pathology were based on the humours. Thus, in relation to Praxagoras, the pseudo-Galenic work *Introductio sive medicus* has: 'There are those who attributed to humours alone what is related to a state in accord with nature and what is related to a cause contrary to nature.'[43] Steckerl writes: 'Praxagoras made health and disease depend, in the last analysis, on the humours. The humours were the basis of all his medical thinking.'[44] There is some discussion about the extent of Praxagoras' subdivision of the four basic humours. Galen, in *De facultatibus naturalibus*, remarks:

And I have written to some degree in another work about the humours according to Praxagoras, son of Nicarchus. For if he particularly makes ten apart from the blood, so that the blood itself would be an eleventh humour, he does not depart from the teachings of Hippocrates. Rather, he divides into kinds and *differentiae* the humours spoken of by that man first of all, along with the proper demonstrations.[45]

Apart from the humours, other significant components in his analysis of disease causation were 'innate heat' and '[innate] *pneuma*'. Paucity of information again precludes detailed knowledge of Praxagoras' ideas on the precise origin and nature of these two entities, particularly to what extent the origin was external or internal in each case. Steckerl, on the basis of what information there is, attributes to Praxagoras the concept that when there

---

[41] For Vallance's comments see OCD, p. 470. The fragment in question is #176 in van der Eijk (2000), vol. 1, pp. 282–7. See also the latter's commentary in van der Eijk (2001), vol. 2, pp. 321–34.

[42] See Caelius Aurelianus, *Acute Diseases* III, Drabkin (1950), p. 402.

[43] *Introductio sive medicus* XIV.698K. See also Steckerl (1958), #46, p. 70.

[44] Steckerl (1958), p. 10.   [45] *De facultatibus naturalibus* II.141K.

is 'balance' (*summetria*) of the innate heat, food is appropriately changed into blood, whereas when there is 'imbalance' (*ametria*) the change is to various humours.[46] He also states: 'Only if the amount of heat coming from outside fits the nature and constitution of the animal, will the food be changed into blood; otherwise there will be abnormal digestion and more or less harmful humours will develop.'[47] In examining the fragments specifically about causation, i.e. those beginning '[disease] *aitia* . . .', the factors inculpated, while predominantly humours, also include cooling of the innate heat, inflammation, swelling and 'bubble' (*pompholyx*) formation.[48] Finally, it is worth noting Steckerl's claim that Praxagoras favoured a reductive analysis of disease, '. . . basing the manifold diseases on a comparatively small number of fundamental morbid conditions'.[49] This is not dissimilar from Galen's own approach.

(viii) Herophilus

Identification of Herophilus' position on causation generally, and on the role of causal explanation in dealing with disease, is uncertain. Evidence, again in no small part dependent on Galen, remains fragmentary and somewhat conflicting. Thus, in *De causis procatarcticis* Galen apparently quotes Herophilus as having said: 'In fact cause, whether it exists or not, is by nature undiscoverable, it being by judgement that I think I am cold, or hungry, or filled with food and drink.'[50] It is on this basis that Galen accuses him of 'timidity'.

Amongst modern commentators, three more or less distinct positions may be discerned. At one extreme, von Staden places him firmly within the Dogmatic tradition and committed, therefore, to causal explanation. In his summary for the OCD he writes: 'In his physiopathology, he appears to have accepted the traditional notion that an imbalance between humours or moistures in the body is a principal cause of disease, but he insisted that all causal explanation is provisional or hypothetical.'[51] Expanding on this, von Staden, in his collection of Herophilean fragments, has this to say: 'For all Herophilus' emphasis on the provisionality and hypothetical nature of causal explanation, the evidence presented in this chapter (especially

---

[46] See Steckerl (1958), p. 11. Steckerl uses only the term *summetria*, whereas Galen also uses *ametria* – see I.4c above.
[47] Steckerl (1958), pp. 11–12. .
[48] The fragments in question are #57, #62, #64–72, #74, #75, #77–9.
[49] Steckerl (1958), p. 16.   [50] *De causis procatarcticis* XVI.198.   [51] OCD, p. 699.

T205–T225) leaves no doubt that Vindician is right, at least to the extent that Herophilus engaged in causal explanation not only for physiological but also for pathological purposes. While Herophilus' cautious, sceptical strain breaks through in his statement that people sometimes suffer from fever although there is no antecedent (i.e. proximate) cause, Pliny confirms that "Herophilus established examining the causes of diseases" . . .'[52] Of ancient authors, both Galen himself and Pliny as above can be cited in support of this view. In *De compositione medicamentorum secundum locos* Galen writes: 'As one knows following Apollonius of the Herophilean sect, Herophilus throughout enjoined the doctor to be acquainted with what kind and how great the cause of a disease was, and by what means particularly it prevailed so as to make the treatment most appropriate for each.'[53] Further, in the pseudo-Galenic *Introductio sive medicus*, Herophilus is listed among the Rationalists.[54]

At the other extreme is the view expressed by Kudlien, that Herophilus can 'lay claim to a place of honour in the history of medical empiricism'.[55] Opposing this claim, and indeed taking an intermediate position generally, is Hankinson who, in his commentary on Galen's *De causis procatarcticis*, writes: '. . . it seems that Herophilus was not the straightforward medical sceptic that Kudlien . . . discerns. Herophilus, after all, held that all living creatures are regulated by four faculties . . . which seems paradigmatically Dogmatic in tone.' At the same time, Hankinson also takes issue also with von Staden's opinion.[56]

In conclusion, it does seem on balance more probable that Herophilus did acknowledge the importance of causal analysis and that it is correct to attribute to him support of Aristotle's dictum, 'first the *phainomena*, then the causes or principles'.[57] The exact understanding of this statement as a basis for Aristotle's, and subsequently Herophilus', methodology is not uncontroversial, however, as Lloyd has pointed out.[58] Certainly what evidence exists does show that he studied the phenomena, particularly the anatomical phenomena, in some detail, and that he did attempt causal analysis, whilst remaining aware of the often provisional nature of such analyses (*ex suppositione*).[59]

---

[52] von Staden (1989), p. 302. The reference to Pliny is *Natural History* XXVI.14.
[53] *De compositione medicamentorum secundum locos* XII.619K.
[54] *Introductio sive medicus* XIV.683K.
[55] Kudlien (1964), p. 13 – cited by von Staden (1989), p. 117.
[56] See *De cansis procarcticis*, Hankinson (1998), pp. 270–81.
[57] Following von Staden (1989), p. 118. The reference to Aristotle is *Parts of Animals* 639b3 ff.
[58] See Lloyd (1993) for a discussion of this issue.
[59] See *Ars medica* I (I.305–9K) for Galen's statement on Herophilus' tripartite division of medicine and also von Staden (1989), pp. 103–5, for a partial translation and analysis of this.

(ix) Erasistratus

With his fellow Alexandrian Herophilus, Erasistratus shared the distinction of having contributed significantly to the important advances in medicine made at the time, particularly in anatomy and physiology, although the two men shared also the lasting opprobrium associated with their presumed human vivisection. In terms of theories, particularly pertaining to causation, Erasistratus had more in common with his successor Asclepiades (considered below), in that they both held a concept of structure based on atomist theories, and both advanced a reductive account of disease causation. Once again, with Erasistratus there are difficulties due to the absence of extant works and dependence on the reporting by others often opposed to his ideas, such as Galen. In fact, in various considerations of his views on disease causation based on what information there is, there are definite differences.[60]

First, on the issue of structure, it does seem clear that he rejected any theory involving qualities – considerations of hot and cold were more relevant to the bath-house attendant than to medical practice[61] – and to have embraced a particle/void-based theory. Thus Longrigg, relying on Diels' earlier work, relates Erasistratus' views to the theories of Strato, writing: 'Like Strato, then, Erasistratus conceived of his particles as very small, imperceptible, corporeal entities surrounded by a vacuum in a finely divided or discontinuous condition.'[62] Two other aspects of importance in Erasistratus' basic physiology were the important role of *pneuma*, thought to be derived from inspired air and distributed through the arteries after passage to the heart, and the principle of *pros to kenoumenon akolouthia* (*horror vacui*), which may also have been derived from Strato.[63]

On the causation of disease, matters are also somewhat complex. It could be argued that Erasistratus shared with Asclepiades a commitment to a radically reductive account of disease causation, based by the former on *paremptosis*,[64] and by the latter on particle/void theory (see below). Galen's attitude to *paremptosis* is dismissive. In *De causis procatarcticis* he writes:

[60] Compare, for example, Dobson (1927), Garofalo (1988) and von Staden (1989).
[61] See *De methodo medendi* X.109K = Hankinson (1991), p. 58.   [62] Longrigg (1993), p. 214.
[63] See, however, Longrigg (1993), p. 256, n. 179, who writes: 'Wellman, however, maintains, again in opposition to Diels, that Erasistratus' doctrine of *horror vacui* was derived not from Strato but from Chrysippus, who, he believes, had in his turn derived the theory, from Philistion of Locri . . .'
[64] The nature and pathological consequences of *paremptosis* are well described by Vallance (1990), pp. 126–8.

For it is not possible to show how *paremptosis*, that is a 'falling' of blood into the arteries, has been brought about in a man who is overheated, fatigued, angry or sad. Here, therefore, they make this argument involved, and trying to be sophistical they trick the young people who come with the hope of learning an art that is good and useful in life. In fact, what comes to them through the trickery of those people is contrary to that which they sought.[65]

Von Staden, however, in his summary for the OCD, writes that, '. . . Erasistratus introduced several causes of diseases, all ultimately instances of different forms of matter (blood, pneuma, various liquids) that normally are rigorously separated, somehow not remaining separated,'[66] although he describes only the process of *paremptosis*. If, however, we take the diversion of blood from veins to arteries (*paremptosis*) with the resultant disruption of the distribution of *pneuma* as the supposedly 'final cause', the issue then becomes, at least for inflammation and fever, the actual causal mechanism linking *paremptosis* to these manifestations of disease.

In summary, it is not difficult to see why Galen was at odds with Erasistratus on the issue of causation. First, there was the fundamental difference of structural concepts, although from available material it is difficult to see how Erasistratus related his causal analysis of disease to his concept of particle/void structure. One obvious consequence, however, of rejection of the continuum theory of structure was the tendency to downplay the importance of factors such as hot and cold, whether internal or external. Secondly, Erasistratus' apparently radically reductive analysis of causation was contrary to Galen's own, and this was especially obvious in relation to the effects of external factors. Third, and more fundamental in terms of the concept of causation, were their differences on the issues of causal analysis itself. For a cause–effect relationship to be certainly identified, must the effect invariably follow the cause and must the magnitude of the effect be proportional to the magnitude of the cause?

(x) Asclepiades

Without question, Asclepiades occupies an especially important position in any consideration of early theories of disease causation. Primarily this is because he, like Erasistratus, attempted a radically reductive approach, founded on a clearly articulated theory of basic structure which was a form of particle/void theory. As discussed earlier, reductive theories of disease causation had been advanced, for instance in the Hippocratic treatise *On*

---

[65] *De causis procatarcticis* XI.139–40.   [66] OCD, p. 553.

Breaths, just as extreme reductive theories on the basic structure of matter had been advanced since the beginning of Greek philosophy. What, arguably, distinguished Asclepiades' theory[67] is that by limiting disease causation to a single mechanism, therapy could be simplified and be, at least potentially, radical. And, indeed, Asclepiades' therapeutic methods were simple, just as they were no doubt attractive to the patient owing to their essentially benign nature, however successful or unsuccessful they might have been.

The essence, then, of Asclepiades' theory was that under normal conditions, the particles or corpuscles (*anarmoi onkoi*), whatever their precise nature, moved through imperceptible channels (*poroi*) within the body. If this movement was interfered with (*entasis*), disease ensued. A further possible component of disease causation was the movement of particles to inappropriate places. Whether this latter could invariably be attributed to blockage (*entasis*) is not altogether clear. Thus, in the pseudo-Galenic treatise *Introductio sive medicus* there is the following: 'According to Erasistratus and Aesclepiades, there is altogether only one cause in the case of every disease; according to the former *paremptosis* of blood into the arteries, whereas according to the latter extension of particles in the crevices (i.e. pores).'[68] Soranus, however, writes:

Similar things have also to be said against Herophilus and against Asclepiades who is wrong in his concept of the elements and about causation also. Besides, he says that obstruction is not the actual cause of all, but of most diseases, because ravenous hunger, dropsy, and fever from exhaustion are produced by another cause.[69]

Two other aspects of Asclepiades' views on disease causation that are important in the present context are, firstly, his awareness of the significance of a *locus affectus*, and secondly, that it seems clearly to be these views that receive specific consideration in the works here being studied, particularly *De causis morborum*, rather than the Methodists' later development of them.

It was suggested above that there is a connection between Erasistratus and Asclepiades in their approach to disease causation, and this is certainly reflected in the quotation from the *Introductio sive medicus* given immediately above. What is common is the attempt at a reductive account; what is different is the theoretical basis underlying these accounts and hence the

---

[67] The important issues of the postulated nature of his particles and void and the identity of those who influenced his theoretical formulations are not considered here – see Vallance (1990), particularly chs. 1 and 2, pp. 7–92.

[68] *Introductio sive medicus* XIV.728–9K. Vallance (1990), who gives the text for this excerpt, has *entasis* in place of *ektasis* which appears in Kühn.

[69] Soranus, *Gynaecology* III.4, translation after Temkin (1956), p. 131.

specifics of the accounts themselves, although both may be included under the broad rubric of particle/void theories. The matter of the relationship between the two men is, in fact, a complex one. Vallance, who considers this particular issue in some detail, provides a useful summarizing table.[70] As to Asclepiades' successors, among the Methodists who embraced his theories a clear distinction may be discerned between the more doctrinaire members, particularly Themison and Thessalus, the latter a target of some severe criticism by Galen, and those of a more moderate bent such as Soranus who were much less hardline in their attitudes on the nature and relevance of disease causation.[71]

(xi)   Athenaeus

In examining concepts of causation in disease, it is particularly unfortunate that the writings of Athenaeus of Attaleia have been lost.[72] As discussed earlier, he is thought to have worked in Rome in the first century BC and to have founded the Pneumatic sect, although details are uncertain. It is, however, generally agreed that he based his physiology and pathology on a continuum theory of structure involving elements, qualities and humours, with the addition of an important role for *pneuma* as the 'fifth element'. Health and disease were then explained in terms of *eukrasia* and *dyscrasia*, as with Galen himself.

There are two fragments of particular importance in the present context. The first, from the pseudo-Galenic work *Definitiones medicae*, links Athenaeus with the concept of *prokatarktic* causes – see section 1.4b above. The second, from the *De causis contentivis*, a work considered more fully below, is included here *in extenso*:

As for Athenaeus the Attaleian, he founded the medical school known as that of the Animists. It suits his doctrine to speak of a cohesive cause in illness since he bases himself upon the Stoics and he was a pupil and disciple of Posidonius. But it does not suit the theories of those other doctors who hold different views to look for a cohesive cause in every illness nor to try to find it in the *homoiomeres* in their natural state and they cannot say, as Athenaeus did, that there are three types of primary cause that are ultimate in their class. Athenaeus' three types are

---

[70] See Vallance (1990), ch. 4, particularly pp. 122–30. The table is on p. 130.
[71] For examples of Galen's criticism of Thessalus see *De methodo medendi* X.4K ff., X.38K and X.51–3K. For a more even-handed treatment of the Methodics see, for example, Celsus, *Proemium* 62–73. For a more conventional account of causation by a Methodist see Soranus IV ('On Difficult Labour'), Temkin (1956), pp. 175–84.
[72] For fragments see Oribasius, *Veterum et clarorum medicorum graecorum opuscula* and Wellmann (1895).

as follows: first that of the cohesive causes, then that of the prior causes while the third type comprises the matter of the immediate causes. This latter term is applied to externals *whose function it is to produce some change in the body, whatever this change may be.* If what is thus produced in the body belongs to the class of what causes disease, then, while it has not yet actually given rise to a disease, it is known as a prior cause. Alterations are produced in the natural spirit by these causes together with those that are external, leading to moisture, dryness, *heat or cold*, and these are known as the cohesive causes of disease. For, in Athenaeus' view, the spirit, having penetrated the *homoiomerous* parts of the body, changes them through its own change and assimilates them to itself. Often, he says, the cohesive cause is produced directly from the immediate without an intermediary, though sometimes it comes through the medium of the prior cause.[73]

There then follows consideration of some specific examples. The relationship of these ideas to those of Galen himself is obvious.

The range of views on the causation of disease existing immediately before and during Galen's time is apparent from a consideration of the so-called medical Schools. These were discussed in outline in chapter I.3 and a summary of the ideas on causation of the main members of each has been given above. It is obvious that the divisions between Schools were based primarily on the interrelated factors of concepts of fundamental structure and concepts of disease mechanism and causation. These differences were necessarily reflected in their approaches to diagnosis and therapy, at least in theory. It remains, however, an interesting and unresolved – possibly indeed unresolvable – question just how important and how sharp the demarcations actually were between the Schools in terms of practice.[74]

Certainly there was a major division on the basis of structural concepts – particle/void versus continuum (elements, qualities, humours). This division does not, however, of itself entail membership of a particular medical as opposed to philosophical school. In either case, a sceptical or empirical stance could be maintained with regard to causal explanation in the complex multifactorial situation of disease. Similarly, it would be theoretically possible to attempt a reductive analysis pertaining to a particular theory and, on the basis of this, to pursue hidden causes as potential keys to the

[73] *De causis contentivis* II. Translation by Lyons (1969) from the Arabic (the italics are his). In the Latin version the three types are given as follows: 'prima quidem coniunctarum, secunda vero antecedentium, tercia autem in procatarcticarum materia continetur.'

[74] An interesting example put forward by Galen himself focuses on the differing therapeutic approaches to the bite of a rabid dog – see *On the Sects for Beginners*, Walzer and Frede (1985), ch. 4, pp. 7–8. For a discussion of this issue see also *De causis procatarcticis*, Hankinson (1998), pp. 41–3. Galen's point is that, despite the marked theoretical differences, the actual treatment method is quite similar for members of the individual Schools.

understanding of specific diseases. In our own time, the highly sophisticated development of particle/void theory currently predominant is an article of faith in medical science. Nonetheless, causal analysis of individual diseases is pursued in most cases without reference to this theory, and involves particularly what Galen and his contemporaries might identify as *prokatarktic* or *proegoumenic* causes. So, in summary, the post-Hellenistic division of doctors into Schools, largely on the basis of their views on causation, could be simplified by recognizing two broad groups. There were those who saw causal analysis (beyond what was obvious) as fruitless regardless of commitment to a particular structural theory and without necessarily denying the existence of causes. And there were those who pursued causal analysis as far as possible, including hidden causes, on the grounds that this type of analysis was indispensable in practice for successful treatment.

In this somewhat skeletal survey on theories of disease causation and their main protagonists prior to Galen, several individuals of undoubted relevance have been omitted. In particular, Mnesitheus, Themison and Thessalus, Olympicus, Soranus and Rufus have received less than adequate attention owing to constraints of space. To no small degree, of course, the perceived importance of a particular individual from the perspective of the present time will depend on the extent of preservation of his writings. On this point, as has been stressed on several occasions, the disproportionate dependence on Galen as a source of information is itself a reason for caution. Nonetheless, despite the omissions and uncertainties, the range of views on disease causation is clearly apparent. Against the background of the above considerations of causation in general and causation of disease specifically, I shall now outline Galen's own views on causation before concluding this section with some reflections on the fate of Galen's ideas about disease causation down to the present time.

1.6C   GALEN ON CAUSATION

(i)   Preliminary remarks

The first point to make is that Galen was clearly committed to the importance of causation in general and to the application of causal analysis to disease in particular. The second point is that his views are complex and hard to summarize. It is, in fact, difficult to be sure that he had a consistent view. There are several aspects to this problem:

1. His views on causes and causation are scattered throughout his vast *oeuvre*. Further, in particular works not ostensibly about these matters

there may be significant digressions embodying important statements on the subjects – an example is *De symptomatum differentiis* I.6.

2. His arguments on causation are characteristically purpose-directed. They are usually either *ad hominem* (e.g. against Erasistratus in *De causis procatarcticis*), or *ad rem* (e.g. about biological structure in *De usu partium* or disease in *De causis morborum*).

3. His use of terminology is variable, as discussed in section 1.4b above. For example, it is argued there that he uses the terms *aitia, aition* and *prophasis* interchangeably in the treatises under examination and that his use of adjectival qualifications for *aition* are inconsistent and unimportant in these works. Despite his several digressions on terminology he is, in fact, using 'cause' in the unqualified way it is used in much of current medical writing – for example, in statements like 'cigarette smoking is a/the cause of lung cancer'.

What I shall do below is consider separately four aspects of his position(s) on causation, employing somewhat arbitrary divisions – (i) causation in general; (ii) his works specifically on causation; (iii) causation in biology/physiology; (iv) causation in diseases and symptoms, with further division into physical and psychical. I have not considered separately the question of the causal status or relevance of the so-called six non-naturals which are discussed briefly in 1.4c above.

(ii) Causation in general

I shall briefly consider here some observations which Galen makes on the general nature of causes and causation in three works: *De locis affectis, De methodo medendi* and the four treatises on diseases and symptoms. In the first of these works the focus is primarily on anatomical aspects of disease. Galen does, however, make several interesting and relevant, albeit brief, observations of a general nature bearing on the temporal and spatial requirements for establishing a causal connection. In the first instance he writes:

It is, therefore, always necessary to begin from the organ of damaged function, then to seek in turn what the manner of damage is to it, and whether in fact the condition is stable or is still coming about and is not yet stable. And if it is coming about, whether the cause effecting the state is retained in the part itself, or passes through it.[75]

Also on the temporal relation of cause to effect, he writes:

75 *De locis affectis* VIII.22K.

For sometimes a state arises from a certain cause, but does not yet have a condition that is stable if the cause is removed. Sometimes it has already come about and sometimes it is still coming about. Often, however, when the cause has gone, what has come about abates, whereas the condition is already stable.[76]

On the matter of the spatial relationship between cause and effect, he observes:

For if some sort of affection occurs to us when we are in contact with something, but ceases immediately when we withdraw, all people believe this to be a cause. In this way, then, fire is believed to be the cause of burning us and a sword of cutting us, and each of the other things in like manner. Therefore, one must presume the evacuated humour to be the cause of the condition that has occurred whenever it is retained in the part.[77]

The final interesting observation, made in relation to the affection of teeth and gums termed *haimodia*, is that, in general, similar effects follow similar causes, although Galen may be attributing this observation to Archigenes here.[78] In fact, he himself makes the more or less opposite observation that a particular effect may follow various different causes, exemplified by indigestion.[79]

Turning to the *De methodo medendi*, although this work does not contain a systematic attempt to identify, analyse and illustrate causes of diseases in the way the four books under primary consideration do, it does, nonetheless, include important observations on disease causation. In addition, unlike the books under study, Galen in this work does relate variations in causal concepts to different individuals. Terminological issues are also raised, although again not in a systematic fashion.

An early and important statement on the universality of the causal relation and some comments on the definitions of terms, both essentially assumed in the treatises on causes of diseases and symptoms, is as follows:

. . . an axiom incapable of proof, although agreed by all in that it is clear to thought. And what is this? That nothing happens without cause, for if this is not accepted we would be unable to seek the cause of damage to vision or its complete destruction. But since this is clear to thought, having postulated that there is some cause of damage, we proceed to look for it. With respect then to this cause, it makes no difference, at least to present considerations, whether you wish to call it some condition of the body or the body being somehow affected. In all cases then you will either say the disease itself is this [cause], or if the disease is a damage of function, the damaging condition is the actual cause of disease.[80]

---

[76] *De locis affectis* VIII.25K. In these two statements about the temporal relationship between cause and effect, examples from eye disease and dysentery are given respectively.

[77] *De locis affectis* VIII.24K.   [78] *De locis affectis* VIII.86–7K.

[79] *De symptomatum causis* III, XII.2.   [80] *De methodo medendi* X.51K.

Subsequently, Galen proceeds to develop a division of what might be called the 'components' of disease which, although framed differently, is conceptually in agreement with the position advanced in the four books under consideration. He lists four such 'components' which he speaks of as *genera*, and which are, in summary, as follows: (i) the body itself; (ii) its functions which may be *kata phusin* or *para phusin*; (iii) causes bringing about either of the preceding conditions; and (iv) a condition in bodies either *kata* or *para phusin* which neither helps nor harms functions.[81] Having distinguished these four *genera*, he then makes the following remarks of particular relevance to causation:

So, if someone should wish to, let him call a condition of bodies contrary to nature, whenever it harms some function, a disease, and the actual damage of function some outstanding symptom of disease. All those things that otherwise occur, such as colours, these let him, if he wishes, call symptoms, although let him distinguish those of damage of functions, and if he terms these outstanding symptoms of diseases, let him call these particular or specific and those apart from these neither particular nor specific, if he wishes, but occurring through some chance. Let there be placed, in addition to these, a fourth *genus*, that of causes of diseases, and of these let him call those that arise in the actual body of the animal *proegoumenic* and those that befall [it] from without *prokatarchontic*.[82]

Later, in the initial sections of Book II, he again lists the four things 'contrary to nature' as (i) impaired function; (ii) the condition that brings about impaired function; (iii) the cause(s) of the condition; and (iv) the symptoms that follow of necessity. Causes are exemplified by excess and deficiency.[83]

In summary, the *De methodo medendi* presents an essentially identical view of disease causation to that given in the four books under consideration. The distinguishing features of the former is that the discussions of causation are somewhat scattered and less systematic, they are more general in that there is no attempt to give an exhaustive description of the causes of diseases and symptoms, there is consideration of other schools and views, and, finally, Galen indulges his predilection for vigorous attack on those whose views he finds uncongenial.

In the four treatises under examination there are several passages related to the general nature of causation which I would like to bring into focus here. The first, referred to on several occasions, is found in *De symptomatum differentiis* I.6 (VII.47–9K). Here Galen begins by offering a general definition of cause as, "that which, from its own nature, contributes some

---

[81] *De methodo medendi* X.63–4K.   [82] *De methodo medendi* X65–6K.
[83] For the list see *De methodo medendi* X.78K and for the exemplification X.86K.

part of the genesis by its occurrence . . .", and then lists five classes of cause rather similar to Aristotle's four causes with one addition. He also introduces the concept of 'those not without' (not 'necessary causes' in the usual sense) which are things that do not actually contribute directly to the effect but are nonetheless required for it to come about. Finally, he considers sequential causal relationships, clearly exemplified by the 'domino effect'. The finger which pushes over the first stone/domino is the primary (*per se*) cause of that stone/domino falling and the secondary (*per accidens*) cause of the subsequent stones/dominoes falling.

In *De causis morborum* II.3b he raises the question of why the same apparent cause does not invariably result in the same effect, an issue considered at some length in the *De causis procatarcticis* discussed below. The answer, in short, is that there may be variation in the magnitude of the cause or, where this is not present, in the state of the affected body. This is an argument that clearly holds in the medical situation. In the later parts of *De symptomatum causis* Galen briefly raises two further matters. The first concerns what might be called the 'bi-directional' nature of causation, insofar as the causative agent, in bringing about its effect, is itself affected by the affected material. Thus, the sword which cuts flesh is to some extent (however slight) dulled by the flesh in effecting the cutting.[84] The second matter is whether a particular effect is only brought about by a single identifiable cause or whether the one effect can have a number of possible causes. The second situation is exemplified by the symptom of indigestion. In this context Galen reflects on the application of the epithet necessary.[85]

(iii) Works on causation

Galen wrote two works specifically about general aspects of causation – *De causis contentivis* and *De causis procatarcticis* – both of which became isolated from the main body of his work as collected in the Kühn edition. They were subsequently recovered, in the first case from an Arabic version and in the second case from a fourteenth-century Latin version.[86] In *De causis contentivis*, Galen deals with what correspond to the Greek *aitia*

---

[84] See *De symptomatum causis* IV.2–3 where other examples are given.
[85] See *De symptomatum causis* XII.1–3.
[86] *De causis contentivis* appears in CMG Supplement O.II, Lyons (1969), with an Arabic text and English translation. An earlier Latin version, due to Kalbfleisch (1904) is given in the same volume. *De causis procatarcticis* appears in Hankinson (1998) with a Latin text and English translation. It is also available in CMG Supplement II, prepared by Bardong (1937) in Latin and Greek versions.

synektika, usually rendered in English by 'containing' or 'cohesive causes'. This is a concept which he attributes to the Stoics, but which he identifies as developed subsequently by Athenaeus. He starts by attempting to clarify the meaning of the term. As Galen presents it, the *synektic* (cohesive) causes are what bring about union of *homoiomeres* in the body, whilst the 'cohesion' of the *homoiomeres* themselves is due to spirit or *pneuma*. In non-biological terms, *synektic* causes are equivalent to glue, nails, pegs etc. in structures made from pieces of wood. In Athenaeus, however, Galen interprets the term entirely in relation to disease, as will be discussed below.

Galen then addresses the issue of the relationship between theories of basic structure and the concept of *synektic* (cohesive) causes. His conclusion seems to be that whilst the Stoics may have grounds for postulating such a cause for the coherence of the elements of basic structure, other views – specifically those of the Atomists – do not permit such a postulate. Furthermore, without an underlying concept of basic structure, there can be no view about *synektic* (cohesive) causes. The identified target here is those doctors who '. . . say that a knowledge of the elements is unnecessary for medical science . . .'[87] He goes on to make the important general statement:

> If you make a thorough examination, I think you will find that every cause is the cause not of *primary* existence but of generation. For generated existence . . . does come first, since the process of generation is as it were a path leading to existence. For that reason it is only *what has been generated* that has a cause which has produced it, and if there is anything that has not been generated, then it has no cause.[88]

The point he is making appears to be that causation, specifically *synektic* causation, is necessary for generation, for change but not for existence alone – that is, for an enduring state. It is necessary, then, for 'what comes into existence' but not for 'what is extant'. As he points out, the requirement for 'every extant thing' to have a *synektic* cause leads to an infinite regress of causes.[89] The distinction is exemplified in biological terms by the pulse and the artery respectively, and more problematically in general terms by running water and still water. Much of what follows in the treatise deals with *synektic* causes in disease, to be discussed below. Galen does, however, have this to say about the role of such causes in structure:

> In the healthy body this position is, as I said before, that if a part is *homoiomerous*, it cannot be said to have a cohesive cause. But where it is an organic compound, that term can be used of what connects and combines the primary simple substances

[87] *De causis contentivis* 7, pp. 62–3 (all translations from this work are after Lyons).
[88] *De causis contentivis* 7, pp. 62–3.   [89] *De causis contentivis* 6, p. 61.

of which it is compounded. As for the Stoics, I have said that they claim these primary *homoiomerous* substances also to have a cohesive cause in the pneumatic essence.[90]

In summary, then, in this short work Galen is arguing that *synektic* causes are to be understood as applying to what comes into being rather than to what exists. In his view they 'hold together' the components of the generated structure like ligaments, tendons and cartilage in biological structures or, to use some of his own examples, like nails, glue and pegs etc. in non-biological structures such as chairs, ladders and ships.

In the second work, *De causis procatarcticis*, there are two main components. The first is a statement of Galen's own views on causation and the second is his vigorous opposition to those who deny *prokatarktic* causes, in this instance Erasistratus. Galen uses the first as a launching pad for the second. Two more minor, but nonetheless significant, components are issues of terminology and the position of Herophilus in the causation debate. Included are two apparent direct quotations from Erasistratus and one from Herophilus. With respect to these, uncertainty of ascription, particularly in the hands of an avowed opponent such as Galen, is, it must be reiterated, a problem. In addition to these identified major and minor components there are several examples of specific situations presenting particular difficulties in causal analysis.

Galen's statement about his own concepts of causation, at least in the context of this work, extends from VI.56 to VII.90. Here, following a series of more or less stock examples, including going to the marketplace and constructing a bed, he lists the number of causal categories as follows:

These two are, in fact, the primary and most basic of causes: the purpose for which things are made and the maker by whom they are made. The causes that are third and fourth in terms of importance are, of course, the instruments 'through which' and the material 'from which'.[91]

The next section begins with a statement which relates to Aristotle's causal categories. The importance of the conjunction of 'agent' and 'patient', another Aristotelian point, is stressed. Galen concludes his analysis, after presenting further specific examples, with the following statement: 'Certainly for me the whole discussion which concerns causes is brought to completion, how many there are, what kind and how they differ from each other and from those that are *per accidens* (incidental) and those 'without which not' (necessary).'[92] Galen then proceeds to the next main

---

[90] *De causis contentivis* 9, p. 69.
[91] *De causis procatarcticis* VI.67.   [92] *De causis procatarcticis* VII.90.

component, the attack on Erasistratus. In essence, what he is attacking is the latter's position on the causation of fever, at least as reported by Galen himself. This is taken to be that if there is not an invariable relation between putative cause and observed effect, as well as proportionality in magnitude between the two, then the supposed cause is disqualified from a causal role. The following apparently direct quotation from Erasistratus states the position against which Galen is arguing in relation to the cause of fever:

For certainly very many, both now and in the past, have sought the causes of fevers, wishing to hear and learn from the sufferers whether the origin of the illness occurs due to cooling, or exhaustion, or repletion, or from some other cause of this kind, seeking the causes of diseases neither according to truth nor usefully. For if cold were the cause of being febrile, the one who is made more cold would be more febrile. This, however, is not so, but rather there are those who are saved after coming to extreme danger from cold who remain without fever from this. Likewise, the same is so in exhaustion and repletion. For many who have been troubled with far greater fatigue or repletion than those who are febrile escape illness.[93]

In the case of fever, then, if two people are exposed to the same 'dose' of the presumed cause (for example, sitting in the sun at the theatre) there are, theoretically four possibilities:
1. Both develop an equal degree of fever.
2. One develops a fever and one does not.
3. Neither develops a fever.
4. Each develops a different degree of fever.
According to Galen, Erasistratus' view is that unless outcome 1 holds, the agent is not causal. Galen's own position is that all four are possible, depending, in general terms, on the state of what is being acted upon. To deny a causal role to things like heating and cooling is, moreover, to fly in the face of common sense, as he believes his various examples attest.[94] Erasistratus' alternative view, attributing fever to the sequence described above involving *paremptosis* and inflammation, is sharply criticized. In several places Galen lists the kind of causes he is concerned with as *prokatarktic*, most completely in XV.195 where exhaustion, heat, cold, repletion, sleeplessness, anger and grief are specifically mentioned.

The issue of terminology is, again, a somewhat complex one. To begin with, Galen speaks of, "... id quod est de preinceptivis et procatarcticis ..."[95] These are problematic terms, neither of which is listed in standard Latin

[93] *De causis procatarcticis* VIII.102–3.   [94] See *De causis procatarcticis* V.36–45.
[95] *De causis procatarcticis* I.4. See also Hankinson's (1998) note, p. 154.

dictionaries. The translation of the latter as 'antecedent' is also unsatisfactory, as has been argued in I.4b above. The causes Galen includes in
the varying list referred to in the previous paragraph are a mixed bag,
incorporating things that can be external and/or bodily states, bodily states
alone (themselves presumably consequent upon some cause), and emotional states which could be anatomic or acting through induced bodily
states. Galen does not make this connection, nor is it without significant
problems itself in terms of causation. Shortly after these initial statements,
Galen equates these causes with *occasiones*, translated by Hankinson and
others as 'revealing causes' in the sense of bringing out effects dependent on
the presumed causal agent acting on a 'prepared substrate'.[96] The specific
examples illustrating difficulties of causal analysis[97] will not be considered
here, whilst the issues Galen raises in the final section on Herophilus have
been dealt with above.

(iv)   Causation in biological systems

In this subsection translations are given of key passages on causation from
three different works: *De usu partium, De causis pulsuum* and *De causis respirationis*. What links these three excerpts is that each offers a causal account
of a basic biological phenomenon – the formation of anatomical structures
in the first case, and, in the other cases, two obviously essential and for
the most part regular functions, pulse and respiration. The common aspect
of these functions that distinguishes them from disease – although each
may itself be involved in disease – is that under normal circumstances (*kata
phusin*) they are invariably present, uniform and regular, so are arguably
more susceptible of comprehensive causal analysis than a sporadic and, in
many instances, apparently random phenomenon such as a disease. What
differentiates them in Galen's descriptions is the quite disparate nature of
the causal accounts given. Some reflections on the reasons for this variation
will follow the passages below.

(a) ***De usu partium***: The primary cause for all things created, as Plato has also
shown somewhere, is the object of function. Accordingly, to someone asking the
cause of coming to the market, it is not permissible to give some better reply,
leaving aside this cause. For it would be ridiculous for someone to say, rather than
that he had come to buy some article or a slave, or to meet a friend, or to sell

96 See *De causis procatarcticis* I.6, 7 and particularly Hankinson's (1998) note, pp. 156–7 where he
discusses, *inter alia*, Bardong's (1937) back translation of *occasiones* as *prophasis*.
97 Three examples of particular interest are the killing of an old woman by a trained gladiator (XI.145–
52), the death of Clytemnestra (XIV.178–82), and the prescription of a harmful drug (XIV.83–90).

something, leaving aside these things, that he had two feet which were easy to move and got a firm footing securely on the ground, and that with these, placing each of the aforementioned feet alternately, he had come to the market. He has, perhaps, stated a certain cause, but it is not truly the cause, not the primary cause. It is, rather, a cause 'not without which' and not the main cause. In this way Plato correctly distinguished the nature of causation. Let us agree, so that we will not seem to be using extreme subtlety about terms, that there are many classes of causes: a first and most important one on account of which something comes about, a second by which, and a third from which, and a fourth due to which, and a fifth, if you will have it so, in accordance with which. And we shall take into consideration these with reference to each class in giving an account of all the parts of an animal, if we are properly natural philosophers. For if people ask why the nature of the vessels of the lung is changed, the vein being made arterial and the artery vein-like, we respond correctly with the primary cause, that it is better in this internal organ alone for the vein to be strongly covered but the artery thinly.

(b) *De causis pulsuum*: Of the causes changing the pulses, some are the causes of their genesis, some of change alone. Those of genesis are the use for which they occur, the capacity by which they occur, and the organs through which they are distended. All the rest are causes of change, both those called internal antecedent (*proegoumenic*) and those called external antecedent (*prokatarktic*) which precede the former. Certainly the threefold class of causes is not in the pulses alone, but also in all other things. There is one that is primary and most controlling, which they call connecting (*synektic*), so named from the holding together of the substance of these, which, as was said before, is the cause of genesis. The other two classes are not causes of the occurrence but are causes of change in what has occurred. At any rate, thickness of humours, or abundance, or viscidity or acridity, are not able to effect pulses, but are able to change [them]. Thus, a cold or hot bath, and winter and summer, and cold and warmth in general, are causes of change of pulses, but not of genesis. Those, then, now being spoken of are called *prokatarktic* (external antecedent), whereas those spoken of before these and related to humours are *proegoumenic* (internal antecedent). To speak generally, those that are outside the body but change something in it are called *prokatarktic*, for certainly they are in advance of conditions in the body. These same conditions, whenever the *synektic* [causes] change, become *proegoumenic* causes of these. Now, by cold falling upon it from without, the skin is thickened, and through the thickness of this, the transpiration according to nature is held back and, being held back, is concentrated together until in this way it stirs up a fever. On account of this the use of the pulses is changed, and through this also the pulses, in this case the *prokatarktic* cause being the external extreme cold, and all other things *proegoumenic*, right up to the use of the pulses. The *prokatarktic* causes, through the mediating *proegoumenic* causes, alter the use of the pulses, which is one of the *synektic* causes and so changes the pulses themselves. For it is not possible to change some *synektic* cause, it being unchangeable in itself.[98]

---

[98] *De causis pulsuum* IX.1–3K.

(c) *De causis respirationis*: To speak in brief, there are three causes of respiration: the purposive capacity, the organs providing service to the purposive [capacity], and with respect to these the use due to which we need the causes set out. Use is the most essential of the causes of respiration, constantly guarding the balance of the innate heat and also nourishing the substance of the psychic *pneuma*. Purpose orders and, as it were, makes regular the respiratory functions. The form of the organs is diverse and various, for some are devoted to the carrying of the *pneuma*, whereas some receive the air, and others are what set in motion those that move.[99]

The main point I wish to make in relation to these three passages, linked in that they offer explanations of basic, normal structures and functions, is the variation in Galen's causal accounts. In the first case, where he is clearly wedded to a teleological explanation (indeed this is the dominant theme of the whole work), the nature and authority of an essentially Aristotelian analysis of causation is most suitable for his purpose and is employed. In the second instance, his purpose is to consider what is a fundamental physiological function and give an account of what changes occur in it under different circumstances insofar as these are of considerable diagnostic importance. Here he employs the tripartite division of *synektic, proegoumenic* and *prokatarktic*, the background of which has been considered in earlier sections. Since he wants to separate the factors that are responsible for the unaffected pulse from both external and internal (bodily) factors that bring about changes in the pulse, this scheme is very suitable. In the third example his aim seems simply to give a brief general account of a basic function which does not demand elaborate causal analysis.

(v) Causation in physical disease

In the *De causis morborum* Galen purports to give an exhaustive account of the causes of diseases. This he does on the foundation of his basic tripartite structural division (*homoiomeres*, organic parts, whole body), the ultimate components of all structures being the elements, qualities and humours. Here he forgoes consideration of the alternative particle/void theory which he did include in the preceding book on disease classification. His account of causation is essentially practical. Thus, he does not deal in depth with the question of how causes, either in general or specifically, give rise to

[99] *De causis respirationis* IV.465–6K. I am uncertain about the precise meaning of *proairesis* here. Furley and Wilkie (1984) have the following note: 'This refers to the traditional distinction between voluntary and involuntary motions, for which see Aristotle, *De motu animalium* 11.' On this basis they render the word as 'choice'. Although, of course, there is an element of choice in respiration, it is not strictly speaking a voluntary function.

their effects. He does, however, consider two general points. The first is the recurring issue of why something identified as a cause does not invariably produce the alleged effect. The usual example is the causation of fever. Galen attributes the variability to three possible factors: the magnitude of the cause, the duration of its action and the state of the affected body. He does not specifically consider contiguity although this is, perhaps, implied in magnitude. The second is the vexed issue of terminology. He provides what amount to definitions of *prokatarktic* and *proegoumenic* as follows:

> It was, I think, proposed to speak completely of the *proegoumenic* causes of each of the simple diseases, and of the *prokatarktic*. For it is no bad thing to follow those who have distinguished the terms in this way for the sake of clarity. They then call either conditions pertaining to the animal itself or movements contrary to nature, *proegoumenic* causes of diseases, and those things that befall [the animal] from without and greatly change or alter the body, *prokatarchontic* or *prokatarktic* causes.[100]

Considering first *homoiomeric* structures, Galen identifies ten *dyscrasias* – four mono-*dyscrasias* (hot, cold, dry and moist), four 'regular' combined *dyscrasias* (hot and dry, hot and moist, cold and dry, cold and moist), and two 'irregular' combined *dyscrasias* (hot and cold, dry and moist). With regard to the specific causes of the mono-*dyscrasias*, he gives considerable attention to those involving heat, and then, with progressively diminishing attention, to cold, dry and moist respectively. The actual causes given are listed in Table 4. In essence, all the factors identified are external and, indeed, in the section on *dyscrasias* of heat he presents illustrative inanimate examples. These factors may be summarized as falling into three categories: activities/ways of life, ingested materials, and contact with external factors.

When he turns to the combined *dyscrasias*, both regular and irregular, Galen introduces the additional causative factor of inflow of material into the affected part, which may act in addition to primary changes in the elements, qualities or humours themselves. The potentially inflowing materials are identified as the humours (blood, yellow bile, black bile and phlegm). In considering this pathological mechanism, he speaks of three of the capacities dealt with at length in *De facultatibus naturalibus* (attractive, retentive and separative), and puts forward his concept of superfluities (*perissomata*) passing from 'stronger' to 'weaker' areas, weakness being due to deficiencies of initial formation, subsequent damage, or specific design, as with the skin.

---

[100] *De causis morborum* II.5.

Galen

Table 4 *Causes of mono-*dyscrasias

Dyscrasia	Cause
HEAT	Increased movement
	Putrefaction
	Proximity to hotter body
	Constriction
	Foods with necessary capacity
COLD	Idleness
	Disproportionate movement
	Proximity to colder body
	Constriction and rarefaction
	Foods with necessary capacity
DRYNESS	Increased activity + sweating
	Low food intake
	Dry external conditions
	Thinking too much
	Staying awake too long
	Dry foods and fluids
MOISTNESS	Excess of fluids
	Excess of baths
	Luxurious way of life
	Gladness of heart
	Moist foods

The causes of diseases of organic bodies are divided into four groups, the categories being form (conformation), number, size and arrangement. The causes of diseases for each category are summarized in Table 5. Considering each of the four groups in turn, the causes of change in form (conformation) are something of a mixed bag. Grouped together are congenital abnormalities, external physical causes, diseases themselves, alterations of cavities and channels (e.g. compression, collapse etc. with little consideration being given to the causes of the causes), and changes of consistency (excessive roughness or smoothness) which are attributable to the effects of humours and other fluids. Within this category he does make a distinction between primary (*per se*) and secondary (*per accidens*) causes, the former exemplified by the diseases *elephantiasis* and *phthisis*, and the latter by abnormal tension due to scarring. Abnormalities of number are basically related to direct physical causes, whilst those of size are given the most cursory consideration. In discussing abnormalities of arrangement, he simply provides a list, as shown in Table 5. It is difficult to regard this list as exhaustive.

Table 5 *Causes of organic diseases*

Abnormality	Examples
FORM	Congenital abnormalities (abnormal sperm)
	Post-natal deformities (improper handling)
	Limb fractures (improper treatment)
	Excessive or deficient filling
	Distorting forces (paralysis, spasm, scarring)
	Changed configuration of cavities and channels (enlargement, reduction, obstruction)
	Changes in roughness and smoothness (due to humours, medicines etc.)
NUMBER	Loss/reduction (cutting, burning, putrefaction, cooling)
	Addition/increase (congenital, acquired)
SIZE	Reduction (as number)
	Increase (of useful material, strong capacity)
ARRANGEMENT	Trauma, e.g. fractures/dislocations
	Violent movement, e.g. dislocations
	Dilatation of channels, e.g. hernias
	Erosion, e.g. displacement of choroid with corneal erosion

With respect to terminology, Galen's usage throughout the discussion is certainly not consistent or systematic. Thus, apart from the differentiation of primary (*per se*) and secondary (*per accidens*) in relation to causes of abnormal form, he uses the term *prophasis* twice in relation to burning that causes an abnormality of number, and violent movement that causes an abnormality of arrangement, both obvious external factors. In fact, in cataloguing the causes of abnormal arrangement, he groups these all under the rubric of *prophasis*.

Finally, he introduces his third class of diseases, applicable to both *homoiomeric* and organic structures, which he terms 'division' or 'dissolution of continuity'. The distinction between this group and some components of the previous group is not entirely clear, as discussed in section I.5b above. It may be just the fact that both types of structure can be affected, and that the normal conformation, size and number are essentially maintained whilst the interrelationship with adjacent structures is also not disturbed. The examples given – for bone, fractures; for flesh, ulcers and wounds; and for both, crushing – are, in terms of mechanism, applicable to both. In this third group, Galen divides the causative mechanisms into the obvious external factors and internal factors, the latter being abnormal humours or fluids producing erosion. Again, in determining the effect of a particular cause, he refers to both the nature of the external agent and the state of the affected body.

De symptomatum causis is an even more obviously practical work than *De causis morborum* in that it is basically a catalogue of the causes of various symptoms. It is systematic in the division of functions (sensory, motor, authoritative) and of the structures subserving these functions, but not systematic in its treatment of causation as such. Having apparently dealt to his satisfaction with issues of terminology, definition and mechanism, Galen now recounts what he identifies as the specific causes of specific symptoms. In general, in the three books of this treatise the precise mechanism of causation in the various instances is not analysed.

There are, however, in the three books of *De symptomatum causis* some important issues of terminology which I shall briefly consider. First, in his description of pupillary dilatation, not only does Galen speak of *synektic* causes but conflates this term with *synechon* and *prosechon* thus: 'Therefore the *synektic* cause, or *synechtic* or *prosechtic* or however someone might wish to term it, is some such condition in the nerve as to impede the capacity being sent down from the *arche*.'[101] In this case the cause is the abnormal tension within the choroid membrane and might be seen as structural in the sense of the degree of coherence between the constitutive components of the membrane. Taking the causal analysis back one step, this change of tension is attributed to a disturbance of flow of capacity (*dunamis*) from the *arche* via the nerve. This raises, of course, the interesting issue of the physical nature of this capacity and its usual role in maintaining normal tension (*kata phusin*).

Subsequently, in speaking of the use of cooling in the treatment of tetanus, Galen makes the distinction between a cause which is 'primarily and *per se*' the cause of the final result and one that is *prokatarktic*, with the implication that the latter is not, of itself, sufficient to bring about the result. There then follow several passages in which he uses *prophasis* repeatedly: in relation to sympathetic affections of the stomach (VII.139K), in situations where the same symptom follows opposite *prophastic* causes (VII.184K), in speaking of the relation between fever and rigor (VII.188K),[102] and lastly in discussing the causes of poor digestion (VII.208K). Whilst these specific examples are predominantly external factors, internal factors (e.g. flatulent *pneuma*, phlegm) are not excluded. Finally, on the matter of terminology, he also speaks of 'effecting (*poietikon*) causes' with respect to digestion.

---

[101] *De symptomatum causis* VII.109K.   [102] Here *proegoumenic* is also mentioned.

In summary, the abiding impression gained from Galen's account of the causes of diseases and symptoms in the two treatises on causes is that his concerns are overwhelmingly practical. Certainly he has to set the stage with definitions and classification, which he does with the two preceding treatises in each case, and he feels he must found his analysis on a theory of basic structure, but in the two causation treatises themselves his aim appears to be to set out all causes, and if any are omitted they can be worked out from the ones that are given. In practice, the doctor must know these causes if he is to institute rational treatment. Causal theories and terms are used to some extent but, as has been said already several times, in neither case is the use consistent or systematic.

(vi)   Causation in mental (psychical) disease

Siegel makes the point that '. . . none of Galen's surviving treatises was specifically designed for the description of nervous and mental diseases',[103] although he did, of course, write on the effects of bodily states on the soul and also gave consideration to what would be called mental diseases in a number of more general treatises. At times, these considerations included what might more properly be called abnormal or aberrant behaviour, or exaggerated forms of normal emotional states such as anger, although the borderline between the extremes of normality and the frankly pathological can be hard to identify.[104] In the treatises translated here, all the nervous and mental abnormalities are included in the two works on symptoms, for reasons which will be made explicit below, and in these two works conditions that are obviously pathological (e.g. delirium, mania) are joined with 'normal' behavioural and emotional variations (e.g. fear, anger).

From the point of view of causation in nervous and mental disturbances, there are several important, indeed fundamental issues, some of which still remain matters of contention. Most obvious is the mind–body relationship itself in all its ramifications. Clearly, views on the causal interaction between *psyche* and *soma* in disorders or diseases will depend on views as to what causal relationship exists between the two conceptually separate components under normal circumstances. In addition, particularly in Galen's own time, there were issues of the location of the soul, of whether it was

---

[103] In his 1973 work, p. 231.

[104] With respect to Galen's view on this matter, Garcia-Ballester (2002) writes: 'He saw in his clinical practice . . . that there is a continuum between body and soul, both in the case of mental illness (e.g. dementia, frenzy, melancholia) or in disorders of a moral nature, but he left in the dark the answer to the question of exactly "what" continuum.'

corporeal or incorporeal, and if the former, what its substance (*ousia*) was, and of whether it was immortal or otherwise – all of these bearing on the analysis of causation in disease states.

In modern times, the doctor accepts that neural and mental events occur in the nervous system, that there is at least a moderately clear understanding of the structural basis for these events, and hence of the substance of the *psyche*, that there is a reciprocal physical interrelationship between mind and body, albeit a complex and quite poorly understood one. Further, it is recognized that this interrelationship can be of causal significance, not only in frank disease, but also in mental and physical variations that fall within the range of normal. The philosophical issues alluded to, while they are of undoubted interest, are accepted as being of no immediate relevance to quotidian issues of medical practice. This robust practical position was, in its essential elements, that which Galen adopted. The following two statements, the first from *Quod animi mores corporis temperamenta sequantur* and the second from *De propriis placitis*, serve to exemplify his standpoint.

I have found the proposition to be true and invariable that the capacities of the soul follow the mixtures of the body, and not once or twice but very often, and not from my own experience alone which is extensive, but from the beginning through my teachers and subsequently along with the very best philosophers. Moreover, this is beneficial to those who wish to bring order to their own souls.[105]

But whether this is because the corporeal substances incorporate themselves or this does not happen except only in their qualities, so I say that the knowledge of these things is not necessary and I have no opinion on it. But I see that it is more plausible to accept the statement of him who says that the mixture is of the qualities. But as to the soul whether it is immortal, by the fact that it governs animals by its mixture with the substances of the body I am not sure of this knowledge, nor whether it is a substance existing by itself. But what is clear to us is that when it is disposed in bodies, we find natures which are generated, as I have mentioned, from a mixture of the four elements. And I do not see that it harms anyone in the art of medicine not to know the way in which the disposition of life runs.[106]

It was, it seems, clear to Galen, as it is clear now, that states of the *soma* affect states of the *psyche* and vice versa. Moreover, states of the *soma* which affect the *psyche* may, in turn, depend on external factors.[107] The doctor's role is, then, to identify where possible the causal relationship between *soma* and *psyche* in each particular case, and to fashion therapies based on

---

[105] *Quod animi mores corporis temperamenta sequantur* IV.767K.
[106] *De propriis placitis* 15 – translation after Nutton (1999), pp. 117–19.
[107] See, for example, *Ars Medica* I.367–9K.

what is identified. To go one step further, if the *psyche* is entirely corporeal, then what might be termed mental diseases and symptoms are no different from bodily diseases and symptoms. Thus Galen's own tripartite division of symptoms into loss of function, reduction of function and abnormality of function would apply to his 'inherited' tripartite division of the *psyche* into the workings of reason, imagination and memory in the same way it does to any other bodily function, all of which are based on a physically identifiable structure. In *De symptomatum causis* II (VII.191K) he writes:

> Perhaps I shall have the audacity to give an opinion about the soul itself in some other work, but for what is now at hand, apart from being audacious, this is also superfluous. It seems, then, that whatever this might be, it is one of two things: either it uses the primary organs for all functions by the *pneuma* or the blood, or the heat in one or both together, or it is in these themselves.

This point is repeated in the later work, *De propriis placitis* already referred to above where he also gives some consideration to the issue of the immortality or otherwise of the soul, writing: 'Just as it is irrelevant to the doctor in treating diseases whether the soul is mortal or immortal, so it does not matter whether its substance is incorporeal, as that one wants, or corporeal, as that one wants . . .'[108] In the practical context of the translated treatises, Galen's position is, however, relatively clear as to the causation of nervous and mental disorders, and the application of his concepts goes beyond diseases and symptoms to mental states like fear and anger, as mentioned above. This position is that all diseases fall into one of three possible categories: *dyscrasias* of *homoiomeric* bodies (either occurring primarily or due to an inflowing substance); structural changes (with division into changes of form, size, number and position); and dissolution of continuity. Operating within this system are changes due to circulating materials, specifically blood and *pneuma*, and changes in 'innate heat'. In the application of this classification, the brain is no different from other organs, i.e. the tissue of the brain is taken as *homoiomeric*, blood reaches the brain and the *pneuma* circulates through the brain within the ventricular cavities in a specific form, the *pneuma psychikon*, and is also in communication with the outside air. Diseases of the brain, which must fall into one of the three categories listed, when they involve the *hegemonical* component will manifest themselves through the symptoms of a disturbance of one of the three subdivisions of this – memory, imagination or reasoning, or some combination of these three – on the account which Galen gives. From the

---

[108] *De propriis placitis* 7 – translation after Nutton (1999), p. 79.

point of view of causation, then, *hegemonical* functions are altered by whatever alters the components of the *hegemonical* structure, or by whatever
produces an abnormal state of the psychic *pneuma*. The actual nature of
the causative mechanism is the same irrespective of whether *soma* or *psyche*
is involved.

1.6D CONCLUSIONS

In summarizing this chapter on Galen's views on causation of diseases
and symptoms, it may be said in general terms that they were influenced
most obviously by the Hippocratic Corpus and by the Stoics among more
ancient sources and were consistent with mainstream Dogmatic thinking,
with significant correspondence to the views of Athenaeus and a healthy
leavening of Empiricism. That is, he sought causes for all diseases, believing
that a causal account was possible for all diseases and symptoms and, more
generally, for all changes in the condition or state of the body. It was, he
believed, a correct causal analysis that offered the best prospect of successful
treatment.

He faced quite considerable challenges to this basic position during his
own lifetime, something which the strongly polemical nature of many of his
works reflects. First, on the philosophical front, there was the continuing
challenge of the Sceptics who, in broad terms, denied causation. Second,
on the medical front, there were both the challenge of the Empiricists who
applied the causal concepts of the Sceptics to medicine, and the challenge of
those who applied particle/void theories of basic structure to medicine. This
latter found its definitive formulation in the medical theories of Asclepiades
and the Methodics. Such a theoretical foundation did not, of course, entirely
preclude causal analysis, as Galen obviously recognizes in the translated
treatises, but the Methodics did, in effect, almost entirely discount the
value of causal analysis.

It is against the background of these challenges that Galen's account of
causation in medicine must be viewed. Unquestionably the views of Galen
and like-minded colleagues prevailed, at least in the realm of causation.
What can be said with certainty is that doctors continue to seek causes for
individual diseases on the assumption that a successful search will lead to the
best treatment, not to mention possible prevention and accurate diagnosis.
The merits of such an approach have been empirically demonstrated over
and over again. It is true also that doctors, particularly in recent times,
seldom concern themselves with the major philosophical issues that still
bedevil concepts of causation. Galen was unusual in his own time for his

strong advocacy of the importance of philosophy to medicine, and would have been even more so now. Speculation on causation was one aspect of this interest in philosophy.

This is not to say that there were not further challenges over subsequent centuries – there were. And, in fact, they were the same basic challenges, albeit in somewhat changed formulations. First, in philosophy, beginning with the writings of Hume, there was a rebirth of the basic sceptical challenge to the foundations of causation. Amongst Hume's positivist successors of the last century, Russell, with his penchant for the memorable phrase, wrote in 1917: 'The law of causality, I believe, like much that passes muster among philosophers, is a relic of a bygone age, surviving, like the monarchy, only because it is erroneously supposed to do no harm.'[109] Subsequently, Wittgenstein wrote: 'We *cannot* infer the events of the future from those of the present. Belief in the causal nexus is *superstition*.'[110] Second, in natural philosophy, there has been the apparent triumph of particle/void theories of structure, the elaborations of which not only raised again the issue of how perceived causes acted on the fundamental structures but also brought forth additional arguments undermining the very concept of causation. Thus Heisenberg, writing in 1930 in relation to the emission of electrons from the Radium atom, claimed that '. . . Kant's arguments for the *a priori* character of the law of causality no longer apply.'[111] Third, major advances in physiology, most notably the discovery of the circulation of the blood, greatly changed the way causation in medicine could be interpreted. With regard to these three aspects, however, it may be said that the positivist assault on causation has not been sustained just as the sceptical assault was not two millennia earlier; that the further developments of particle physics do not allow an abandonment of causation;[112] and that, whilst the details of causal explanation have undoubtedly changed with the developments of physiology, pathology and microbiology, the principles of the endeavour are essentially the same.

The point is, then, that although the catalogue of causal agents has changed and increased considerably, and there has been significant development in understanding how many causal factors operate, the overall approach to clarifying causation in disease is very similar to that proposed

---

[109] Russell (1917), p. 132.
[110] *Tractatus Logico-Philosophicus* 5.1361 (translated by Pears and McGuinness (1961) – the italics are the translators').
[111] Heisenberg (1930), p. 58.
[112] Thus Smolin (2001), writing very recently on the ramifications of modern physics, states that, 'it is causality that gives the world its structure . . .' and also claims that the most important relation between two events is causality.

by Galen in the translated treatises. Before finally enumerating the essential points of Galen's analysis, I shall mention very briefly two recent works
on causation in disease. The first, *Causation and Disease*, is more practical whilst the second, *The Logic of Medicine*, is more theoretical, the two
corresponding to the two facets of Galen's own approach.[113]

The first of these works is the closer in nature to Galen's works here studied. The main difference is that it is predominantly about microbiology:
seven of the eleven chapters with one chapter on the related matter of
immunology. There is also one chapter on what are called 'occupational
diseases' – essentially environmental factors producing disease. What this
work and those of Galen have in common is that they are largely about
external causes. What is different is the nature of the external factors reflecting particularly the great development of microbiology beginning in the
early nineteenth century. The other common factor, and the one I wish
to emphasize here, is the restatement of the 'Erasistratean problem'. Thus
Evans writes: 'A major riddle in infectious diseases is why some individuals develop clinical illness as a result of infection while others do not.'[114]
In an attempt to solve this riddle Evans introduces what he terms the
'third ingredient', which is essentially an elaboration of Galen's much earlier explanation: the efficacy of the supposed causal agent depends on its
magnitude and duration of action, the possible role of other external factors
and the state of the affected body. Indeed, in a table of 24 factors given by
Evans,[115] at least 10 would be clearly recognized by Galen. Likewise, Evans'
summarizing statement that causation is recognized as '. . . a multifactorial
and complex phenomenon with different sets of risk factors operating in
different settings' would be entirely acceptable to Galen. It is particularly in
the host factors, the state of the affected body, that very recent developments
in the understanding of things like genome segments controlling antigenic
activities, the production of antibodies and cell-mediated immunity and
its genetic control, have been significant.

The second work is, as its title would suggest, predominantly theoretical.
Murphy's book is the kind of work that Galen, with his avowed interest in
philosophy, might have written but did not – at least as far as we know.
It is a work less restricted to a particular time in that in the relevant sections it is about theoretical aspects of causation and not the recognition
of specific causal agents and mechanisms – although the more complete

---

[113] The two works are by Evans (1993) and Murphy (1997), respectively.
[114] Evans (1993), p. 208.   [115] Evans (1993), table 11.1, p. 208.

the range and understanding of specific examples so the more complete the theoretical account that is possible. Here I shall simply mention four points that emerge from Murphy's analysis that seem to me to have relevance to Galen's own work. The first is the importance of recognizing the role of the 'conjunction of causes' – clearly corresponding to the *sunaitia* and *summetaitia* of the ancients. Consideration of this 'conjunction of causes' is, however, refined by the introduction of the concept of *paratasis*, a factor which may prevent a satisfactory causal analysis, whether by deduction, induction or computation, unless 'every material factor can be identified in every case'.[116] Secondly, there is the observation that even in apparently simple causal situations – infections, Mendelian disorders, specific intoxications and vitamin deficiencies are mentioned – other factors may have an important influence. The third aspect is Murphy's discussion of the reasons for failures of causal analysis and his ideas on 'longitudinal' and 'transverse confounding'.[117] The important point is that failed causal analyses are likely to be discarded, perhaps prematurely, on empirical grounds. Finally, and of particular interest, is the linking of causal analysis to basic concepts of structure, an issue certainly addressed by Galen, and the fact that different structural concepts may be applicable in the causal analysis of different diseases. On this point Murphy writes: '. . . the structure of the world may be seen as ranging from the indestructible singularity, the billiard ball with an infinitely high ontological density, to what I suppose we might call ontological "dust" or "miasma", stuff so finely divided and so pliable that it might be treated as a continuum.'[118]

The relevance of these ideas to Galen's deliberations on causation is obvious. In conclusion, then, I shall enumerate the main points of these deliberations as follows:

1. The most fundamental point is that Galen believed that every change in the condition or state of the human body, whether identified as a disease, a symptom or an affection (*pathos* or *pathema*), was causally determined.
2. These determining causes could be ones that were external to the body (the most obvious being heat and cold) or internal within the body (for example, the movement of humours) and were either antecedent only or both antecedent and co-temporal with their effects.
3. A complete analysis of causative agents acting to bring about a particular effect was, in theory at least, possible.

---

[116] See Murphy (1997), pp. 240–4.   [117] Murphy (1997), pp. 234–9.
[118] Murphy (1997), p. 245. See also his table 12.1, p. 246.

4. One of the ultimate aims of medical science was to give a complete causal account of each disease, symptom or affection and to couple this with an exhaustive classification of these conditions. This, in fact, is the aim of the translated treatises.

5. His own causal account of diseases, symptoms and affections was given in terms of a continuum theory of microstructure and a tripartite division of macrostructure into *homoiomeres*, organs and the whole body, although such an account could be based on an alternative theory of structure – the *anarmoi/poroi* theory of Asclepiades is the example given. That is, causal analysis is in a general way independent of theories of structure.

6. Causal accounts of what might be called 'mental' diseases, symptoms and affections are of the same type as those of these bodily conditions – i.e. mental conditions are to be explained on a physical basis.

7. In a causal interaction the affected body or substance acts back in a causal way on the identified causal agent although the reciprocal relationship is likely to be markedly asymmetrical. This is an important, if somewhat neglected, concept in medicine.

8. His approach to terminology in causal analysis in medicine is somewhat laissez-faire. He clearly accepts *aitia* and *aition* as interchangeable with each other and possibly both as interchangeable with *prophasis*, although the last may carry the implication at least of being prior and/or readily apparent. As to qualifying terms, I take Galen to mean, by *prokatarktic*, causes that are antecedent and external to the body, by *proegoumenic*, causes that are antecedent and internal within the body, and by *synektic*, causes that are internal and activated by the two '*pro*' forms of cause. His usage of this tripartite division is, however, variable and his employment of it rather than alternative classifications and his exact interpretation of meaning in each case are matters for debate.

9. His approach to causal analysis in the case of condition changes such as characterize diseases is different from that in the case of fixed structures, for example the structure of particular organs, and that in the case of universal and regular physiological functions such as the pulse and respiration.

10. Causal analysis of condition changes is open to correction or re-evaluation on empirical grounds.

11. The particular value of an accurate and comprehensive causal analysis in diseases is that it provides a secure and rational basis for allopathic treatment and, if correct, guarantees its success, at least in theory.

12. Variations in the relationship between putative cause and apparent effect, especially in the case of external factors – what might be called the 'Erasistratus problem' – are entirely explicable on the grounds of variations in the 'dose' or magnitude of the cause and variations in the prior state of the affected body.

What is, finally, most striking is that if one substitutes current concepts of basic structure and physiology for those employed by Galen, and eschews the now abandoned qualifying terminology (although not necessarily the concepts behind the terms), this could well be the *credo* of a currently practising doctor on the matter of disease causation.

PART II

Translation

Introduction

As noted earlier, the translations of these four treatises have been made from Kühn's Greek text with its accompanying Latin version (VI.836–80K, VII.1–272K). The Kühn text as a whole has been much criticized for its supposed inaccuracy, not least by those using it as a basis for translation, but is, in the case of these four treatises, the only post-sixteenth century Greek text available. There are three other possible sources of the text: (i) early manuscripts, as listed by Diels;[1] (ii) Arabic versions; (iii) Latin versions, as catalogued by Durling.[2] In the present case, the Florentine manuscripts Laurent. plut. 74.16 and 74.12 have been examined,[3] but no significant changes to the Kühn text have been made on the basis of this. The Latin versions used, apart from that included in Kühn, are all those listed by Durling other than the anonymous one. Whatever the precise relationship to the original, the text as presented in the Kühn volumes contains very little that is uncertain or unclear to the extent that textual emendation seems mandatory. Certainly, the preparation of a new Greek text in the form of the estimable, but only very gradually accumulating, CMG series would be a most worthwhile endeavour. This, obviously, is not what is attempted here. Points of apparent textual difficulty are indicated in the footnotes as they arise, as are sentences difficult of comprehension – although these are arguably as likely to be due to Galen's style, also a target of criticism by some, as to errors in transmission of the text. Within each of the six books of the four treatises the chapter numbering follows that in Kühn. The subsections within each chapter generally correspond to those in the Copus/Valleriola Latin edition although some changes have been made on the basis of uniformity of subject matter.

---

[1] Diels (1905), pp. 78–80.
[2] See Durling (1961), where the Latin versions of the four treatises are listed in summary and in order as #65 (p. 287), #64 (p. 287), #113 (p. 291) and #112 (p. 291). There are four versions in each case.
[3] I am grateful to the University of Florence library for providing a microfilm of these manuscripts and to the Document Services department at the University of New England for obtaining this.

On the question of style in the translation itself, there is, as always, a decision to be made as to whether to take literalness or close correspondence to the original as the important criterion rather than ease of reading in the language of the translation and modernity of phrasing. That is, assuming these objectives are mutually exclusive. This translation is consciously based on the former criterion. The treatises are, after all, medical texts. Clarity in the presentation of ideas or the detailing of factual information is therefore of paramount importance, with stylistic grace a secondary matter. Undoubtedly this applied in Galen's time as it applies now. The aim, then, is to present a translation as close to the original as possible and which captures something of the style of the original without sacrificing clarity of expression.

CHAPTER II.I

On the Differentiae of Diseases

SYNOPSIS

I.1 Outlines the objectives in this book: to define health and disease and to enumerate in full all 'simple and primary diseases' and the combined diseases arising from these.

II.1 Initial definitions of health and disease in both structural (*kataskeue*) and functional (*energeia*) terms. Introduction of the terms *kata phusin* and *para phusin* – in accord and not in accord with nature.

II.2 Health and disease identified as 'balance' (*summetros*) and 'imbalance' (*ametros*) respectively.

II.3 The issue of what is or is not in balance is raised. Galen recognizes two possible structural concepts: (i) *poroi* and *anarmoi*; and (ii) the four 'qualities'.

II.4 Discussion of the difficulties of accounting for degrees of health or disease ('more or less') on the basis of impassible, immutable elements.

III.1 Galen's scheme of three levels of structure: (i) *homoiomeres*, e.g. arteries, bones etc.; (ii) organs, e.g. heart, lungs etc.; (iii) the whole body.

IV.1 Diseases of *homoiomeres* on the *poroi/anarmoi* hypothesis are two in kind: an imbalance due either to an excess of constriction, or to an excess of dilatation. Two additional states are described: an imbalance in either direction not yet sufficient to constitute disease (i.e. harm function), and an extreme imbalance causing destruction of the part.

IV.2 On the basis of the hypothesis of elements/qualities which Galen favours, there are four primary diseases consisting of imbalances involving heat, cold, dryness and moisture respectively.

IV.3 Diseases of compound structures (organs) are common to both hypotheses and comprise four classes:
1. Formation: destruction or disturbance of normal form; acquisition or loss of a cavity or channel; abnormal roughness or smoothness.
2. Number: deficiency or excess.
3. Magnitude: some part greater or less in size than it should be.
4. Mode of combination: change in relation of parts to each other.

IV.4 Divides organs into primary, secondary, tertiary and quaternary. Primary organs are those formed by union of *homoiomeres* for a single function, secondary by combination of primary and so on.

IV.5 Identifies a further class of disease affecting all compound bodies (primary, secondary organs etc.), which is a breakdown of combination (dissolution of continuity).

V.1 Recapitulates basic subdivisions according to 'first hypothesis' (*poroi/anarmoi*), i.e. imbalance of pores: (i) constriction: subdivided into 'collapse' of body into itself and obstruction of *poroi* themselves; (ii) dilatation: subdivided into outward expansion of all parts and expansion of *poroi* themselves.

V.2 Recapitulates basic subdivisions according to 'second hypothesis' (elements/qualities): (i) *dyscrasia* due to change in one of the four 'qualities' in a *homoiomeric* body; (ii) *dyscrasia* due to inflow of material bringing one of the four 'qualities'. Gives examples of changes in heat causing a 'hot mono-*dyscrasia*'.

V.3 Gives examples of changes in cold causing a 'cold mono-*dyscrasia*'.

V.4 A digression on terminology, particularly the distinction between disease and symptom.

V.5 Gives examples of changes in moistness and dryness giving a 'moist mono-*dyscrasia*' or 'dry mono-*dyscrasia*'.

V.6 Introduces the idea of 'debility' (*atonia*) exemplified by poor digestion in the stomach. He seems to be saying that this is not a separate class from the imbalance of either *poroi* or 'qualities' already spoken of as affecting *homoiomeres*.

VI.1 Introduction to diseases of organic parts. A distinction is made between parts that are entirely the cause of function and parts that 'assist' the part responsible for function. Makes a distinction also between diseases as whatever of themselves hinder function, and causes of disease which hinder function through hindering the primary organ of function. A reiteration of the fourfold division (form, number, magnitude, arrangement) in the light of this distinction.

VII.1 Examples of abnormalities of form with recognition of congenital and acquired defects.

VII.2 Examples of abnormalities of form involving cavities or channels. He makes the point that when a body is swollen so as to hinder function this is one disease, whilst if the swelling obstructs channels also hindering function, this is a second disease from the same process.

VII.3 Exemplification of the situation of dual diseases in relation to liver and intestines. Again a distinction is made between the condition that primarily damages function, which is the disease, and what causes that condition, which is the cause of the disease.

VII.4 Abnormalities of form due to abnormal roughness or smoothness exemplified by the respiratory passages.

VIII.1 Abnormalities of number (of parts) are divided into those where there is excess, and those where there is deficiency. Examples are given of excesses with the distinction again being made between what primarily harms function (a disease) and what harms function through damaging the part that carries out the function (a cause of disease).

VIII.2 Examples of deficiency/loss of number.

VIII.3 A return to the distinction between parts that themselves serve a function, and those that provide a service to those that function. Damage to the former hindering function is a disease whilst damage to the latter hindering function by way of the part being assisted is a cause of disease. In some instances a single part has both roles (Galen gives the uvula as an example), so damage to it can be both a disease and a cause of disease.

VIII.4 Further examples of abnormalities of number. Galen also raises the question of whether the two classes, number and magnitude, could be collapsed into one class – quantity – but decides against this.

IX.1 Examples of diseases that are abnormalities of magnitude.

X.1 Examples of diseases that are abnormalities of arrangement.

XI.1 Consideration of what Galen calls the 'fifth class of disease' – dissolution of continuity. This can occur in either *homoiomeres* or combined parts. Examples are given.

XII.1 The final two sections (XII and XIII) consider combined diseases. In *homoiomeres* these will be, on the basis of the 'first hypothesis' (*anarmoi/poroi*), a combination of abnormal dilatation and abnormal constriction and, on the basis of the 'second hypothesis' (that of elements and qualities), a combined abnormality of two qualities (hot and dry, hot and moist, cold and dry, cold and moist). As with the mono-*dyscrasias*, these can be due to a primary change within the affected structure, or to inflow of a substance.

XII.2 Considers other forms of combined diseases in simple bodies particularly involving dissolution of continuity in conjunction with a *dyscrasia*.

XIII.1 Consideration of combined diseases in organs – for example, a limb that is simultaneously inflamed and dislocated. A distinction is also made between primary and *per accidens* (secondary).

XIII.2 Further exemplification of combined diseases with reference to the eye. There is also further consideration of what are regarded as diseases *per accidens*.

XIII.3 Further discussion of diseases affecting multiple parts of a single organ and how to classify them. Again the eye is used as an illustration.

ON THE DIFFERENTIAE[1] OF DISEASES

I.1 [VI.836K] It is necessary, first, to state what it is we call a disease so it is clear what this work is concerned with; second, and following this, how many simple and primary diseases there are altogether and are, as it were, elements of the others; third and next, how many diseases there are that are combined from these.[2]

II.1 And here one must accept the agreed principle (*arche*) that all men, whenever they have the functions[3] of the parts of the body faultlessly directed to serving the actions of life, persuade themselves they are healthy whereas, whenever they are damaged in any one of these [functions], **[VI.837K]** they consider themselves to be diseased in that part. If this is so, one must seek health in these two things: either in functions which accord with nature, or in the constitutions[4] of the organs by which we function, so that disease is equally damage of either function or constitution.[5] But also when we are sleeping, or otherwise passing time in darkness or silence, or often just lying at rest, we neither move any part nor sense anything external at all, yet we are no less healthy. From this it is clear that to be healthy is not to function but to be able to [function], and we are able to function from the constitution that accords with nature. Being healthy, then, inheres in this. Constitution now will relate to function as cause so that whether you wish to call health a constitution of all the parts in accord with nature, or the cause of the functions, both statements amount to the same thing. But if health is this, then clearly disease is the opposite, i.e. either some constitution contrary to nature, or a cause of damaged function. It is clear,

---

[1] The term *differentia* is used in preference to 'difference' to render *diaphora*, both in the title and in most instances in the text, to reflect the taxonomic nature and Aristotelian spirit of this enterprise.

[2] Galen stresses the importance of this endeavour in several places in the *De methodo medendi*. For example: 'Let us then be done with these people and go back again to what was proposed. It was put forward as foundational that if someone does not find out methodically the total number of diseases then he will take a major fall at the very start of the therapeutic method' (X.115K). He is also cognizant of his predecessors in this proposed undertaking – Hippocrates, Plato, Aristotle and Theophrastus – see *De methodo medendi* X.15K, 118K.

[3] The term *energeia* is rendered throughout as 'function' in the sense of bodily or biological function unless otherwise indicated.

[4] *Kataskeue*, rendered as 'constitution', is seen by Galen as interchangeable with *diathesis* in his definitions of health and disease although the former term does, perhaps, carry more of a structural connotation. Latin versions include *constitutio* (Copus) and *structura* (Kühn). See also *Anonymus londinensis* III.

[5] This is Galen's initial definition of disease. The term *blabe* is consistently used by him in the sense of injury, harm or damage in broad terms. The distinction between structure and function remains important throughout these books. He returns to this definition in *De symptomatum differentiis* IV.9.

in fact, that if you also speak of a condition[6] contrary [**VI.838K**] to nature, you will be using an old term but you will be signifying the same thing.

II.2 If we were to find out the number of ways that bodies are hindered in functions when they are changed from an accord with nature, we would then find out the number of all the simple diseases. And here the agreed principle (*arche*) is that what accords with nature is balance, not only in an animal but also in a plant or a seed or anything living,[7] whereas, conversely, what is contrary to nature is imbalance. Health would then be a balance and disease would be an imbalance.[8] Next one must consider what things disease is an imbalance of.

II.3 Is it not clear that disease is an imbalance of the very things which health is a balance of? Thus, if health lies in a balance of the pores, disease will arise in an imbalance of the pores.[9] If health lies in a *eucrasia* of heat and cold and dryness and moisture, disease will necessarily follow in a *dyscrasia* of these.[10] In the same way, if health were to lie in a balance in some other class, clearly also disease [**VI.839K**] would arise in an imbalance in that class.

II.4 Let us consider this same point again more dialectically. If a body is simple and exactly one, it would never admit of more or less, nor would it be in that class where one thing is better or worse than another. On the other hand, if it is combined from many things, in this way at least, many modes of combination[11] could occur in it, both better and worse, whilst

---

[6] *Diathesis* has been consistently rendered as 'condition' and *kataskeue* as 'constitution' throughout (see n. 4 above re the latter). *Diathesis* is a somewhat problematical term which has remained in medical use in varying senses to the present time.

[7] 'Living' is taken to be an appropriate rendering in the present context of the term *organos* which has a wide range of meaning in Greek.

[8] The idea of 'balance' as a determinant of health dates back to Alcmaeon. In the fragment in question (recorded in Aëtius) the contrast is between *isonomia* and *monarchia* with reference to pairs of opposites exemplified by hot and cold. Health is defined as '... balanced mixture (*summetron krasin*) of qualities (*poios*) – see D–K, vol. 1, pp. 215–16. The same view is expressed by other later writers, for example Hippocrates in *On Ancient Medicine* XVI. Galen makes particular use of the paired terms *summetros/ametros.*

[9] The term *poros* has a considerable range of meaning, both biological and non-biological. Within the biological there is also variety. The pores referred to here are the 'theoretical' pores of Asclepiades, a concept which Galen elsewhere rejects – see, particularly, Vallance (1990). Galen himself uses the term to refer to both perceptible and imperceptible channels. I have generally used 'channels' for the former and 'pores' for the latter.

[10] The term *krasis,* in the sense of blending or mixing, is of central importance in medicine in relation to the continuum theory of elements/qualities/humours. I have retained the Greek terms throughout for the two possible states of *krasis*, i.e. balanced mixing or *eukrasia* and unbalanced mixing or *dyscrasia.*

[11] The sense of *sunthesis* here corresponds to Aristotle's usage in *Parts of Animals* 645a35 and 646a12 where the example of the house is used in the former and the specific application to the body made in the latter. See also Lloyd (1968), pp. 171–5 for a discussion of this and related terms.

in this way too the components themselves could be stronger or weaker. What is combined best would be the best of all the things of the same class. Is it the case, then, that in the bodies of animals there is more or less, so as to say that one is in perfectly good health,[12] one simply in good but not perfect health, one healthy but not in good health, another somewhat unhealthy and another already diseased, and of this [last] there is mildly or dangerously, moderately or severely? Or are we all equally affected when diseased or healthy? One cannot say this. It is not the case, then, that the body of animals is one thing, like the atom of Epicurus or one of the *anarmoi* [VI.840K] of Asclepiades.[13] It is, therefore, in all respects composite. But if it is composed from atoms or *anarmoi* or entirely from impassible[14] things, it will have the more or less in the quality of its combination, as when a house is built from impassible stones, but not in the structure if it is put together in every respect correctly. But if stones were themselves also passible,[15] there would at least be greater variability in the more or less with respect to the house. And if the actual elements of our bodies were in their nature mutable and passible, then not only in the combination and, as it were, the conformation[16] of the parts, but 'through their own entirety' (δι' ὅλων ἑαυτῶν). would more and less be allowed. Moreover, it is clear where there is disease 'through their own entirety' there will be as many forms of disease, simple, primary and, as it were, elements of others, as there would be things that are combined.[17] This 'through their own entirety' is not in impassible elements for it is not possible for an atom itself to be affected. Rather the affection (*pathema*) is in the combination or conformation.

---

[12] *Euektikos* is taken as 'good health' but, as Galen's sequence here shows, implies more than just being healthy, being perhaps equivalent to the 'rude health' of idiomatic English. See for example Plato, *Laws* 684c and Galen, *De alimentorum facultatibus* (VI.662K) for the association with *eukrasia*.

[13] Galen, as here indicated, is quite opposed to the various formulations of atomic theories. Of course, there is considerable variation among these theories. Asclepiades' version, our understanding of which is itself significantly dependent on Galen's accounts, has been considered in detail by Vallance (1990).

[14] The sense of *apathos* as an adjective here is taken to be more than insensible or impassive (see e.g. Aristotle, *Metaphysics* 991b26, 1019a31 and *Topics* 148a20). In the present context it seems that 'not susceptible to change' is also meant – cf. e.g. Gale (1677), *Contra gentiles* IV.253, where God is spoken of as 'eternal, inflexible and impassible'. See also Galen, *De atra bile* (V.122K).

[15] As the converse of 'impassible' Galen uses the infinitive of the verb *pascho*, in the sense employed in later Stoic philosophy – see Arrianus, *Epicteti dissertationes* I.2.3, I.18.1.

[16] *Diaplasis* has both a specific medical meaning in relation to the setting of a dislocated limb and a more general meaning as here.

[17] This sentence is somewhat obscure in the Greek. I have taken it to mean that where the primary component parts are susceptible of change there will be as many primary diseases as there are primary parts. This conforms to Galen's basic classification of four simple or single (mono-)*dyscrasias*.

III.1[VI.841K] Combination and conformation in the bodies of animals are threefold:[18] first of the so-called *homoiomeres*,[19] i.e. arteries, veins, nerves, bones, cartilages, ligaments, membranes and flesh; second of the organs, i.e. brain, heart, lung, liver, stomach, spleen, eyes and kidneys; third of the whole body. Each of these organic parts is compounded from certain other parts that are simple in terms of sense perception, and each of these from the primary elements. Thus the *differentia* of flesh itself, *qua* flesh, is only in the combination of the primary elements; *qua* where it is part of an organ, it is on account of conformation and magnitude. And the *differentiae* of the organs themselves are also in these things. Therefore, when we have set out the number and kinds of all the diseases of *homoiomeric* bodies according to the first hypothesis, we shall pass on in order to the other,[20] which proposes that the whole substance is susceptible to change and alteration throughout itself.

IV.1 [VI.842K] There are two primary affections (*pathos*) – a dilatation of the pores (*eurutes*) and a constriction (*stegnosis*). As the underlying primary elements are impassible, the affections (*pathema*) are in combination alone, i.e. the aforementioned *differentiae* of the whole combination.[21] Consequently each of the *homoiomeres* is necessarily made strong whenever the balance of its pores is preserved, whereas, when this is destroyed, there is a change from what accords with nature. But since the *differentia* of the whole balance is twofold, for there is excess and deficiency, it is clear that the primary diseases of simple bodies will also be two in number, one a dilatation of the pores and the other a constriction. And, in fact, with respect to bone, flesh and each of the other bodies that are simple in terms of sense perception, if they are more constricted or dilated than what is balanced, we shall say they are in a bad state. If, however, they are midway between each extreme so as to be particularly suited to their uses, under

---

[18] In this scheme of organization there is some variation depending on whether the 'elements' are listed first, as in Aristotle (*Parts of Animals* 646a and *Generation of Animals* 715a9), or omitted as here, and also whether the whole body is included or not. See also Peck (1942), pp. xlvii–xlix.

[19] I have retained the Greek terms, *homoiomeric* and *anhomoiomeric*, due to Aristotle, with respect to the apparently uniform and non-uniform parts – see Peck (1942). Valleriola (1548), pp. 36–40, considers the issue of variation in Galen's own use of the term, particularly in relation to arteries and veins which are here included.

[20] The two hypotheses referred to here and subsequently are that of Asclepiades, whom Galen treats in a much more temperate manner here than elsewhere (e.g. *De elementis secundum Hippocratem* II.3,4), and that of the elements susceptible to change within themselves, which is the theory that Galen himself espouses.

[21] I have taken Galen to be using the terms *pathos* and *pathema* interchangeably and have translated both as 'affection' while signalling which one is used in each instance. Galen himself discusses these two terms at some length in *De symptomatum differentiis* I.

these circumstances we shall say they are healthy to the highest degree. On the other hand, we shall say small deviations from perfect balance in each direction are not yet diseases [**VI.843K**] if they should not yet bring about perceptible damage of any function. Often in these there is more or less, as there would be a sufficient interval between the imbalance of disease and the balance of perfect health. In this whole range lie the *differentiae* of health. In the range beyond this, that of perceptible imbalance, lie the diseases, until they should come to that imbalance which already brings about destruction of the part. For it is certainly not natural for the bodies of animals to be constricted or dilated completely, but rather there is here a certain limit beyond which it is impossible for them to go without dissolution and destruction. This, then, is the hypothesis of impassible elements.[22]

IV.2 Those who postulate that the elements are passible and, in fact, act reciprocally, and are mixed in their entirety, will necessarily say that there are as many primary diseases as they would suppose there to be primary elements. Well then, there are four primary elements, heat, cold, dryness [**VI.844K**] and moisture, and when these are mixed with each other in due proportion the animal is healthy, but when not in due proportion, diseased. There will, then, also be four primary diseases: the first when heat is beyond the balance that accords with nature, the second cold, the third moisture, and the fourth dryness. And these are the diseases of the so-called *homoiomeric* bodies according to the second hypothesis, which in fact appear absolutely simple.[23]

IV.3 The diseases of the organs that are combined in us are common to both hypotheses. Let us, then, also recount these briefly, demonstrating first this very point, i.e. how they are common. Certainly it is necessary

---

[22] The critical aspects of this statement of the 'first hypothesis' are that the atomic components, whether Asclepiadian *anarmoi* or otherwise, are incapable of undergoing change in themselves, so disease is dependent on changes in the pores which must be in one or other direction, either dilatation or constriction. It is not clear, however, whether the pores themselves constrict to cause obstruction or the 'particles' obstruct the pores, in which case 'stoppage' would perhaps be a better rendering of *stegnosis*. The same uncertainty applies to *eurutes*, where 'opening up' might be better. The almost complete loss of Methodist writings makes definitive resolution of this point impossible, although Galen himself attempts some resolution in V.1. Further, although only Asclepiades is mentioned by name here, the section is best seen as a general statement of the Methodist position. Vallance (1990) addresses these issues particularly on pp. 140–3. See also Tecusan (2004). It is interesting to contrast Galen's relatively even-handed consideration of Methodist concepts of pathology here with his intemperate attack on Thessalus in relation to the same matter in *De methodo medendi* – see X.5K ff.

[23] This is, of course, Galen's own position following the Hippocratic identification of the primary elements as set out, for example, in *De natura hominis* and Galen's commentary, *De elementis secundum Hippocratem*.

that the whole perceptibly combined body, which in fact they also call *anhomoiomeric*,[24] if it is going to function well, should not be formed from such parts as happen to be simple, nor from some number or magnitude of parts that is not fitting, nor that the mode of combining be by chance. In these four classes there will be the diseases of all the organs. The *differentiae* in relation to each class are as follows. It is in the specified first [class] **[VI. 845K]** whenever the proper form of the part is destroyed, or the shape is not as it should be, or the part has acquired a cavity or channel,[25] or lost one of those that should be present. Of this class too are inappropriate changes in either the roughness or smoothness of the part.[26] In the second class, that relating to the number of simple and primary parts, the *differentia* of diseases will be twofold; either a deficiency of what there ought to be or an excess of what there ought not to be. Furthermore, in the third class, that relating to magnitude, the *differentia* of diseases will likewise be twofold. Thus, if something becomes greater when it ought to be less, or again something is made less when it ought to be greater, the whole organ would not be right. In the remaining class of diseases, that relating to combining, *differentiae* will arise when either the position that accords with nature or the relationship of the parts to each other is changed.

IV.4 Just as each of the primary organs combined from simple bodies is formed either correctly or defectively, and from these very things there is health and **[VI.846K]** disease, so again from these same primary organs, the secondary organs arise. For a muscle, a vein and an artery are of the primary organs, whereas a digit is of the secondary [organs], and a foot still more than this, and a leg more than a foot.[27] For, in general, whatever arises from the union of *homoiomeres* for the purpose of a single function will be numbered among the primary organs, whereas those combined from these in turn, even if they should carry out predominantly the one function of the whole organ, will be classified among the secondary [organs]. And there will also be

---

[24] *Anhomoiomeric*, a term coined by Aristotle (see n. 19 above), applies to parts that are non-uniform, i.e. broadly, organs as opposed to tissues (*History of Animals* 486a7, *Generation of Animals* 722b31), the specific examples being tongue, hand and face.

[25] This is the other use of *poros* indicating a macroscopic 'channel' – see n. 9 above.

[26] The paired terms are used in relation to anatomical structures by both Plato and Aristotle. The causes of roughness and smoothness are considered in the next book (*De causis morborum* VII.33K).

[27] Galen here, and in what follows, appears to recognize some variation in terminology. His definition of *to organon* in *De methodo medendi* is as follows: 'I call an organ a part of an animal that is an effector of a complete function, for example the eye of seeing, the tongue of speaking and the legs of walking. In this way too an artery, vein or nerve is both an organ and a part of animals. And this usage of terms was not determined by us alone, but also by the Greeks of old. Thus the eye will be called a part of an animal as well as a division and an organ whereas the external coat is a part and a division but not an organ' (X.47K). So for Galen a primary organ is also a *homoiomere*.

the same diseases of these organs as were spoken of in relation to the primary organs. But with respect to the *differentia* of organs, it has been determined in another work which ones it is appropriate to designate entirely as primary, and which among them are secondary, tertiary or quaternary.[28] Some are susceptible of two interpretations in their distinguishing features, so as to seem to be both primary and secondary. The present discussion, at least, does not require such precision, although I think it is worthwhile to consider this one point; whether the part is simple or combined in relation to sense perception. [**VI.847K**] For what are called primary diseases are of what is simple, being distinguished by a difference of the physical elements, whereas the secondary [diseases] are of what is combined, and are common to both hypotheses. There is no class of disease, either in simple or combined bodies, which is peculiar to either, for the method of division shows this to be impossible.

IV.5 But there is still one [disease] common to all bodies, including those that are combined, whether these are primary, secondary or tertiary organs, which will now be spoken of. Its method of discovery is also through its being common to all the parts discussed, for if there is something common to them in their being in accord with nature, as providing some certain function or use to the animal, presumably when this is altogether destroyed some disease common to them will arise. What is it that is common to all? It is the union of the particular parts of which each partakes, and is said to be one, and to perform one function or use. And if this were in some way to break down, the disease is also of this part. What sort [**VI.848K**] of designation this disease acquires in relation to each of the parts, we shall speak of a little later when we divide the *differentiae* of the previously mentioned classes into kinds in order.[29]

V.1 And indeed, let us now address this matter again starting from the first hypothesis. In this there are two diseases of *homoiomeric* bodies arising in an imbalance of pores, one a dilatation and the other a constriction. The *differentia* of each of these is twofold. Of constriction there is either a collapse of a body into itself from all sides or an obstruction of the pores

---

[28] Galen provides a detailed account of the organs from differing viewpoints in *De anatomicis administrationibus* (II.25–731K) and *De usu partium* (III.1–931K). May (1968), in her translation of the latter work, uses 'instrument' rather than 'organ' to render *organon* because, as she notes, '. . . Galen frequently applies the word to parts now not ordinarily spoken of as organs . . .' (p. 67, n. 3).

[29] Having completed the general outline of the taxonomic project, Galen now provides the details of the classes, considering first *homoiomeric* bodies, then organic bodies and finally the diseases common to both, which fall under the heading of 'dissolution of continuity'.

themselves, whereas of a dilatation there is either an outward movement into every part of the body or a kind of expansion of the pores themselves through a falling away of the elements, which in fact they also quite properly say are called bodies that are simple and primary,[30] for things combined from these they call compound.[31]

V.2 In the case of the second hypothesis, the differentiation of diseases happens also to be twofold in that sometimes, in fact, the *homoiomeric* bodies are changed in their qualities alone, whereas sometimes a certain substance flows into them **[VI.849K]** which has the qualities spoken of. Certainly the second form, bringing about a swelling around the bodies, is obvious to all doctors. For the *erysipelata*, inflammatory swellings (*phlegmonai*), swellings (*oidemata*), tumours (*phumata*), glandular swellings (*phugethla*), scrofulous swellings (*choirades*), *elephantiases*, *psorai*, *leprai*, *alphoi* and indurations (*skirroi*) are of this class, and can escape no one.[32] The diseases arising in a *dyscrasia* of the qualities themselves alone are harder to detect, unless at this time a major turning aside of the part towards what is contrary to nature occurs. Under these circumstances it will be readily known by everyone that when heat prevails in the whole body it is termed fever, although sometimes it is also clearly manifest in the parts. Certainly the legs, in those who walk more than is customary, and the hands, should someone work particularly hard with them, say by rowing, or digging, or doing something of this sort,[33] clearly seem warmer, both to those who are themselves affected, and to those who touch them from without. If, of course, a large swelling is added to the parts when some hot substance flows into them, **[VI.850K]** this will be from the second *differentia* of diseases. From the first there are all those things just now spoken of, whether involving any one part whatsoever, or the body of the animal in its entirety, or

---

[30] This statement addresses in part the issue raised in n. 22 above, i.e. what exactly is the process which results in a change of patency of the Methodist pores? Thus in the two possibilities (i.e. constriction and dilatation) there may be, in each case, an actual change in the overall dimensions of the pore-containing body such that the pores themselves are secondarily affected. This is the first *differentia*. The second *differentia* is less clear. With 'constriction' it appears to be an obstruction by the 'elements' whereas with 'dilatation' the process seems to affect the pores directly.

[31] The term *synkrima* meaning a compound body is used in a physical sense by Epicurus (Fr. 75, Usener (1987), p. 345) and in an anatomical sense by both Soranus (1.22) and Galen himself (*De dignoscendis pulsibus* VIII.928K and *De uteri dissectione* II.899K).

[32] A number of these terms have been transliterated only, in view of the varying meaning over time. What is significant here is that they all represent conditions in which there are visible superficial changes affecting the skin or immediately subcutaneous structures, these changes being attributed to inflowing material. See the list of diseases and symptoms given in the section on terminology (I.4d).

[33] Galen also uses the first of these examples in his discussion of causation in *De causis procatarcticis* when considering the same matter – see Hankinson (1998), pp. 126–7.

from the burning effect of the sun, or the remaining condition arising from
the heat beside a fire, such as those who are called feverish and pyrexial.³⁴

V.3 When there is a disease of cold, which is the converse of heat, a
condition often arises which visibly involves the extremities so that these,
having necrosed,³⁵ also fall off. On the other hand, when the condition
involves the whole body, it is like what happens to those travelling in
extreme cold. For there are many of these, both those who die on the actual
journey, and those who first come to a lodging house before reaching home,
obviously half dead and frozen. Often, also, such a condition occurs with
apoplexy, epilepsy, tremor and spasm (convulsion). And of those dying
through cold on journeys, some are seized by *emprosthotonos*, some by
opisthotonos, some by *tetanos* and some by what is called freezing (*pexis*),
whilst some suffer something akin to apoplexy.³⁶

V.4 Certainly in all such cases in which **[VI.851K]** some symptom supervenes, it draws the attention of many to itself, so that they think the symptom is the disease, whereas the disease itself is the cause of the symptom.
Of course, in the case of those by whom damages of functions are believed
to be diseases, on the same basis they also call spasms (convulsions), anaesthesias, numbnesses and other such things diseases. But we addressed the
issue of nomenclature at the outset in order to point out that in all such
things the disagreement is not in the matters themselves, but in the names.
Certainly, one should only censure those who do not maintain their own
hypothesis consistently but who think they are doing something intelligent
when really they have erred. So it is that one hears them sometimes making
a distinction and asserting that if a spasm (convulsion) occurs in the case
of an inflammation, this is both an epiphenomenon and a symptom of the
inflammation, whereas if in the case of a *dyscrasia* alone, it is a disease. In
fact, they also do the same in the case of a fever, whenever a perceptible
condition of some part supervenes, thinking it a symptom, but if otherwise

---

³⁴ The distinction made here in the two *differentiae* is that between those in which a direct effect on
the components of the part changes a *eukrasia* to a *dyscrasia*, and those in which something flows in
from without, effecting the same change.

³⁵ The verb *nekro*, as used here, is rendered by its derived technical usage in English. It is also used by
Galen in relation to a part affected by fever in *De curandi ratione per venae sectionem* (XI.265K).

³⁶ The association of several of these symptoms with cold was recognized by Hippocrates (*Aphorisms*
V.17–21). I have retained the Greek terms *emprosthotonus* and *opisthotonus* for stiffness in flexion and
extension respectively since the latter remains in use. Further definition of these terms is to be found in
De tremore, palpitatione, convulsione et rigore VII.641K and in the pseudo-Galenic works, *Introductio
sive medicus*, XIV.737K and *Definitiones medicae* XIX.414K. Of the last three manifestations, the first,
tetanus, is mentioned by Hippocrates. The second, 'freezing' is my translation of *pexis*, which is used
by Plato (*Philebus* 32a) to indicate an unnatural hardening due to cold but elsewhere by Hippocrates
to indicate the freezing that occurs in water (*Airs, Waters, Places* VIII). It remains unclear precisely
what the third is.

they call it a disease or an affection (*pathos*).[37] One must, then, censure those [**VI.852K**] who do not await refutation from without, but fall into discord among themselves. Certainly both those who propose to call damages of functions diseases and do this in every case, and those who look at things wrongly in some other such way, must be thought of as being mistaken in names, not as erring in the matters. More has been said on all these medical names elsewhere, so if someone wishes to use them correctly, let him read that treatise.[38] Since it is my purpose now to look at the matters themselves following the aforementioned agreement on names, let us proceed to these in due order.

V.5 So, then, there has been discussion of hot and cold conditions apart from material flowing. In the same way, moist and dry diseases will arise when there is a change in the entire nature of bodies but they receive no external substance into themselves. Then small changes are difficult to detect, whereas large changes are clearly seen, particularly in parts that are necrosed. For some of these appear as if preserved by salting and [**VI.853K**] are exceedingly dry, although this is rather rare, whilst others seem so 'mossy'[39] and moist to those looking at and touching them that if you also wish to take hold of their parts, they immediately flow away and slip through the fingers like water. So too with decaying bones, there are those that seem like sand, being similar to wood that has become rotten through time, and there are those that are, as it were, 'mossy', of which the excess of the *dyscrasia,* occurring due to moisture or dryness, necroses the whole bone.

V.6 All the other *dyscrasias* of the parts which are slight and escape the notice of most are called by them 'debilities'.[40] When an inflammation or ulcer or something else of this sort exists in relation to the stomach, they seek no other cause of the failure of digestion. If, however, there is none of these things, they say there is a 'debility' of the stomach, as if they are

---

[37] The issue of terminology, particularly the distinctions between disease, symptom, epiphenomenon, affection and condition, is given detailed consideration in the introductory section (I.4a). In these four treatises Galen himself grapples with the terminological distinctions in the opening sections of *De symptomatum differentiis* I.

[38] *De nominibus medicis* – lost in the Greek but surviving in Arabic and translated into German by Meyerhof and Schacht (1931).

[39] The term *bruodes*, which is used by Aristotle to describe a place with thick seaweed (*History of Animals* 543b1) is later used medically in the sense of 'mossy' or 'flabby'. See also Alexander Aphrodisiensis, *Problemata* II.62, Galen, *De methodo medendi* X.195K and Soranus, I.82, 95.

[40] Atonia/atonic remain as medical terms and might be appropriate here, although it seems that a more general sense is intended, hence 'debility'. The point seems to be that the majority who are unaware of the precise nature of the condition describe it using an imprecise term. The word is used by Hippocrates in *Airs, Waters, Places* XX as a general term in relation to the Scythians, where both Adams (1886), vol. 1, p. 177 and Jones (1923), vol. 1, p. 123 translate it as 'flabbiness'.

saying something other than what clearly has happened, which is that the food has not been digested properly. For what else would someone take them to be saying [in using the term] 'debility' other than that there is a weakness of function? [**VI.854K**] But this is not what is sought, but rather the cause of this 'debility'. For why is the stomach weak in terms of its particular function, when it is not inflamed, indurated, ulcerated, nor has any other such thing? Certainly there is no deprivation of proper digestion without some cause. In all cases then, either an imbalance of the pores or a *dyscrasia* must be taken as causal.[41] From this it is also obvious that none of the primary diseases, such as are specific to the *homoiomeres* themselves, will be able to be treated rationally without due consideration being given to the primary elements. But what is likely in relation to these has been discussed in other works.[42] What must now at least be known is whether a 'debility' of the stomach, or of a vein, artery or muscle, or of any living and vital organ in general, is necessarily accepted as coming about through some imbalance of the pores or through a *dyscrasia*. How such conditions of these [structures] must be recognized is not germane to the present argument, for it is not my purpose to speak of diagnosis but to enumerate the primary diseases themselves. [**VI.855K**] And it seems to me that everything has been said on the matter of *homoiomeres*.

VI.1 What follows is to say what [the diseases] of the organic parts would be. In these, then, it has been shown elsewhere[43] that some one part is entirely the cause of function, all the other parts being created to provide a certain use for this part. The function of the whole organ will be damaged particularly and primarily when there is disease of the actual body which is the cause of function, for now also the more major conditions of all the other parts hinder the function. However many things, then, that not through themselves but through damage hinder the primary organ of this function are causes of diseases, but not themselves diseases. If, however, they are able to hinder function apart from some damage to the primary part of the function, one must now call such conditions diseases. This will be, as we said, when there is a change in the conformation that accords with nature, or when the necessary number of parts has not been preserved, [**VI.856K**] or when each has maintained an inappropriate size, or when their combining is not as it should be. For since it has been shown that none of these [parts] has been created by nature without a purpose, but

---

[41] The verbal adjective, *aitiateon*, as used for example by Plato in *Timaeus* 57c10, 87b5 and *Republic* 379a6, is used only this once in these four treatises.
[42] Valleriola (1548), p. 72, takes this to be a reference to Galen's *De locis affectis* (VIII.1–451K).
[43] Primarily in *De usu partium*, as discussed by Valleriola in his commentary on this section (pp. 72–4).

in all cases for the better or safer functioning of the whole organ, it is altogether necessary also that injuries of these, either those that entirely prevent function, or those that merely hinder it, are thought of as diseases, whereas those that carry over to an injury of the primary part responsible for the function are called causes of diseases, as has been said just now.[44]

VII.1 Because of this, then, those who are splay-footed, or bandy-legged, or have flat feet,[45] function less well with their limbs owing to a fault of proper form. In the same way too, those having an improperly set fracture do not function well with the limb. Those who are distorted by a very large joint,[46] or by fractures of the articular rim where the joint readily passes over it and is dislocated,[47] or [**VI.857K**] by excessive growth of chalkstone[48] in relation to it in such conditions, the whole joint being hard to move owing to the narrowness of the space, also [function] badly. These, then, are acquired defects[49] of form. Congenital [defects][50] arise in every part of the body in relation to a hindrance of the primary formation while still *in utero*, rendering the animal diseased in that part. For the form of the heart, lung, stomach, brain, tongue, spleen, kidneys and all other parts must be preserved, since when some damage occurs around these, of necessity it makes the specific action of the whole organ worse.

VII.2 Furthermore, if the size and number of all cavities in the parts are not preserved, function would also necessarily be damaged because of this. There are many such diseases, some arising through a certain coalescence, some through the obstruction of viscid and thick humours, some again when bodies are dried up, or when surrounding [structures] are narrowed by something falling in on them and causing compression. Sometimes,

---

[44] This is an important distinction for Galen. As he says in *De methodo medendi*: 'It has been shown that there are three conditions in the body that are contrary to nature – causes, diseases and symptoms. Causes are exemplified by excess and destruction, diseases by inflammation and ulceration, and symptoms by discoloration and thinness' (X.86K).

[45] The adjective *blaisos*, applied to the limbs, is taken to mean either 'splay-footed' or 'knock-kneed' – see Hippocrates, *On Joints* LIII and LXXXII respectively. I have taken *raibos* to mean here 'bandy-legged' – see Galen, *De usu partium* III.9. For *leiopous* as 'flat-footed' see Galen, *In Hippocratis de articulis librum commentarii* XVIIIA.613K.

[46] It is not clear whether the term *arthritis* here refers non-specifically to an increase in the size of a joint (Hippocrates, *Affections* XXX) or to gout specifically, which is the meaning given by Durling (1993) for its use by Galen (p. 71).

[47] This process is described in greater detail in relation to the arm in *De usu partium* – see I.119H and May (1968), p. 151.

[48] For the specific orthopaedic use of the term *poros* see Aristotle, *History of Animals* 521a21 and the several occurrences of both noun and verb in Galen listed by Durling (1993), p. 281.

[49] This rendering of *epiktetoi kakiai* depends on the use of the former as 'acquired' in relation to a deformity (see Paulus Aeginata VI.29), and of the latter, although most commonly used with moral or behavioural connotations, as a physical defect.

[50] See Galen, *De sanitate tuenda* VI.3K.

[VI.858K] also, the substance of the actual bodies that have such channels, when it is indurated (*skirromene*), or inflamed (*phlegmone*), or gangrenous (*sphakelizousa*), or suppurating (*diapuiskomene*), or swollen (*oidiskomene*), or in any other way whatever acquires an added magnitude, having poured the swelling into the internal cavities, obstructs the channels. These are different from those pores which the proponents of the prior proposal postulated as occurring in relation to the coming together of the primary and impassible elements.[51] We clearly see all these large and obvious channels, those of the intestines, veins, arteries and all other such organs. If, however, sometimes such a channel escapes detection by the senses owing to its small size, it is still not from the same class as those pores which the first of the proposals postulated. Certainly, in all such conditions in which, when the bodies themselves have been swollen into some mass,[52] it happens that the channels are closed up and constricted, there will sometimes be one disease alone, the obstruction damaging the function, and sometimes not only this but also **[VI.859K]** the condition of the bodies bringing about the obstruction. Thus, when the body that has acquired the swelling has no specific function, there will be one disease relating to the obstruction, whilst the condition of the body having the swelling is the cause of this but is still not a disease.

VII.3 For if it should happen that the tunic of the vein in the concavities of the liver[53] is affected in such a way that it is constricted in the channel from which the vessels in the convex parts of the liver take up blood, there would be in this way two diseases; one of the affected vein itself and one the obstruction involving the channel. At all events, the condition of the vein hinders the generation of useful blood, whereas obstruction hinders its distribution,[54] each of these being a function necessary to the animal. Clearly

---

[51] As indicated in n. 9 above, the distinction between macroscopic pores and the 'theoretical' pores of the Methodists is signalled by using 'channel' to translate *poros in* the first case, although there is no distinction in the Greek. The term *sunodos* has a wide range of meanings, even within its specifically biological usage, which Galen avails himself of – see, for example, *In Hippocratis de natura hominis librum commentarii* XV.47K and *De usu partium* IV.391, XiI.8. Plato uses the term in the *Timaeus* both in relation to the coming together of bodies (58b) and the condensation of the earth (61a). Aristotle applies it to the coming together of form and matter, if one accepts Jaeger's emendation (*Metaphysics* 1033b7). Interestingly, the Latin translation by both Copus and in Kühn uses 'concursus', again a word with a wide range of meanings, but used in the present sense, for example, by Lucretius (I.384, 685).

[52] See Valleriola (1548), pp. 82–5 for a detailed consideration of Galen's concept of this process.

[53] *Simos* is taken as referring to the concave lower surface of the liver – see Galen, *De locis affectis* VIII.35IK and *Ad Glauconem de medendi methodo* X1.93K.

[54] For Galen's concept of blood formation in relation to the inferior surface of the liver see *In Hippocratis librum de alimento commentarii.* XV.387K. I have translated the term *anadosis* as 'distribution', although at least in some instances it may imply more than that – see, for example, Brock's (1916) translation of *De facultatibus naturalibus*, p. 13, n. 5. May (1968), in her translation of *De usu partium* preserves the Greek term – see particularly pp. 232–9.

conditions which primarily damage functions should themselves be said to be diseases. Of course, when the vein itself is not affected, if distribution is damaged owing to some viscid or thick humour being impacted in the channels, this would be a case of the obstruction alone being a disease in the viscus. In the same way, in the intestine, if there is obstruction alone, there will be one disease, **[VI.860K]** whereas when the intestine is inflamed, and because of this is closed off with respect to the space within preventing the superfluities from going downward, there would be two diseases. For often a disease arises from a disease, as is the case in matters previously spoken of, whenever also in inflammations (*phlegmonai*), *erysipelata*, *herpetes*, pustules (*anthrakes*) or some other such thing, a fever supervenes. Sometimes what is brought about is damage of function, and it is necessary to call this an affection (*pathema*) or a symptom, its cause clearly being a disease, just as obstruction is the cause of food no longer being distributed, or cooling is the cause of impaired sensation, these being the diseases related to the symptom. Whenever the condition itself primarily damages function, although its cause does not damage [function] primarily, it is necessary, on the one hand, to term the condition a disease and, on the other, to term what brings it about, the cause of the disease, as in the case of viscid humours and obstruction. For the obstruction itself is the disease, whereas the humours are the causes of the disease.

VII.4 Thus, all the diseases occurring in relation to cavities, whether those of obstruction **[VI.861K]** or those of disproportionate extension, are to be subsumed under the class of conformation of the part, for in all these the natural conformation is in some way hindered. But, in fact, even smoothness and roughness are not themselves without purpose in the natural conformation of the parts. Here too, at any rate, diseases involving all the parts will arise when what is by nature smooth becomes rough, or again, when what is by nature rough becomes smooth. To doctors the most obvious examples of these [situations] are those occurring in rough and smooth bones and the roughness of the throat that brings about coughing. And here too it is necessary to know that sometimes, when the form of the part is damaged, it harms at the same time some channel in it. Something of this sort is seen to occur in the nose whenever, by a violent blow, it is both bent upwards and the channel within it is constricted to such a degree that one either cannot breathe at all through it, or only with difficulty. It is clear, then, that in such conditions the constriction of the channel is the disease (for this primarily hinders the function of breathing) and the bending upward of the nose is the internal antecedent (*proegoumenic*) cause of this, being damage of the form that accords with nature in it. **[VI.862K]** Certainly it is in the class of conformation when there is departure from

what accords with nature to such a degree as already to harm function, that
the aforementioned *differentiae* of diseases will arise.

VIII.1 In relation to the number of simple parts from which each of the
organs is formed, the primary *differentiae* of diseases will be twofold: one in
which a certain part is lacking, and one in which it is in excess. In each of
these there are others. For, of the excesses, there are those from the class of
things in accord with nature, as when a sixth digit occurs in someone, or a
pterygium in the eye, or an eruption of flesh[55] in the nose, or any other such
thing whatever in relation to some other channel. Certainly, some of these
will themselves be diseases, like a pterygium, in that it obstructs the eye
whenever it is increased sufficiently, casting a shadow over the pupil, whilst
others will be causes of diseases, like the eruptions of flesh which obstruct
channels, in that the obstruction is primarily the disease since that is what
primarily damages function. Some [of the excesses] **[VI.863K]** are in the
whole class contrary to nature, like helminthes and ascarides,[56] a stone in
the bladder, a chalazion in the eye, a cataract (*hypochyma*), pus (*puon*), warts
(*akrochordones*), cysts (*melikerides*), fatty swellings (*atheromata*), sebaceous
swellings (*steatomata*), *alphoi, leprai, leukai*, chalkstones in joints (*poroi*)
and all those things found in abscesses (*apostemata*).[57] That we shall call as
many of these as primarily hinder function, diseases, as with cataract, and
call those that don't, causes of diseases, is clear to everyone.

VIII.2 Of the deficient parts, there are those where the whole [part]
is completely destroyed, and those where it is as if up to a half is cut off
or 'docked'.[58] It is clear to everyone that, in fact, many such things occur
during primary genesis. Among the newborn, often whole bones are taken
out in relation to fingers, limbs, head or thorax. Sometimes a finger, or
foot, or hand,[59] or lower part of the leg,[60] or the forearm is taken away.

---

[55] This term, *blastema*, which is used non-specifically in Hippocrates' *Humours I* to mean a growth or
excrescence – translated by Jones, vol. 6 (1931), p. 65 as 'growth' – appears to indicate here a nasal
polyp – see Valleriola (1548), p. 90, and his references to Paulus and Aëtius.

[56] The Greek terms are retained to avoid unwarranted assumptions of equivalence to the varieties of
intestinal worms now recognized. See Aristotle, *History of Animals* 551a8–10, and Peck's note e to this
(Peck (1970), p. 173). See also Hippocrates, *Aphorisms* III.26.

[57] There is some overlap between this list of lesions which, owing to 'excess', hinder function and the
earlier list in V.2 which is of lesions that are *dyscrasias* due to some inflowing substance.

[58] 'Docked' is preferred to 'mutilated' for *kolobo/kolobos*. See Valleriola's (1548) discussion of the term
(p. 92).

[59] *Cheir* could be the lower part of the arm or the hand specifically. For example, in his translation of
Plato's *Protagoras*, Lamb (1924) uses the former whilst Guthrie (in Huntington and Cairns, 1989)
uses the latter. See also Xenophon, *Institutio Cyri* VIII.8.17.

[60] Again it is uncertain precisely which part, in this case of the leg, is indicated here – see for example
Iliad IV.147. In *De ossibus ad tirones* Galen uses the term to refer specifically to the tibia (II.774K).

[Sometimes, also,] varicose veins, or indurated glands, or decayed teeth are taken away, as are, indeed, the windpipe, omentum, foreskin and part of the penis itself, in fact, often the whole [VI.864K] penis, and in the same way the testes. Someone recently, who clamped his teeth in a great spasm of the whole body, bit off the tip of his tongue. Then, when he was saved from the spasm, he was unable to speak in the same way. Of this class too are the so-called 'dockings' of lips, noses, ears and such of the other fleshy parts as have been violently torn away, or being decayed, are completely cut off. In all such circumstances, the number of the parts that accords with nature is not complete, either one or two or many being missing, having been destroyed altogether or removed in part.

VIII.3 Certainly, however many such things as hinder functions by reason of themselves are placed in the class of diseases. Those which either cool some other part that effects functions, or those which distribute nutrition deficiently, are causes of diseases. Some combine both and so have the place not only of cause but also of disease. For example, the uvula,[61] whenever it has been cut to its base, both damages the voice and cools the [parts] relating to the lung [VI. 865K] and the thorax. So when you learn in the considerations of functions and uses, that of all the parts of the animal, some accomplish a certain function useful to the whole animal, and some do not themselves function, but rather provide a certain service to those functioning, it is clear that also in respect to damages of these, you will speak of those that make differences directly to function as primarily diseases of the parts of the animal, and those [that make a difference] to some service as causes of diseases. Thus, with those parts that fulfil two functions or two uses, sometimes in respect to one injury there will be a twofold relation, of disease and of cause. If some part effects both service and function at the same time, as seems to some to be the case with the uvula, destruction of this part will be, according to one relation, a disease, but according to the other, a cause of disease. It is clear too that the disease is in what remains and is preserved, and not in what no longer exists. For in relation to that part of the open space of the mouth, of which there is now an affection (pathos), you will say there is a part called the pillar[62] or uvula. [VI.866K] Whenever this is destroyed, something is missing in the space, and so with

---

[61] Although the term gargareon has other uses and may indicate the trachea (Aristotle, History of Animals 492b11) or a disease of the uvula (Hippocrates, Affections IV), Galen seems to reserve the term for the uvula as a structure. For his ideas on the dual functions of the uvula see De usu partium (II.146H ff.) where there is reference also to the lost work, De voce – see also May (1968), vol. 1, p. 279 and vol. 2, pp. 525–7. There is a definition in the pseudo-Galenic Definitiones medicae XIX.368K.

[62] Galen uses kion as an alternative term for the uvula, although it may indicate other anatomical structures – see for example Rufus, Peri onomasias XXXI – in addition to its more general meaning.

respect to the whole, one disease occurs, since it was agreed at the outset that it is of what remains that the whole function is damaged by disease. It must be shown, then, either that speech, inspiration and expiration are not one function of the animal, or, if this is the case, clearly, that destruction of the uvula brings about a disease in the roof of the mouth.

VIII.4 In the same way too, destruction of a tooth is a disease of the mouth. If it is of those adapted to chewing, the damage relates to mastication, whereas if it is of the so-called incisors, the hindrance extends to eating and speaking. In like manner also, if half the tongue is cut off, the unnatural 'docking' is in the part remaining. The same also applies to the omentum, and to the penis, and to all things affected in this way. And if someone does not wish to call this a disease but an affection (*pathos*) or an affection (*pathema*), he will be disputing about the name and not about the matter itself. Clearly, as in the tongue, and in the omentum, and in the penis, and in general in all such [VI, 867K] 'docked' organs, there is some reduction of size in all the diseases spoken of. The reduction will not necessarily be apparent in the animal itself so that it is obviously 'docked', but some number of parts will be taken away; that is to say, arteries, veins, nerves and sometimes skin as well as fat, membranes and flesh are taken away in such conditions. Of course, in the case of the uvula or varicose vessels being cut out, also some number of the parts of the organs themselves is taken away. Furthermore, all such things are classified by the number of parts changed whereas, when some of the amount of organs is taken away, but parts are not taken out, these are, in fact, assigned to both classes. For what is deficient in the animal is either the number of simple parts or the magnitude of the combined organ; what is 'docked' is the whole. Furthermore, it is clear to everyone, I imagine, that both classes, that pertaining to number and that pertaining to magnitude, can be subsumed under another higher category, that of quantity. That is to say, there is a discrete form of quantity [VI.868K] which is properly called quantity, and a continuous form which is called magnitude. But in the present [treatise] it seemed to me clearer to divide things thus – that is to classify one difference of quantity as number and the other as magnitude.

IX.1 But since the diseases pertaining to this class have been spoken of, let us proceed to a consideration of those pertaining to the size or magnitude of the parts, or whatever one might wish to call it. This is not the same as that previously spoken of. For when the form that accords with nature remains in the part whilst the magnitude is destroyed, whenever some function is damaged, what happens as a result of this will be a disease of the part – as for example if the tongue becomes so large at the time of its first formation that it cannot turn in the mouth owing to its size, or so small that it does not touch all parts of it. Increases contrary to nature occurring in parts already formed are not **[VI.869K]** very frequently seen, whereas reductions in size are, in fact, often seen, and the disease is called in some cases atrophy (*atrophia*), and in others wasting of the part (*phthisis*).[63] Increases of the parts occur in exuberant ulcers (*helkē*) and in so-called priapism. Nicomachus the Smyrnaean's whole body was excessively increased and he was not able even to move himself, but Asclepius cured him.[64] We have seen someone's tongue increased in size to the greatest extent without any pain, so there does not seem to be swelling (*oidema*), induration (*skirros*) or inflammation (*phlegmone*). There was no indentation on pressing, no loss of sensation, and no feeling of pain, but this very thing alone, an inordinate increase in the size, there being no damage to the actual substance of the part. In the same way too, either one or both testes, or one or both breasts, are disproportionately increased in size. And so-called scrofulous swellings (*choirades*)[65] are of this class, producing not a little disturbance in functions whenever there is excessive increase. Furthermore, the excessive increases of the canthi are of this class also, an increase being called **[VI.870K]** a tumour (*enkanthis*), and a decrease, a discharge (*ruas*).[66] Certainly such things are also among the *differentiae* of this class of diseases.

X.1 When the combination that accords with nature is changed, diseases occur. In terms of position, [this is seen] in dislocations (*exarthresis*), subluxations (*pararthresis*), intestinal hernias (*enteroplokele*) and so-called hernias of the omentum (*epiplokele*). In terms of the association of adjacent parts not being in accord with nature anywhere, laxity, tension or rupture of a ligament hinders the movement in that part of the articulation. In this class

---

[63] The term *phthisis* appears to have three distinct medical meanings: a chest disease, the term having come to be associated with tuberculosis (Hippocrates, *Aphorisms* V.15, pseudo-Galen, *Definitiones medicae* XIX.419K); a contraction of the pupil of the eye (pseudo-Galen, *Definitiones medicae* XIX.435K); and general wasting. Although Durling (1993) lists only the first two usages, it is clearly the third which is intended here (see Hippocrates, *On Joints* I and also Valleriola (1548), p. 103). In fact, both terms, *atrophia* and *phthisis*, also have a specific ophthalmological application (pseudo-Galen, *Definitiones medicae* XIX.435K).

[64] In their *Aesculapius*, Edelstein and Edelstein (1945) list this under 'Undeterminable Cases'.

[65] This seems to be the most suitable translation for *choiras* – see Hippocrates, *Aphorisms* III.26.

[66] The first of these terms, *enkanthis*, seems to be specific to a tumour involving the inner canthus of the eye (see Galen, *De tumoribus praeter naturam* VII.732K), whereas the second, *ruas* or *roias*, has several meanings, but is here used to indicate a weeping discharge from the eye (see Galen, *De methodo medendi* X.1002K and pseudo-Galen, *Definitiones medicae* XIX.437K). A definition of both terms, with Greek names preserved, is given in Celsus, *De medicina* VII.7.5 for the first and VII.7.4 for the second, which Spencer (1938) takes to be a lacrimal fistula (vol. 3, pp. 330–1).

also are the excessive bands, both those of the tongue and those of the penis, in which the tongue is hindered enough to involve speaking and chewing, whilst the penis, in the dispersal onwards to the womb, is unable to send forth the sperm directly because the channel is distorted. Furthermore, the unnatural coalescences of ulcerated lips, eyelids, fingers, anus [**VI.871K**] or some other such [part] are of this *differentia*. Such are the kinds of diseases of the class pertaining to the combination of parts.

XI.1 There remains a fifth class of disease, the dissolution of union, whether this occurs in one of the simple parts termed *homoiomeric,* or in the combined parts, which is why we also made mention of this a little earlier in the common diseases of each of the two [kinds of] part.[67] Thus, where a ligament or artery is avulsed, the affection (*pathema*) is common to both the whole organ and the avulsed part itself. Each has had dissolution of continuity, the whole in that its parts are no longer joined together and united, and the avulsed part itself in that it no longer remains one but has become two. If, however, it has not been completely avulsed, but [only] from a certain part, this is no longer a disease of the whole organ, unless it is *per accidens,* in that part of it is affected, but only the affected part specifically [**VI, 872K**] and singularly. The dissolution of continuity in bone is called a fracture (*katagma*), and in all the fleshy parts generally an ulcer (wound – *helkos*). Breakage (*regma*) and rupture (*spasma*)[68] are of the same class, the one arising in a fleshy part, the other in a sinewy part, when the fibres in these are torn apart by some violent crushing or a sudden and overwhelming stretching. What are called severings (*apospasmata*)[69] are specific affections (*pathemata*) of the organic parts alone. These are all the *differentiae* of simple diseases.

XII.1 It is now time to pass to the combined [diseases], beginning again from the *homoiomeric* bodies. According to the first hypothesis, there will be

---

[67] Galen here returns to the final class of diseases initially discussed in section IV.5 There is, however, some variation in terminology, *lusis tes enoseos* and *lusis tes sunecheias* respectively, although the same type of abnormality seems to be indicated. Galen speaks of the equivalence of the two terms in *De constitutione artis medicae ad Patrophilum* (I.238K).

[68] The two terms, *regma* and *spasma*, are used in conjuction by Hippocrates in *Airs, Waters, Places* IV where Jones (1923), translates them as 'ruptures' and 'strains' respectively (vol. 1, p. 79). Galen indicates here that the same process is being referred to, although affecting different tissues. This differs from his description in *De constitutione artis medicae ad Patrophilum* (I.238–9K) where the tissues are muscle and flesh respectively. The terms are also defined in pseudo-Galen, *Definitiones medicae* (XIX.462K and 413K respectively).

[69] I have used 'severings' here because the process seems to be different from the 'avulsions' involving principally ligaments – see Galen, *De methodo medendi* X.232K and *In Hippocratis de articulis librum commentarii* XVIIIA.736K.

a combined disease from dilatation and constriction of the pores, although it is not the case that each of the pores suffers both in turn. But when bodies are constricted and dilated alternately, there is neither more dilatation of pores than constriction **[VI.873K]** to be implicated in relation to the whole *homoiomeric* body, nor is there some perceptible part of it in which there is only one, but always all that is affected is affected by both. According to the second hypothesis, owing to the qualities alone departing from what accords with nature, in each of the *homoiomeric* bodies there will be four combined diseases: hot and dry, hot and moist, cold and dry and cold and moist. When a certain substance flows into these [bodies], there are likewise four other [diseases] having the same conjunctions of qualities.

XII.2 Since the division[70] of continuity happens not only in compound organs but also in simple bodies, this too will be implicated sometimes in the combined diseases now spoken of in relation to both hypotheses, as well as in the simple diseases written about right at the start of the whole work. For it is not impossible for a part to be ulcerated and, at the same time, also more dry than accords with nature, or more moist, or more cold, or more hot, nor to be ulcerated and, at the same time, **[VI.874K]** more moist but not to be more hot at all. Therefore, parts that are simultaneously ulcerated and inflamed depart from what accords with nature in three ways: owing to the ulceration there is destruction of the unity of the specific parts, whilst because they are inflamed they are made hotter and more moist than is natural. Of course, the swelling in these [parts], whenever it has taken on such a size as to harm function of itself, must be thought of as being now a disease. Otherwise it is only a symptom or affection (*pathema*), just as pain also is. Therefore, all bodies that are simultaneously inflamed and ulcerated are necessarily diseased in three ways, and sometimes in four. For what we now call inflammation is clearly not the kind of 'burning heat'[71] of the parts which was customary among the ancients, but a red, firm and painful swelling. In this way also, ulcers sometimes occur in the *erysipelata*. In pustules (*anthrakes*) it cannot be otherwise, whereas intermediate in nature between these are the *herpetes* and cancers (*karkinoi*), many **[VI.875K]** occurring accompanied by ulcers but sometimes also apart from them. All such diseases are, at any rate, combined, even if they occur without an ulcer. In one way, all these diseases are creations of superfluous fluid whether hot or cold: *erysipelas* of yellow bile, cancer (*karkinos*) of black

---

70 *Diairesis* is used here instead of *lusis* as in XI.1 above.

71 It is not clear precisely how *phlogosis* differs from inflammation. See, for example, Thucydides II.49 where Smith (1919) translates it simply as 'inflammation' (vol. 1, p. 345). The difference from ancient terminology is also mentioned by Galen in *De difficultate respirationis* (VII.853K).

bile, inflammation (*phlegmone*) of blood, and swelling (*oidema*) of phlegm. In another way, because of the aforementioned humours, even if in form they are all moist, in capacity they are not moist, for black bile is dry and cold, and yellow bile is dry and hot, whereas moist and cold is of phlegm, whilst the blood is moist and hot. In a third way again, because all these are combined with each other, it is also rare to find any one of them in a pure state. Thus, often in inflammations, some *erysipelas*, swelling or induration is mixed in, whilst in *erysipelas* some inflammation, swelling or induration [is mixed in], and likewise in each of the others. Therefore, all such diseases are compound in many ways. More will be said **[VI.876K]** about these in the treatise on the causes of diseases, and in the work following that on the symptoms of diseases and, in addition to these as well, right through the therapeutic work,[72] for the sake of which all this is written.

XIII.1 Now, since we have spoken of the manner of combination of these [simple diseases], let us proceed forthwith to the diseases of organs and show how they too become combined. First, it is necessary to recall what was said at the outset – that there are some [diseases] of primary bodies which are *homoiomeric,* and some of organs which are combined, inflammation (*phlegmone*) being of primary bodies and dislocation (*exarthrema*)[73] of organs. Thus, whenever a limb is dislocated and inflamed at the same time, the dislocation is primarily a disease of the whole organ itself, whereas the inflammation is neither primary nor specific but *per accidens.* For since the inflammation is a disease of each one of the parts of the limb, it may also be *per accidens* a disease of the whole organ.

XIII.2 Furthermore, *ophthalmia*[74] is, on the one hand, an inflammation of the **[VI.877K]** membrane adherent to the cornea and sclera[75] and, on the other, *per accidens* a disease of the eye. It happens sometimes, when there is a deep ulcer (*helkos*) of the cornea and it is subsequently completely destroyed, some part of what is called the choroid falls forward with it, whilst the

---

[72] The reference is to the remaining five books here translated and to *De methodo medendi* (X.1–1021K).
[73] The two different terms for dislocation used here and in the following sentence (*exarthrema* and *exarthresis*) seem to be interchangeable – see Hippocrates, *On Joints* LVIII and LIII for both used in close association and pseudo-Galen, *Definitiones medicae* XIX.460K for the former. A limb is taken as an organ(ic part).
[74] Ophthalmia appears to be a general term to characterize an inflammation with discharge – see Hippocrates, *Epidemics* I.5 and also Celsus, *De medicina* VII.7.15. For a consideration of ophthalmological terminology in ancient times, in which ophthalmia is equated with conjunctivitis, see Mettler (1947), pp 1006–11.
[75] Terminology is somewhat confusing here. *Keratoeides* appears to refer to cornea plus sclera and *keratoeides chiton* to the cornea alone – see Galen, *De usu partium* III.771K, 773K and Celsus, *De medicina* VII.7.13, particularly Spencer's (1938) note (vol. 3, p. 346).

pupil is drawn aside, and each of these three is considered an affection (*pathema*) of the eye. And yet the ulceration and destruction is of the cornea alone, the prolapse is of the choroid, and the drawing aside is of the pupil. But, as has been said, diseases of *homoiomeric* bodies are *per accidens* diseases of the whole organ. Therefore, whenever a combined disease afflicts any one of these, this will also be a disease of the whole organ *per accidens*. Whenever more [parts are afflicted], but each is occupied by one disease, there would in this way be a combined disease of the whole organ. For let it be the case – and this is not an impossible supposition – that in the eye there should happen to be simultaneously a pterygium, *ophthalmia*, erosion[76] of the cornea and sclera, prolapse of the choroid, and the start of the formation of a cataract (*hypochyma*). That this is neither **[VI.878K]** a single nor a simple disease is clear to all. One person will call it a combined disease of the eye, whereas another will say it is not one combined [disease] but several diseases in relation to the eye, arising in different parts of it. It has no bearing on the diversity of the therapeutic indications, which is why we investigate all such things, whether it be one combined [disease], or many requiring contending remedies. Quite clearly, more will be said on these matters in the writings on therapeutic method [*De methodo medendi*]. It is enough for the purposes of the present argument at least, to have pointed out and explained such a thing, which would be to present what both parties would plausibly hold; i.e. those who assume there to be many diseases in relation to the eye, and those who consider that, just as there is one affected organ, so there is one disease which is combined whenever, as has been said, more parts are affected in relation to it.

XIII.3 Just as, then, in the case of simple diseases, the disease was primarily of the whole organ itself like a cataract (*hypochyma*), or was so *per accidens*, like ulceration of the cornea and sclera, so too of combined diseases there will be (a) those specific **[VI.879K]** to the whole organ greatly troubling several parts of it at the same time, and (b) *per accidens*, combined diseases existing in relation to some one part in it, like *ophthalmia*, which is an inflammation of the adnate membrane.[77] Inflammation was shown to be a combined affection (*pathos*). When an ulcer (*helkos*) exists as well, in relation to this same membrane, it would be much more the case that the

---

[76] *Diabrosis* the noun, which in general indicates an 'eating through', has been rendered here as 'erosion'. In Galenic usage the term is particularly applied to a vessel – see *De locis affectis* VIII.262K.

[77] This 'closely applied' membrane is listed in LSJ as the conjunctiva, with reference to Galen's *De symptomatum causis* VII.101K. In fact, the term 'adnata tunica' was not applied to the conjunctiva until much later – see Mettler (1947), pp. 1022–3. This structure is not, however, included in Galen's detailed description of the anatomy of the eye in *De usu partium* X, particularly section 2 (III.762–9K). See also May's (1968) note, pp. 467–8.

part is implicated in a combined disease, although it could equally be said
that the whole eye itself is affected by a combined disease. Certainly such
things are *per accidens* combined diseases of whole organs. Those through
which several parts are affected at the one time are primarily combined
diseases of the organs themselves, and especially if also each of the simple
parts is not involved *per accidens,* but the disease is primarily of the whole
organ, as with pterygium, cataract (*hypochyma*) and discharge (*ruas*) in the
eye. For each of these is a specific disease of the eye, and when all occur
at the same time, they bring about a specific combined disease of the eye.
Someone who would use such a method might discover all the combined
diseases of [**VI.880K**] all organs. It seemed to me superfluous to discuss
and bring together all [these diseases] because anyone who has learned all
the simple diseases and the manner of their combination would be competent to train himself in these things severally. So to read once only what
is written in this book is of no benefit if one does not intend to train still
further in these things.

CHAPTER II.2

On the Causes of Diseases

SYNOPSIS

I.1 A statement of aim – having catalogued and classified all diseases, to identify the causes of each. For simple (*homoiomeric*) parts, on the 'first hypothesis' (that of *anarmoi/poroi*) all diseases are either (i) a disproportion of pores, or (ii) a dissolution of continuity. On the 'second hypothesis' (that of elements and qualities) there are four 'simple' *dyscrasias* and four 'combined' *dyscrasias*.

II.1 Listing of 5 causes of excessive heat: (i) movement; (ii) putrefaction; (iii) proximity to another hot body; (iv) constriction; (v) food with the 'necessary capability'. Examples are given in each case, using inanimate objects.

II.2 How excess heat comes about from these five causes.

II.3 A consideration of why a putative cause does not invariably produce the same effect. The explanation lies in variations in the magnitude and duration of the cause and in the state of the affected body. Again, inanimate examples are given.

II.4 Further consideration on the variability of the relationship between presumed cause and expected effect.

II.5 A distinction is drawn between *proegoumenic* and *prokatarktic* causes. The former are either 'conditions pertaining to the animal itself or abnormal movements' (internal antecedent causes) whilst the latter are external factors (external antecedent causes).

III.1 Enumeration of six causes of excess cold: (i) contact with cold things; (ii) certain foods and drinks; (iii) constriction; (iv) rarefaction; (v) idleness; (vi) disproportionate movement.

III.2 As in II.2, an elaboration of how these causes produce abnormal cold, again illustrated with inanimate examples.

III.3 Examples of causes of contact with external cold and their observed effects clinically. Examples also of things ingested that bring about abnormal cold.

III.4 A consideration of why extreme constriction causes cold diseases (*dyscrasias*), given in terms of its effects on blood vessels and innate heat.

III.5 A discussion of why, with only moderate constriction, the effects will be different, not only quantitatively but also qualitatively. This may, in fact, produce a fever.

III.6 Consideration of rarefaction as a cause of cold *dyscrasia*, acting through dispersal and dissipation of the innate heat.

IV.1 A brief consideration of the causes of excessive dryness: (i) hard work with perspiration; (ii) eating little; (iii) eating things dry in capacity; (iv) thinking too hard; (v) staying awake too long; (vi) contact with dry external conditions, either air or water; (vii) taking medicines dry in capacity.

V.1 An even briefer consideration of the causes of excessive moisture: (i) abundance of moist foods; (ii) excess of drinks; (iii) luxurious way of life; (iv) gladness of heart; (v) numerous drinks; (vi) an idle life; (vii) moist external conditions; (viii) moist medicines.

VI.1 A brief statement that the causes of combined diseases are themselves combined.

VI.2 When a body is acted on by a group of causes, including those that are opposite in capacity, superiority in number, magnitude and duration of action determine which are effective. Sometimes opposite causes both have an effect simultaneously, producing an 'anomalous' *dyscrasia*.

VI.3 Reiterates the distinction between *dyscrasias* due to a primary change in one or more of the four qualities of a body itself, and those due to the inflow of material (fluxion) altering the balance of qualities in a body. Summarizes the qualities of potential inflowing material – yellow bile, black bile or phlegm – with some examples of diseases due to these.

VI.4 Considers that inflow of material is due to what is superfluous in one part being set aside to a less important part. Galen raises the issue of why or how this happens.

VI.5 He speaks of four capacities: attractive, alterative and separative, the last being subdivided into two. He then considers the gradation of the parts of the body from stronger to weaker with skin as the weakest, having no function as such. The flow of superfluities is from stronger to weaker.

VII.1 Starts the consideration of the causes of diseases of organs following the classification in the previous book. This section deals with disorders of conformation and why certain instances of these occur, focusing on those apparent at birth or arising in early life.

VII.2 Further examples of diseases of conformation, due to improper wrapping by nurses, or to unsatisfactory healing in fractures and dislocations due to incorrect treatment, or to other trauma.

VII.3 Examples of diseases of conformation due to excessive filling, or lack, or to distortion due to spasms or paralyses.

VII.4 The causes of diseases of conformation due to changes in the configuration of cavities or channels.

VII.5 Causes of the final subclass of diseases of disordered conformation – those due to abnormal roughness or abnormal smoothness.

VIII.1 Diseases of organs due to reduction or increase of the number of parts, and why these occur in a number of instances.

IX.1 Diseases of organs due to change in the size of parts, whether increase or decrease.

X.1 Causes of diseases of organs due to alterations in arrangement, exemplified by dislocations, internal and external hernias, and other, predominantly trauma-related causes.

XI.1 The third class of diseases common to *homoiomeric* and organic parts – dissolution of continuity. Galen sees this as a new class of diseases first identified as a class by him. Again trauma is the main causative agent and may affect bones or fleshy parts.

XI.2 A subclass of diseases of dissolution of continuity in which there is preservation of surface structures but dissolution of continuity within. Causes include sudden, irregular or violent movements, especially in unprepared tissues.

XI.3 A summary of causes of diseases of this class. They are either external (wounding, crushing) or internal (abnormal movements, abnormal humours causing erosion).

ON THE CAUSES OF DISEASES

I.1 [VII.1K] All diseases whatsoever, in divisions according to kinds and classes, simple and combined, have been set out in the other book.[1] Next should be to go through the causes of each of these, starting from the simple and so-called *homoiomeric* parts of the animal, then passing in turn to the combined and organic. Since, therefore, it was shown that according to those who suppose the underlying substance to be a unity and to be changed in coming into being and destruction, **[VII.2K]** every disease of a body that is *homoiomeric* and simple to sense perception is either some *dyscrasia*, or a dissolution of continuity of its parts. On the other hand, according to those who think [the underlying substance] is not a unity, but that also some empty space is interwoven into the whole combination of the body, a disease is an imbalance of the pores or a dissolution of the perceived unity. Let us begin now to consider the causes of each of the diseases of

---

[1] The previous book, *De morborum differentiis* (VI.836–80K).

the first hypothesis, which we certainly believe to be true.[2] There were, I
believe, four simple and four combined [diseases]: sometimes when it [the
body] receives an excessive increase of heat or cold alone, or of one of those
of the other opposition, in relation to dryness or moisture, and sometimes
also to a conjunction of those things increased, as when the disease is hot
and dry at the same time, or cold and dry, or hot and moist, or cold and
moist.

II.1 Let us now consider, then, what the causes are of the genesis of each
of the aforementioned diseases, making a start from the *dyscratic* disease
in relation to excessive heat.[3] **[VII.3K]** Certainly it seems that in the case
of all other bodies, however many become hotter than they normally are,
the increase of heat is either from some movement, or from putrefaction,
or from proximity to another, hotter body, or from constriction,[4] or from
a food with the necessary capability. [It is] from movement in the case
of those exercising in any way, or the rubbing together of stones with
each other, or wood, or the fanning of flames. [It is] from putrefaction in
the case of all other things, but especially of seeds or faeces. At any rate,
I too have sometimes seen the putrefying faeces of pigeons kindle into
flame.[5] Furthermore, that things coming near are heated by association
with hotter bodies is obvious to anyone who calls to mind the bath-house,
or the summer sun, or any conflagration. In the same way too, if you light a
fire in a large house in winter but obstruct its outlets, you will accumulate
the heat within, whereas, if you allow it to be opened to all sides, you
will have none left. Then too, both bath-houses and furnaces accumulate
heat within themselves in the very same way. From this it is clear that a
constriction is sometimes a cause of increased heat. It is also clear **[VII.4K]**
from firewood, insofar as reeds that are dry readily give rise to an intense fire,
whereas green wood, especially if you were to greatly heap it up on itself,
goes as far as to weigh down very considerably and, as it were, suffocate the
fire, although eventually it does increase.

[2] Both theories are given extended treatment in the previous book. Here Galen again declares his
allegiance to the continuum concept of structure as opposed to the atomic. Valleriola ((1548),
p. 127), lists as other prominent adherents of the former Plato and Aristotle among philosophers
and Hippocrates, Galen, Paulus, Aëtius and Alexander among doctors. As adherents of the latter, he
lists Democritus, Mnesitheus and Asclepiades.
[3] The various examples of excess heat, particularly in relation to fever, are given detailed consideration
in *De methodo medendi* IX (X.599–660K). See also Valleriola, pp. 129–31.
[4] Here and in what follows, Galen uses *stegnosis* in the general sense rather in specific relation to the
poroi.
[5] The incident to which Galen is presumably referring is described in detail in *De temperamentis* III
(I.657K). In fact, a similar consideration of various examples of change in the four qualities in relation
to inanimate objects is given in that work.

II.2 How then, in the body of an animal, is each of these things brought about? Someone who exercises quite excessively is made weary. This is to have excess heat in the joints and muscles more than accords with nature. For these are primarily what move. And if the heat remains there, or comes to be released prematurely before it is distributed to the whole body of the animal, what is generated in this way would be fatigue[6] alone. Conversely, if [the heat] is spread to the whole body, the disease is called fever, which is an excessive heat of the entire animal. In the same way also passion, which is a seething of the heat around the heart,[7] when it is distributed due to excess movement, sometimes stirs up a fever involving the whole body. Furthermore, those things that putrefy in the body of the animal are those that produce an excess heat in the actual parts in which they putrefy, **[VII.5K]** just like the *erysipelata*, the *herpetes*, pustules (*anthrakes*), inflammations (*phlegmonai*) and glandular swellings (*phugethla*) and those that having made the whole body hot like themselves[8] give rise to a fever. The third cause of excess heat is, then, already clear from these things, i.e. how it arises in animals, and from so-called heat-strokes (*enkausis*).[9] For in the case of swollen glands (*boubones*), inflammations (*phlegmonai*), the *erysipelata* and all diseases that are hot in this way, invariably what is touching and the part contiguous to this, first get the benefit of the heat, and thereafter may also transmit it to what is adjacent, and in turn to what is adjacent to that, and so, when a *dyscrasia* comes upon the *arche* of the innate heat,[10] the whole body rapidly partakes of the affection of the *arche*. Long periods of time spent in sunny places sometimes excessively heat the whole skin of those who are naked but the head alone of those who are clothed. This is heat-stroke. If it were to be distributed to the whole body, in this way a fever would occur. The fourth class of cause which kindles the innate heat excessively is seen to occur in coolings and contractions. **[VII. 6K]** For if someone is extremely cold or has swum in water which has astringent qualities,[11] or partakes of some other such capacity, the skin contracts and

---

[6] For *kopos* as 'fatigue' generally see Hippocrates, *Ancient Medicine* XXI, and specifically in relation to exercise, Galen, *De sanitate tuenda* VI.190K.

[7] The concept of anger as a seething of blood around the heart is formulated by Aristotle in *On the Soul* 403a25 ff., although here *orge* is spoken of. A similar concept relating to *thumos*, but without the anatomical specificity, is found in Plato, *Republic* 440c.

[8] See Hippocrates, *Regimen* II.66 and also Galen, *De differentiis febrium* VII.387K.

[9] The third cause is proximity to hot objects. For heat-stroke see Dioscorides, *De materia medica* V.13.

[10] The concept of 'innate heat' is spoken of by Hippocrates (*Aphorisms* 1.14) and elaborated by Aristotle (see e.g. *Meteorologica* 355b, 379a). See also section on terminology.

[11] The term *stupteriodes* indicates 'alum-containing' or 'astringent' – see Hippocrates, *Airs, Waters, Places* IX, and the pseudo-Aristotelian *Problems* 937b23. See also Galen, *De sanitate tuenda* VI.35K.

thickens and closes up the air vents[12] within. These things, if there should happen to be a concentration of smoky material, give rise to fever. The pungent and hot qualities of foods are the fifth kind of excessive stirring up of heat, [those of] garlic, leeks and onions and however many other such things there are. Furthermore, the occurrence of a rather excessive use of these things sometimes provokes a fever. Certainly people are feverish when they partake greatly of hot drinks, such as old or bitter wine in a weak body, or of pungent medicines, both remedies and poisons.

II.3 Why then, they say, is a fever not always kindled in the case of each of the stated causes?[13] It is not only that the magnitude of the effecting cause is unequal but also that the condition established by this in the body has a great difference in terms of more or less. And the whole actual body of one animal may differ greatly from that of another in respect to the ease or difficulty of departing from [**VII.7K**] what accords with nature. So then, you will not be puzzled as to why every movement does not bring about fatigue. But this much, at least, should be clear to you – that if the movement were not greater or stronger than the natural constitution of the joints and muscles, these would not then be fatigued at all. On the same basis, you must know that the actual condition of fatigue, if it is not great and of noteworthy duration, would not be able by itself to cause harm to the whole body. It is not possible for a small movement to bring about fatigue, so how will a small degree of fatigue invariably kindle a fever? Or will movement have its action in [the category of] relative, whereas fatigue will not have? And the bodies of athletes, at least, endure prolonged and very violent movements at the same time without being fatigued whereas those of us ordinary people, even if we toil only slightly more than is customary, are immediately distressed. This is something everyone, even the most stupid, already knows. It is not, therefore, surprising that someone who has exerted himself is not at all febrile. For if the exertion is slight, or of short duration, or less than the strength of the body, or if the exercise of short duration, [**VII.8K**] or not vigorous, or weaker than the natural constitution of the one exercising, it would not then bring about fatigue. On the other hand, fatigue will stir up fever, even if it is slight or of short duration, or weaker than the strength of the affected body. But this, in fact, of all things is seen in the most active fire, as this does not, without time and strength, burn things that are chilled, for sometimes coming from the icy cold we pass our hands through a great fire without harm. Nor will it

---

[12] The concept of transpiration via the skin dates at least from Hippocrates – see *Nutriment* XXVIII.
[13] This question is at the core of Erasistratus' objection to the Dogmatic account of causation. Galen deals with it at length in *De causis procatarcticis*.

readily set alight all firewood. Thus dried reeds are burned immediately at first contact, whereas wood that is wet and green needs a long time and a strong fire in order to be set alight.

II.4 How then, if none of these things is surprising in the case of fire, are you surprised in the case of fatigue, that it needs both magnitude and duration and also a readiness of the body to be heated? It were better for you not to wonder at this, but to consider the kind of body of an animal that is by nature easily heated, and the kind [that is heated] with difficulty. But you will hear about this next. For the present, at any rate, let it not seem to be strange to you, if **[VII.9K]** what is about to act in any way whatever needs time and magnitude, as well as a suitability of what is adjacent, to be affected. For it is not possible for fire to burn, apart from these things, nor for a sword to cut, nor for any other of the most efficacious things to act on what is stronger than itself by nature, without some significant time. You would not, then, pour oil in a concentrated way on a lamp flame, much less water, nor would you attempt to cut stones with a sword, much less adamant, so would you think fatigue, heat, cold and other such things to kindle a fever invariably, even if slight, or brief, or if the whole body were unsuitable to be heated, or not? For what is already hot is more susceptible to being further heated, just as what is cold is more susceptible to being further cooled, whereas it is the converse with what is unsuitable. So, then, the perplexity of those seeking such things is due to stupidity and ignorance.

II.5 With respect to those who readily and recklessly assert that fever never occurs owing to any of the stated [causes], **[VII.10K]** they should either be pitied for their obtuseness or reviled for their contentiousness. Their sophistical arguments have at least been refuted in another book written specifically about *prokatarktic* (external antecedent) causes.[14] But now is not an appropriate time to refute those who have erred, but to set out to teach the truth. Going back again then, let us hold on to what has been proposed. It was, I think, proposed to speak completely of the *proegoumenic* (internal antecedent) causes of each of the simple diseases, and of the *prokatarktic* (external antecedent) causes. For it is no bad thing to follow those who have distinguished the terms in this way for the sake of clarity.[15] They then call either conditions pertaining to the animal itself, or

---

[14] This work (*De causis procatarcticis*) is not included in Kühn. For the Latin text and an English translation see Hankinson (1998). The particular target here is, as indicated, Erasistratus.

[15] The translation of *proegoumenic* as 'internal antecedent' and of *prokatarktic* (or *prokatarchontic* which is taken to be the same) as 'external antecedent' is argued for in the introduction (section I.4b and chapter I.6). Galen does not specify to whom he is referring here but one might speculate that it is the Stoics and perhaps Athenaeus.

movements contrary to nature, *proegoumenic* (internal antecedent) causes of diseases, and those things that befall [the animal] from without and greatly change or alter the body, *prokatarchontic* or *prokatarktic* (external antecedent) causes.

III.1 Well then, we have spoken in general of the causes of a hot disease, [so] let us pass now to cold. The causes of this are great in number, such as the contact of cold things, the quantity and quality of what is eaten and drunk, **[VII.11K]** both constriction and rarefaction,[16] and besides these, idleness and disproportionate movement. For these, in fact, are the causes[17] that extinguish fire itself. Thus, if you place a large amount of snow or ice on a small fire, or pour cold water on it, you will extinguish it immediately. And if the ambient air is extremely cold – a particular example is around the Danube during winter – not only will you see a lamp in the open air immediately extinguished, but also any other small fire. In this way, fire is overcome by the contact of very cold things. On the other hand, it is damaged somewhat by an excess of those things that are of the nature to nourish it, or by a deficiency, or by an unsuitable quality. If you heap a lot of wood all at once onto a small fire, you will suffocate it by the excess of immoderate quantity whereas, if you provide no wood at all, or only a small amount, you will see it die away through a lack, or paucity, of nourishment. In the same way also, I presume, we see a lamp flame diminish and be in danger of extinction owing to excess of appropriate nourishment. For if you either do not provide abundant oil for it, or if you pour it on in a concentrated way, in each case you will disturb it greatly. And if you provide **[VII.12K]** plentiful fuel for it, but what is either of such a nature as not to burn at all, or only with great difficulty, you will also immediately make this flame less, just as if you were to pour oil mixed with water on a fire. Further, if you obstruct the access of the surrounding air to the fire, or rarefy it excessively, you will also see, in this way, the flame quickly diminish and be in danger of being extinguished. It is closed off if you place around it a medical cupping-glass[18] or a stove cover, or some

---

[16] Galen uses *manosis* here as the contrary to *stegnosis*, rather than *eurutes*, as when speaking of *poroi*. For *manosis* as rarefaction in contrast to *pyknosis* see Aristotle, *Physics* 212b3. It is not clear what difference in the physical process is implied.

[17] This is the first use of *prophasis*, rather than *aitia/aition*, either alone or qualified, in this treatise. I have left open the question of whether anything else, such as 'external', is implied. In Hippocrates, *Aphorisms* III.12, where the term is used in a similar context, Jones, vol. 4 (1931) translates it as 'provocative', whilst Adams (1886) has 'slight cause' (vol. 2, p. 231). The matter is considered in the introduction (section I.4b).

[18] A description of this device is given by Hippocrates, *Ancient Medicine* XXII. The adjective 'medical' is used in conjunction with the noun by Plato (*Timaeus* 79e).

other such thing. It is the same if you block up the openings of furnaces. If you set a fire in the hot sun, or in a warm and sunny place, or if you place it beside another stronger fire, you will see, at that time, the lesser flame quenched from the vigorous rarefying and dispersing effect of the external flame, which is stronger. And it is clear that when you fan it, which is a movement, you will increase it if you do this in a measured way whereas, if you fan it excessively, you will break it up and scatter it. So at all events, the streams of air will always be in accord with the magnitude of the fire if they are going to be of some benefit to it. [VII.13K] Those that are greater than this scatter rather than fan it. And it should be clear from this that a fire needs additional movement for its increase, but not that which is excessive. It will grow weak if it is not fanned at all, whereas it is scattered and dispersed when assailed by movement from without.

III.2 Certainly in relation to the first kind of cause due to all the cold befalling [someone] from without, there will be some cold disease, in part from the contact alone, and in part from the strength.[19] In this way, swimming in cold water, or bathing badly,[20] or travelling through freezing places, harms a person. And I know that some have died before reaching home. In relation to the second [kind of cause], some become apoplectic, or epileptic, or are harmed in relation to either movement or sensation, or in some other way are made cold, by inebriation.[21] And yet wine in moderation, in fact, augments the innate heat,[22] being a most suitable nourishment. Furthermore, the excessive intake of what are to the animal the most useful and nourishing foods is a cause of cold diseases. However, many of the things eaten and drunk that are too cold in nature [VII.14K] are also causes of cold diseases. Of such things there are poppy, mandrake, henbane and hemlock,[23] which actually kill through the severity of the cold.

III.3 Extreme constriction, for we certainly established this as the third cause of cold diseases, brings about unconsciousness (karos), coma (koma) and apoplexy. This is also what was said by Hippocrates: that in suddenly becoming mute, stoppages of the veins afflict the body.[24] Like others of the ancients, he called the two classes of blood-containing vessels veins, unlike

---

[19] I have taken *dunamis* to refer to the strength of the cold here.

[20] This is taken to mean bathing in water of unsuitable temperature – see *De causis procatarcticis* V.44 and Hankinson's note on pp. 185–6.

[21] The adverse neurological effects of wine are set out more fully by Galen in *De temperamentis* III (I.660–1K).

[22] See Hippocrates, *Aphorisms* I.14.

[23] Galen provides details of these four agents in Books VII and VIII of *De simplicium medicorum temperamentis et facultatibus* (XII.72–5K, XII.67K, XII.147–8K, XII.55K respectively).

[24] This is not an exact quote. See Hippocrates, *Aphorisms* I.14 where he attributes the sudden loss of speech to descent of phlegm into the veins.

those of recent times who restrict this term to vessels that do not pulsate.[25] Whenever the arteries in an animal are cut off,[26] this is so when they are full of blood, so that no empty space is still left in them into which, by being dilated, they will be able to draw the external air. The innate heat is also choked up by this. Those so affected quickly become immobile and insensible throughout the body. For it was also shown by us in the treatise on the use of the pulses that the arteries pulsate in order to maintain an exactly suitable heat in accord with nature in all parts of the animal,[27] **[VII.15K]** whilst [it was shown] in the treatise on the use of respiration, that this maintains an exactly suitable heat in the heart.[28] So just as if you were to deprive external flames of communication with the surrounding air, whether you put a cover over them, or a cupping-glass, or some other such thing, you will immediately destroy them, in the same way, if you confine and close off the heat in animals so there is no connection with the ambient air, you will quickly kill them. Thus, the heat in the heart communicates through the channel of the 'throat'[29] with the surrounding air, and if you obstruct this [channel], you will immediately choke off the heat and kill the animal. The heat in the arteries in the whole mass of the body breathes to the surrounding air through the heart itself by virtue of its communication with the pharynx, and through the entire skin. It is fanned in expansions and pours out what is sooty[30] in contractions, preserving by both of these its balance in accord with nature. And in particular, when the arteries are stopped up **[VII.16K]** either, as we said a little earlier, by an excess of blood, or by some obstructions occurring in their orifices, so that there is no transpiration at all, the heat is necessarily quenched, and the body acted upon in this way made lifeless.

III.4 Nevertheless, when a moderate constriction occurs, such an affection (*pathema*) involving the innate heat will still not necessarily arise. But if, for example, there is some sootiness or smokiness, the superfluity arising under these circumstances in the body of the animal will be one affection

---

[25] The differentiation of arteries from veins is usually attributed to Praxagoras. For a discussion of the history and significance of this distinction see *Herophilus*, von Staden (1989), VI.6 and VII.4.

[26] Nutton has suggested 'ligated' for *apolambano* in this context.

[27] The work is *De usu pulsuum* (V.149–80K). Although the matter is discussed in general, I am unable to locate this specific statement.

[28] See *De respirationis usu* IV.506K.

[29] The term 'pharynx' presents something of a problem, being used for the throat generally and for the pharynx or larynx/trachea specifically. For Galen's use of the term interchangeably see *De usu partium* VIII.1 and May (1968), vol. 1, p. 385.

[30] The distinctions between the three terms *aithalodes*, *lignuodes* and *kapnodes*, typically applied to superfluities or excretions, are not entirely clear. For purposes of translation I have used 'sooty' for the first two and 'smoky' for the third. See Galen's *Synopsis librorum suorum sedecim de pulsibus* IX.470K and *De methodo medendi* X.579K.

(*pathema*) of the innate heat, whereas, if what is evaporated is only sweet and good, it will be another. Each of these is twofold, the differentiation being thus: whenever the blood in the body is entirely good, and is not made turbid by any troublesome superfluity, a wholesome vapour is stirred up from its being heated which carries along with it nothing fiery or acrid. Certainly such a body, when it is moderately constricted, would either quickly become *plethoric*,[31] or hotter than accords with nature. *Plethora* arises in those who live an inactive life, since those things remain within which ought to be evacuated when working hard, whereas those who do work hard are hotter, as if **[VII.17K]** the innate heat were increased from the movement but not transpired owing to the body having been made dense. In respect of a body that is constricted owing to a smoky superfluity being fostered, either a fever will be kindled, the sooty exhalation being shut up within,[32] or the innate heat will be choked off and quenched.[33] Each of these will be dependent on the quantity of superfluity and the degree of constriction. For if the need for evacuation of the smoky superfluity is great, or the constriction extreme, there is a danger of the choked-up innate heat being quenched by the superfluity, whereas, if the superfluity is small in amount or the constriction slight, a fever will be kindled. It is clear, then, that it is necessary to know both the natural and acquired conditions of the body in which what is transpired is smoky, sooty or vaporous. But this will be discussed in the treatise on the therapeutic method.[34] For now let us go back to what was proposed.

III.5 For just as constriction is often the cause of cooling in the manner spoken of, so too a rarefaction, whenever **[VII.18K]** it disperses and dissipates the innate heat more than is appropriate, makes the body colder. And these things occur in relation to the whole animal, although not in the same manner in each part, whether it is constricted or rarefied. For if the whole body has a particular condition in the case of obstructions or repletions[35]

---

[31] *Plethora*, used as a general term by Hippocrates (e.g. *Regimen in Acute Diseases* XXXVII), came to have a specific pathological meaning for Erasistratus, indicating a superfluity of blood in the veins with consequent spill-over into the arteries – see von Staden (1989), p. 304 and Longrigg (1993), pp. 216–17. Galen also uses the term with reference to the humours – see *De methodo medendi* X.891K.

[32] Here the term *lignuodes* is applied to 'exhalations' (*anathumiasis*) – see also Galen, *De usu partium*. XI.14 (III.901K).

[33] Galen appears to use the verbs *sbennumi* and *aposbennumi* interchangeably. I have translated both as 'quenched'.

[34] These matters are considered in both *De differentiis febrium* (VII.273–405K) and *De methodo medendi* XI (X.734–809K), the latter being the work referred to here.

[35] The term *plerosis* is uncommon in Galen. It is used by both Hippocrates (e.g. *Ancient Medicine* IX and XXI) and Aristotle (*Rhetoric* 1380b3) to describe fullness with food, although see Freese (1926), p. 188, n. b. In the Latin translations *plenitudo* is used both for this term and the much more common *plethos*.

of the arteries, a part may have this [condition] due to the arteries alone being affected in it, making it necessary, I presume, for the part to be diseased to an almost equal degree with it. Furthermore, the remedies applied to it externally, both medicinal and cold fluids, and the surrounding air itself, will be able to produce either constriction or immoderate rarefaction in the part. And certain strong bindings, sometimes when applied to the part itself and sometimes to the part lying above it, will mortify and cool it, depriving it of communication towards the *arche* in the animal, from which both the innate heat flows to it and the motor capacity supplies the arteries.

IV.1 [VII.19K] Enough certainly has been said about the diseases of heat and cold. Let there be discussion next about those of dryness. If someone works quite hard and perspires, or eats sparingly, and of those things that are dry in capacity, being more dry in temperament (*krasis*), he will readily be drawn into a dry disease, particularly if he thinks too much or stays awake too long. Furthermore, dry conditions of the air surrounding us clearly also dry out the actual bodies of animals, as does swimming in water which is alkaline, or sulphurous, or astringent, or full of asphalt, or partakes of some other such quality.[36] Moreover, whatever medicines are dry in capacity, whether employed internally or externally, these also dry. More has been said about these in the works on medicines.[37]

V.1 These, then, are the causes of dry diseases. All the opposites [are causes] of moist diseases: an abundance of foods that are moist in capacity, an excess of drinks, an altogether more luxurious way of life, a gladness of heart,[38] and numerous baths **[VII.20K]** of sweet waters, especially after food. So too is a completely idle life, and lack of labour, many rains, and every moist state, and those medicines that are able to bring this about.

VI.1 It is clear that the causes of combined diseases are undoubtedly combined.[39] For if, on occasion, heat and dryness conjoin at the same time as a cause, the disease will necessarily be hot and dry, and if heat and moistness,

---

[36] For these four kinds of waters, particularly with regard to bathing, see respectively *De simplicium medicamentorum temperamentis et facultatibus* XI.387, 393K; *De methodo medendi* X.387K; *De sanitate tuenda* VI.219 and *De methodo medendi* X.535K; *Hippocratis Aphorismi et Galeni in eos commentarii* XVIIB.657K.

[37] *De simplicium medicamentorum temperamentis et facultatibus* XI.379–892K and XII.1–377K.

[38] For the term *thumedia* in a medical context see Aretaeus' *On Causes and Signs of Chronic Affections* I.5.

[39] I am indebted to Hankinson for pointing out that Galen never uses the common terms for joint causes, i.e. *sunaitia* and *sunergon*. Here he uses the term *suntheta* ('combined') in making the point that the different causes have identifiably different roles in producing the overall effect.

hot and moist. It is the same in the case of the remaining two conjunctions, moistness and coldness, and dryness and coldness.

VI.2 Let us now say what it is necessary to add to and define in the discussion. This is that the body is often changed by all the causes that are of the same kind as each other, or often by those that are opposite in their capacities. Of these, sometimes the greater number prevails, or the longer-lasting, whilst sometimes the stronger prevails, or sometimes the body receives damage from both alike. And even if it seems, in fact, impossible for one and the same body to be made simultaneously more hot and more cold [**VII.21K**] than is natural, or again more moist and more dry, nevertheless this does also occur. This is properly termed an 'anomalous *dyscrasia*', and those things that are appropriate for us to say about this have been said before separately in another work.[40] So it is not necessary now to dilate further on them. Rather, we must pass on to the remaining classes of diseases and consider the causes of these.

VI.3 It is appropriate to recall again here what was said in the work on the *differentiae* of diseases to the effect that sometimes bodies change from what accords with nature in the four qualities themselves alone, no other substance flowing into them from without,[41] whereas sometimes they are filled with a fluxion[42] which is undoubtedly moist in form but not moist in capacity. There has been discussion, both by earlier physicians and by philosophers, about the capacity of such fluids.[43] We have documented this also in certain other treatises and in those on medicines.[44] What from these that is pertinent to the present discussion will be spoken of now. For instance, yellow bile is hot and dry in capacity, black bile is dry and cold, blood is moist and hot, and phlegm is cold and moist. [**VII.22K**] And sometimes each of these humours flows unmixed, but sometimes mixed with others, and the conditions of swollen, indurated and inflamed parts, in consequence, vary still more. Thus pustules (*anthrakes*), cancers

---

[40] The short work *De inaequali intemperie* (VII.733–52K).

[41] The distinction between the two kinds of change of qualities is considered in *De morborum differentiis* V.2 (VI.848–50K).

[42] *Reuma*, translated here as 'fluxion', is a term that has both non-medical and medical usage. Within the latter it may be applied specifically to humours or to discharges more generally. The definition given in the pseudo-Galenic *Definitiones medicae* is: 'A fluxion is a forceful flow of thin fluids (humours) that is uncontrolled and purposeless' (XIX.433K).

[43] Fluxions in a pathological sense are spoken of for example by Hippocrates (*Ancient Medicine* XVIII) and by Aristotle (*Sense and Sensibilia* 444a13). Galen speaks particularly of the views of earlier doctors and philosophers on the subject of capacities in relation to medicines in *De simplicium medicamentorum temperamentis et facultatibus* I (XI.432–4K).

[44] For example, *De temperamentis* (I.509–694K), *De facultatibus naturalibus* (II.1–214K) and *De simplicium medicamentorum temperamentis et facultatibus* (XI.379–892K, XII.1–377K).

(*karkinoi*), *herpetes*, *erysipelata*, gangrenes (*gangrainai*), swollen glands (*phugethla*), cancerous sores (*phagedainai*) and *satyriasis* are from this class. And besides, *alphoi*, gruel-like tumours (*atheromata*), *achores*, cysts (*melikerides*), *ganglia* and sebaceous tumours (*steatomata*) are diseases generated by fluxions. These, and all the others previously mentioned, differ from each other in that some arise from phlegm alone, some from blood, some from yellow bile, some from black bile, and some from another humour not completely contrary to nature. But whatever this may be, it is certainly from one of the previously discussed classes. For it is not possible that this is not hot and dry, or hot and moist, or cold and dry, or cold and moist but inasmuch as it is to the greatest degree thick and cold, it falls outside the form of phlegm that accords with nature and rather seems to be another humour [**VII.23K**] in the whole class contrary to nature. But this is definitely not the case. For if any [humour] is moist and cold in capacity, it is encompassed within the class of phlegm. On the same basis, should any [humour] be dry and hot, it is a congener of yellow bile. More has been said about these matters elsewhere.[45] It is not now necessary to expand further on them as more will be said about all such things in the works on therapeutic method.[46] Let us return again to what is germane to the present description.

VI.4 For all such diseases occur on each occasion when nature sets aside what is superfluous to less important parts.[47] This too has certainly been said before by many others, whereas what the manner of the setting aside is, has not yet been spoken of. We shall be attributing a certain reasoning power and purpose to Nature,[48] if we say that it simply sets aside anything that is not useful from the important to the unimportant parts. But that in diseases the beneficial crises[49] come about through some such capacity is clearly seen. However, what the manner of generation is in these, my predecessors have not explained accurately because, [**VII.24K**] with respect to the physical capacities, which we have gone over in detail in other treatises, they were unable to show accurately how many and of what kind these were, and what the action of each was. But now, at least, there is no difficulty in going

---

[45] In the works referred to in n. 44 above, especially the first two.

[46] *De methodo medendi* (X.1–1021K).

[47] For the distinction between 'important' and 'unimportant' parts see also Galen, *In Hippocratis praedictionum librum primum commentarii* III (XVI.540K) and Aristotle, *Generation of Animals* 772b28 where Platt, in Barnes (1984), translates *kuros* and *akuros* as 'functional' and the converse.

[48] In this context, and in what follows, I have taken 'nature' to be personified – see also *De facultatibus naturalibus*, trans. Brock (1916), pp. 12–13, n. 4.

[49] Galen also speaks of *aristae kriseis* rather than *agathai kriseis* as here, although presumably the meaning is the same. See *De diebus decretoriis* IX.919K for a description.

over all these, assuming for this use the demonstrations throughout those [treatises].⁵⁰

VI.5 There are four capacities, of which every part of both an animal or plant partakes: attraction of what is suitable, retention,⁵¹ alteration, and separation of what is superfluous, superfluity being twofold according to class.⁵² For there is superfluity either in quantity or in quality. Moreover, since all parts of the body are not equal in strength, but the more important parts are from the very beginning made stronger by Nature, it is reasonable that in impure and superfluity-containing bodies something flows to the less important parts. For seeing that the excess is carried off from all the stronger parts, and is able to remain nowhere, it comes to the weakest part of all. Such a part is different in different cases, whether **[VII.25K]** it is made defective immediately in the first formation of the animal, or is damaged subsequently, or is required by nature to be such [a part], like the skin.⁵³ For insofar as this is created for no function, but only for use, it is fitting that it is weaker than those parts having functions. It is like some natural covering or garment of the animal, providing no digestion, no distribution of nutriment, no formation of blood, no pulse, no respiration, no voluntary movement, nor any function at all to the animal. At the same time too, it is situated external to all [the parts], so with good reason it receives the superfluities from the whole body. Right from the beginning, Nature has crafted many organs for the sake of the evacuation of superfluities, and these alone are sufficient for health whenever neither any damage comes upon the animal from what surrounds, nor the whole body is made excessively superfluity-containing from a faulty way of life. Should such a defect occur, and the physical organs be not still sufficient on their own to clear away the great amount of superfluity, **[VII.26K]** fluxions, in this case, rush down to the weaker parts, having been driven out from the stronger. It sometimes happens too, when there is constriction of the cleansing channels, that these flow to other places. These are the actual origins of the genesis of all the diseases previously mentioned. The harm is now increased in the members themselves, as if, when the superfluities have been plugged up and caused to putrefy, in this way they also become worse, and the

⁵⁰ Galen's concepts of the natural capacities or faculties are considered in extenso in his *De facultatibus naturalibus* (II.1–214K) as are the opinions of his predecessors.
⁵¹ *Kathektike* is missing in the Kühn Greek although present in the Latin text (*alia retineat*).
⁵² In translating *perissos/perissoma* I have used 'superfluity' rather than 'excretion' as the term as used by Galen clearly has a more general applicability than would be indicated by the latter. See also Brock (1916) in his translation of *De facultatibus naturalibus*, particularly p. 35, n. 3.
⁵³ In Galen's physiology the skin was an important route of disposal of what was superfluous – see, for example, the pseudo-Galenic *Definitiones medicae* XIX.370K.

humour which subsequently flows, even if it is useful, is at the same time corrupted.

VII.1 But since we have gone through the specific diseases of *homoiomeric* bodies, next in order would be to speak of the diseases of organic [bodies], beginning from the first class among these, that pertaining to conformation. This is when sometimes the form that accords with nature is changed, and when sometimes there is a certain smoothness, or roughness, or destruction of a channel.[54] The causes of a change of the form that accords with nature are, first, an abnormal conformation in what is conceived while still in the womb, when there is abundant material or an unsuitable quality hindering the physical **[VII.27K]** movements of the sperm. The second is that relating to the birth itself or due to a fault in the wrapping in swaddling clothes. For being soft still, and almost fluid, the bodies of new-born infants are easily distorted should the midwife receive them in an incorrect manner during birth, or if the wrapping in swaddling clothes is sometimes not as it should be, or again, if nurses do not pick them up and put them down in the proper manner in the providing of milk, or in washing and wrapping. For in all such instances, if someone does not handle [the infant] suitably, the natural form of each of the limbs is easily distorted and destroyed. Furthermore, it happens that in the whole rearing thereafter, many of the limbs are distorted, some by an excessive filling,[55] others by a defective movement when they are allowed to stand or walk earlier than is proper, or are moved too vigorously, when repletions hinder the physical functions, or when untimely or violent movements agitate the limbs and twist them around as they ought not to be. **[VII.28K]** For the legs are distorted either inwardly or outwardly in relation to the original inclination of the shank[56] from the actual weight of the bodies which are borne. In those whose legs are straighter than is natural, they are more splay-footed (knock-kneed – *blaisos*), and in those whose legs are more curved in, they are bandy-legged (bow-legged – *raibos*). I shall call a bending

---

[54] It is not clear whether the destruction applies to three things, smoothness, roughness and pores, or specifically to the smoothness and roughness of channels. The Kühn Latin text omits any mention of 'channels' whereas Copus translates as if these are three separate terms. Clearly the later section (VII.5) indicates that abnormal roughness or smoothness can apply to structures without channels or pores. See also Plato with regard to the tongue (*Timaeus* 65c).

[55] *Plesmone* generally indicates a filling or repletion with food – see Hippocrates, *Aphorisms* II.4.

[56] There is some variation in the use of the term *kneme*. The early meaning was the part of the leg between the knee and ankle (*Iliad* IV.147) which is also the meaning in Hippocrates (*Fractures* XV). Galen came to use the term to refer specifically to the tibia – see *De ossibus ad tirones* (II.774K), although see also *De usu partium* III.9 (I.154H) and III.13 (I.180H) where he recognizes the dual application. May (1968) in her translation of the latter retains the Greek word (pp. 174, 193).

outward 'splay-footed' ('knock-kneed') and the opposite 'bandy-legged' ('bow-legged').[57]

VII.2 And in the thorax, the parts are often deformed by nurses binding them badly from without in the initial nurture. Particularly do we see such a thing occurring all the time in young girls. For their nurses, wishing the parts around the hips and flanks to be increased so as to become much larger than those around the chest, surround them completely in a circle with bandages, strongly binding all the parts in relation to the shoulder blades and thorax, and thus often, when there is an unequal tension, either the breast shows a prominence to the front, or the opposing parts in the spine are convex.[58] Sometimes what happens is as if the back is broken in half and turned to the sides, so one shoulder blade **[VII.29K]** seems not to have grown and is small and very tucked in, whereas the other is projecting, inclined forward, and in every way bigger. All these defects of form in the thorax arise as a result of the error and ignorance of nurses not knowing how to bandage in a properly balanced way.[59] In the same way also, doctors frequently distort fractured limbs when they do not bind and set them correctly. Again, apart from errors in treatment, when the actual person who suffers the fracture attempts to use the limb before the callus[60] is made completely strong, he is the agent[61] of his own deformity. But also with parts that are crushed like the nose, or shattered[62] like the margins of joint sockets, or sometimes too when bones have been cut off, or there is abundant flesh, and then there is not an equal increase, the natural form is destroyed.

[57] There is some uncertainty about the terms *blaisos* and *raibos*, both of which mean essentially 'crooked' or 'bent'. Galen's description here appears to indicate the specific English terms as used – see also *De morborum differentiis* VII.1 (VI.856K) and also, for example, Aristotle, *Sophistical Refutations* 182a22 and *History of Animals* 526a23 and particularly Hippocrates *On Joints* LIII, LXXXII where the first term is also understood as 'knock-kneed'. See also Galen, *De usu partium* III.9.

[58] I have simply rendered *kurtos* as 'convex' here – see e.g. Hippocrates, *On Fractures* VIII. *Kyphos* is a more specific term for a curvature of the spine outward and is preserved in current usage as 'kyphosis' – see Hippocrates, *Art* XLI.

[59] See Valleriola (1548), pp. 176–8, for a description of the problems attributed to improper early treatment by nurses.

[60] *Poros* has several meanings, both medical and non-medical, the former generally indicating pathology in the form of a 'chalkstone' formed from putrefied blood (Aristotle, *History of Animals* 521a21) or a stone in the bladder (Hippocrates, *Nature of Man* XIV). The verb is, however, used to indicate union of a fracture by callus (Hippocrates, *On Fractures* XLVII) and this is the sense taken here.

[61] *Demiourgos* is taken in a general sense here, although it does have a specific medical usage (Hippocrates, *Ancient Medicine* I) and, of course, particular philosophical relevance (Plato, *Timaeus* 40c).

[62] For the use of *perithrauo* in the sense of 'breaking all around' see the pseudo-Aristotelian *Problems* 935b2. The specific issue of such breakage involving the margins of joint sockets is given detailed consideration by Galen in *De usu partium* III.17.

VII.3 There is another kind of damage of forms which is due to excessive filling or lack, as in those who are very fat or very wasted, whether in some one part or in the whole body. Thus, what are called *elephas* and consumption (*phthoe*) clearly change the shape completely. For the nose is turned up, the lips thick, **[VII.30K]** the ears obviously pointed, and those with *elephas* (*elephantiontes*) become altogether like satyrs. In those with consumption, the nose is sharp, the temples sunken, the eyes hollow and, with regard to the shoulder blades and arms, they seem like wings hanging down from the outside. In all these the natural form is destroyed because of a primary cause. On the other hand, [this occurs] *per accidens* in those who are paralysed, in those with spasms, in inflammations (*phlegmonai*) or indurations (*skirroi*), in divisions involving nerves or tendons, or in those afflicted by tough scars.[63] In all such [instances] the part becomes inclined to one side owing to a different cause at different times. Thus, in those who are paralysed on one side, there is a dragging by the functioning muscles. It is the same in unilateral spasms as a consequence of the spasms.[64] And inflammations (*phlegmonai*), indurations (*skirroi*), tough scars (*sklerai*) and all such affections (*pathemata*) draw what is adjacent towards themselves, and in this way distort the part. Moreover, in severed nerves and tendons, just as in those who are paralysed, the function of those things that are opposing by nature draws the part towards itself, **[VII.31K]** so that these various causes can all be grouped together in one way by the unequal tension which distorts the part. This is enough about the *differentia* of forms contrary to nature.

VII.4 It happens that the cavities within the parts, or their channels, are either destroyed entirely or damaged owing to the following causes: growing together, narrowing, obstruction, compression, collapse or opening up. Sometimes, when the internal surface within the cavity itself is ulcerated and then the ulcerated parts coalesce with each other, destruction of the natural conformation occurs. Sometimes, there is a growing up of flesh or some other unnatural excrescence,[65] or induration (*skirros*) exists, or inflammation (*phlegmone*), or an abscess (*apostema*) occurs in the actual bodies

---

[63] This is the distinction between 'primary' (*per se*) and 'secondary' (*per accidens*) that Galen attempts to clarify in his definition of causes in *De symptomatum differentiis* I.6.

[64] There is again the issue of whether *spasmos/spao* is to be translated by 'spasm' or 'convulsion'. It may be that here Galen is describing the phenomenon now known as Todd's paresis, a temporary paralysis of the affected limbs after a focal motor seizure. However, he could also be referring to the sustained distortion associated with a spastic limb.

[65] Jones (1931), in his translation of Hippocrates' *Humours* I (vol. 4, p. 65), renders *blastema* simply as growth. It is, however, a complex term which also refers to 'sprouts' or 'outgrowths' in botany – see Theophrastus, *History of Plants* I.1.2. In biological/medical usage it has come to mean primitive material with a particular capacity for growth.

of the organs, and then, when an unnatural swelling occupies the cavity within, narrowing occurs. Furthermore, the obstruction of viscid or thick fluids, or of certain stones[66] or clots, brings the cavities to the same condition. Likewise too, if something falling in from without were to compress strongly, the bodies surrounding it are necessarily forced into the internal cavity. [VII.32K] And even if the bodies collapse in on themselves, just as they are drawn together when affected by astringents,[67] or are contracted owing to being cooled, or are withered as a result of being dried, clearly this will constrict the channels particularly, and only then the cavities themselves. And not only are the openings of the channels constricted, but they often also become completely 'blind' in such conditions. But then too, an excessive movement of the so-called retentive capacity, drawing together and compressing the openings of the channels to an extreme degree, itself sometimes becomes the cause of the constriction, just as sometimes an excessive movement of the separative capacity becomes the cause of a rarefaction. On the other hand, often a weakness of the retentive [capacity], or some medicine, or a liquid proper for opening, or some disproportionate abundance of fluid occurring in the organs themselves, or the mixture of what surrounds us, effects a change towards moistness and excessive heat. It is these, in fact, that are the causes of the conditions involving cavities and channels. And it is apparent, as is obvious from what has already been clearly said, that those who wish these sorts of things to be the causes [VII. 33K] of the diseases in *homoiomeric* bodies are those who think these [bodies] are combined from particles and pores.[68] It has seemed to me otiose to make mention of these individually, their whole hypothesis being false.

VII.5 But let us return to the matter in hand and speak of the causes of the remaining diseases, beginning again from the class pertaining to conformation.[69] There remains in it a twofold genesis of diseases, the organs being made either rough or smooth contrary to nature. Indeed, some are made rough that were previously smooth, and some become smooth that were previously rough, the former when washed by acrid humours or medicines,

---

[66] *Poron* is thought here to be *pooroon* (Theophrastus, *On Stones* VII) in the medical sense of 'stone'.

[67] For *stupho* in relation to digestive cavities see Hippocrates, *Airs, Waters, Places* VII, where Jones, vol. 4 (1923) has 'stiffened', which does not seem quite the right term in opposition to 'loosened' in the present context.

[68] Clearly Asclepiades and the Methodists generally are the target here. As indicated earlier, I have attempted to preserve the distinction between *poros* as macroscopic channels and *poros* referring to the 'theoretical' pores of the Methodists by using 'channels' in the first case and 'pores' in the second.

[69] I have translated *diaplasis*, which has a general meaning of 'putting into shape' or 'formation' – see Alexander Aphrodisiensis, *Problems* II.72 – and a specific application to the setting of fractures – see Galen, *In Hippocratis librum de fracturis commentarii* III (XVIIIB.332K) – by the term 'conformation' throughout.

and the latter when wet by oily moisture or viscid humour. These things most obviously occur in bones, sometimes due to doctors themselves not treating properly, or sometimes being set in motion from the very nature of the fluids in the animals.[70] In the eyes and throat roughness is not from these things alone, but also occurs from acrid vapours, dust or smoke, just as, in my opinion, in the gullet, belly and intestines, from superfluities arising in the body itself **[VII.34K]** and from the quality of what is eaten and drunk in which there are also deleterious things. It is clear that each of the roughening causes, when it occurs rather strongly, brings about a certain ulceration or erosion in the fleshy parts, or caries in the bones. These, then, are the causes of the first class of diseases, that pertaining to conformation.

VIII.1 Of the second class again, that pertaining to number, if any of the [parts] which accords with nature is destroyed, then a certain cutting, burning, putrefaction or strong cooling is predisposing.[71] Now the causes of cooling have been spoken of previously.[72] There is putrefaction in some cases due to medicines whose nature it is to putrefy, or superfluities produced in the animals themselves, and in others by a failure to be dissipated by exhalation.[73] Those things that predispose to not being dissipated by exhalation have also previously been spoken of.[74] If something additional arises which is not of those things that accord with nature, it is a disease and one pertaining to the number of parts. But if what arises in addition is of a form that accords with nature, **[VII.35K]** the increased amount is a cause of useful material. If it is of a form contrary to nature, the quality of the material would also be contrary to nature. The capacity in both cases must be strong, otherwise it would neither form what is useful nor get rid of what is abnormal. It acts in the formation of foetuses whenever a sixth finger or something else of this sort is created, and in those already formed whenever it causes excessive flesh to grow in ulcerated parts, like a pterygium in the eyes. It lays down what is superfluous in *ganglia*, cysts

[70] It is not entirely clear what is meant here, whether these are natural fluids or fluids set in motion by nature, and in either case what the fluids are.
[71] It is notable, in light of the discussion of Galen's use of the causal terms *proegoumenic* and *prokatarktic*, that he uses the verb *proegeomai* here in relation to what are clearly external factors.
[72] In section III of this treatise.
[73] The verb here is *diapneio* which has a range of meanings including both intake and output of air, with application to both plants and animals, and the dispersal by exhalation or otherwise of other substances. It also involves the concept of passage through the skin. See, e.g., Aristotle, *On the Soul* 411b9 and *Parts of Animals* 671a20 and Galen, *In Hippocratis librum De alimento commentarii.* XV.377K. For some discussion of the theory of respiration through the skin see Longrigg (1993), pp. 108 ff.
[74] See chapter III.4 above.

(*melikerides*), sebaceous tumours (*steatomata*), fatty tumours (*atheromata*) and all such things.

IX.1 Furthermore, the size of the parts is increased by an increased amount of useful material or by a strong capacity, whereas it is diminished by the opposites, whenever some cutting, burning, putrefaction, or necrosis from extreme cold destroys part of some organ, so that what remains of it is mutilated.[75]

X.1 Some diseases in the class of arrangement[76] have sudden and violent predisposing movements,[77] **[VII.36K]** whereas some occur because of an excess of moisture in the joints, wetting and relaxing the ligaments, and making the whole articulation slippery owing to the viscidity. In some, when the rims around the joint socket are shattered, a ready overlapping occurs in the heads of the limb bones.[78] In some, right from the start the joint sockets are inverted, inclined forward, and altogether superficial. All these particular things, then, are causes of dislocations (*exarthremata*). In the intestinal hernias (*enteroplokele*) and the so-called omental hernias (*epiplokele*), what happens is that the channel which leads from the peritoneum to the testes is altogether dilated and sometimes disrupted, so that the omentum, or some part of the intestine, slips down into the channel itself, or into the tunica vaginalis testiculi.[79] The intestines leave their usual position and, whenever the peritoneum has been divided, they prolapse. Often also a lobe of the lung falls out in wounds of the thorax.[80] And when the cornea is eroded, the choroid membrane is slackened to an extreme degree. Also, if a lobe of the internal organs is sometimes folded[81] in violent **[VII.37K]**

---

[75] 'Mutilated' is used here (and elsewhere) in the sense of removing part of a structure – see Aristotle, *Metaphysics* 1024a13. An alternative reading might be 'docked' (as used earlier), although this would not cover the processes listed here. The Greek term *kolobos* may also mean 'stunted' or 'incomplete' (see Aristotle, *History of Animals* 487b23 and *Generation of Animals* 771a2). In Aristotle's terminology the part from which something is taken is *kolobos* and the part taken, *koloboma* – see also Galen, *De methodo medendi* X.1002K. The latter term is still in use.

[76] The normal anatomical position of structures in the body.

[77] These are presumably the violent movements spoken of previously in relation to *proegoumenic* causes.

[78] For an anatomical description of the rims of joint sockets and their function see particularly Galen, *De usu partium* I.15. With regard to 'overlapping' following fractures and its treatment see Hippocrates, *On Fractures* XV.

[79] The differentiation here refers to the contents of inguinal hernias – see particularly Celsus' detailed account (VII.18) and Spencer's (1938) notes, vol. 3, pp. 391–4, where the 'sheath-like tunic' is also considered.

[80] These two examples refer to situations in which internal structures have become external and suggest observations made by Galen during his days as doctor to the gladiators in Pergamum.

[81] For the use of the term *hypotusso* see Hippocrates, *Nature of Women* VII, and applied to the eye, Galen, *De usu partium* X.9.

falls[82] or crushings, this too would be a disease of position at the same time as being a change of form, occurring as a result of the previously mentioned [causes]. The association between adjacent parts is destroyed, either when some grow together with others in ways they should not, or when some ligament or band is slackened, strained or broken. It is clear that each of these arises from certain causes.[83]

XI.1 It is necessary still to speak of the causes of genesis of one further class of disease common to all parts, whether these be *homoiomeric* and entirely simple, or combined. I am accustomed, then, to call this whole class a dissolution of unity, or a destruction of unity, or a dissolution of continuity,[84] or however else I would hope the argument will be clear to those hearing it. For we have not received any term concerning this, established by those who have gone before,[85] just as in the case of certain forms of this, when there is dissolution of continuity in bone [they speak of] fracture or caries (*teredon*),[86] and ulcer (*helkos*) or wound (*trauma*) **[VII.38K]** in flesh. In relation to the bones of the head, in fact, there are even more terms. For what is like a fracture in other bones is termed a 'fissure' or 'burst', whereas what is due to something sharp falling on them and cutting [is termed] 'gash' or 'cleft' or 'seat'. The term of *teredon* (caries) seems to add the letter *e*,[87] for they believe it to be derived from *trema* (perforation), as if it is some kind of worm.[88] And what happens when [bones] are eroded by acrid humours falls from the beginning into another class of disease. It is called, at any rate, roughness of bone rather than *teredon* (caries). Where a greater *trema* (perforation) occurs, for example when a hole already appears, it is termed *teredon* (caries). Furthermore, crushing is of this class, occurring many times in the fleshy parts, but sometimes also in the bones of the head, especially in children. For what will be crushed

[82] *Kataptosis* may indicate simply a fall (Hippocrates, *On Joints* XLII), or a syncopal collapse (Galen, *De methodo medendi* X.837K), or even a seizure (Alexander Aphrodisiensis, *Problems* II.64).
[83] The use of *prophasis* for 'cause' is to be noted here.
[84] See *De morborum differentiis* XI.1 (VI.871K) and also p. 43 above.
[85] The point here seems to be that Galen sees his novel contribution as the gathering of these and related examples under a single class heading.
[86] I have chosen to translate *teredon* here and below as 'caries', whilst also retaining the Greek in view of the apparent etymological point to follow – see n. 88 below. Potter also retains *teredon* in his translation of Hippocrates, *Diseases II* – see Potter (1988), vol. 5, p. 233. *Teredon* is also a kind of woodworm (see Theophrastus, *History of Plants* V.4.4) and the appearance of bone affected by caries resembles the effects of such creatures elsewhere. See also the pseudo-Galenic, *Definitiones medicae* XIX.443K.
[87] For the use of letters of the alphabet to describe the surface anatomy of the skull, particularly in relation to the sutures, see Hippocrates, *On Wounds in the Head* I.
[88] It is not entirely clear what point Galen is attempting to make here. It is possibly just that the term *teredon* has an added *epsilon* in comparison with *trema* and this is of etymological significance.

must yield into itself in all ways, but must itself be soft and not absolutely hard. Consequently there will be [crushing] of the fleshy parts and of soft bones due to [**VII.39K**] some strong and hard body falling on them from without.

XI.2 Whenever, then, the external visible surface of the part so affected still preserves its continuity, yet in the depths many small divisions are engendered, the disease is called a crushing or bruising. When some cavity appears, which the blow produces in what is bruised, the state is called an 'indentation'. It is, then, necessary that everything in relation to the actual blow is forced in on itself and that what is crushed becomes hollow, otherwise it would not be indented. It is not necessary that the cavity still be preserved after the effecting agent has gone. So, for the most part, everything soft returns to its original state once the striking agent has been removed. If the bone of the head not only gives way internally, but some breakage also happens to it involving the visible surface outwardly, such a thing is already compound, and we have no ancient term established to speak about it. But it is more necessary to make this clear in the discussion than to use foreign terms to an extreme degree, many of which have been discovered by recent doctors. A dissolution of continuity is either a breakage (*regma*) [**VII.40K**] or a rupture (*spasma*), the one existing in a fleshy part and the other in a sinewy part. And the cause of the genesis of these is something sudden, an irregular or violent movement, and especially whenever the bodies precede the movements not conditioned by work, irregular, unheated and unyielding. For in such conditions many of the parts in them are torn asunder.

XI. 3 In summary, all the causes of such a class of diseases are initiated either externally or from the body itself. Those that are external are of the nature of wounding and crushing, whereas those from the body itself are excessive and disorderly movements of the animal, or certain abnormalities of the humours of a nature to produce erosion. Such are the causes of disease common to all the parts, both those that are simple and primary which are called *homoiomeric*, and those combined from these which are, in fact, called organs or organic. It is no longer difficult to discover the causes of combined diseases, combined as they are from those spoken of. So that, since each man who wishes to do so [**VII.41K**] is able to contrive this for himself, it may be time for me to put an end to this discussion here and pass on next to that about the *differentiae*[89] of symptoms.

---

[89] Here as elsewhere I have used the plural of *diaphora* as in the titles and in the Latin versions.

On the Differentiae of Symptoms

SYNOPSIS

I.1 A statement of the same aim for symptoms (i.e. complete classification) as for diseases in *De morborum differentiis*. Everything contrary to nature is either a disease, a cause of disease, or a symptom, this last including epiphenomena.

I.2 Consideration of the term 'condition' (*diathesis*), important for definitions.

I.3 Discussion of the term 'affection' (*pathos* or *pathema*) and its distinction from 'disease'.

I.4 A digression on the general issue of terminology and its relative importance.

I.5 A summary of the distinctions between 'health' (*hugieia*), 'disease' (*nosos*) and 'affection' (*pathos/pathema*) and a restatement of their definitions.

I.6 A definition of 'cause' and an enumeration of types of 'cause' resembling the Aristotelian classification, and also distinguishing between 'primary' (*per se*) and 'secondary' (*per accidens*) causes.

I.7 A definition of 'symptom' (and epiphenomenon) and the distinction from 'disease' and 'cause of disease'.

I.8 Consideration of the distinction between 'symptom' and 'affection' and their possible overlap.

II.1 A division of symptoms into: (i) conditions of the body itself; (ii) damage to functions; (iii) things that follow the former (excess of secretion or retention, abnormal noises). A division of loss of function into 'privation' and 'disorder'.

II.2 Further consideration of the differentiation between 'symptom', 'disease' and 'cause of disease'.

III.1 A statement of the basic divisions of the classification of symptoms: (i) all symptoms into 'psychical' and 'physical'; (ii) 'psychical' symptoms into 'sensory', 'motor' and 'authoritative'; (iii) 'sensory' symptoms into those of sight, hearing, smell, taste and touch; (iv) symptoms of each of the senses into loss of sensation and abnormal sensation with subdivision of the latter into 'indistinctly' and 'falsely'.

III.2 Pain and itch as additional components of symptoms of touch.

III.3 Division of motor symptoms into loss of movement (*akinesia*) and disorder of movement (*dyskinesia*) with further subdivision of the latter.

III.4 Division of symptoms of the 'authoritative' function into those of imagination, those of reason and those of memory.

IV.1 Some general deliberations on 'physical' symptoms with a basic subdivision into those of loss of function, those of reduced function, and those of abnormal function.

IV.2 Relation of 'physical' symptoms to four of the natural capacities (*dunameis*) – attractive, retentive, alterative and separative. A restatement of the division into complete loss of function, deficient function and defective function.

IV.3 Specific consideration of symptoms of the stomach as the organ of digestion – *apepsia, bradypepsia* and *dyspepsia*.

IV.4 Further consideration of gastric symptoms, particularly with respect to the retentive capacity.

IV.5 More on gastric symptoms involving the retentive capacity, including hiccup.

IV.6 Symptoms of the separative or expulsive capacity of the stomach.

IV.7 A general consideration of symptoms related to nutrition.

IV.8 The issue of whether symptoms involving loss or change of colour are due to material (i.e. a humour) flowing into a structure, or to a change in the condition of the structure itself.

IV.9 Diseases are the causes of all the described symptoms.

V.1 The differentiation of symptoms according to the sense modality of their perception, with consideration of each of the five classes: sight, hearing, taste, smell and touch.

V.2 Symptoms understood as the consequences of a *dyscrasia*, and hence of a disease.

VI.1 A division of abnormalities of things expelled from the body into those of the substance itself, those of quality, and those of quantity.

VI.2 Brief consideration of different causes and terms for abnormal expulsions.

VI.3 In the case of expulsions, the need to distinguish what is abnormal, and therefore a symptom, from what is normal and of benefit to the person.

VI.4 Concluding remarks, both on expulsions and in general.

ON THE DIFFERENTIAE OF SYMPTOMS

I.1 [VII.42K] All diseases, of whatever sort and however many there are by divisions according to kind and class, both simple and combined, and as many causes as there are of the genesis of these singly, have been written of in other treatises.¹ What remains is to go through the matter of symptoms so that the discussion of all conditions contrary to nature might be complete.² Every condition of the body which departs from that which accords with nature is, then, either a disease, a cause of disease or a symptom of disease, which some **[VII.43K]** doctors call an epiphenomenon.³ But this is not a very usual term among the Greeks, who customarily call all such things symptoms or affections (*pathema*) or affections (*pathos*).⁴ Not altogether the same thing is signified by these terms, as I shall now distinguish, going through all their relationships with each other in order in the following manner.

I.2 Now disease is spoken of as being any constitution contrary to nature by which function is harmed primarily.⁵ Clearly, for instance, if we were also to speak of any condition contrary to nature by which function is harmed, we shall be saying the same thing. For each thing that exists is in some sense in a condition, whether it be healthy, diseased or neither.⁶ The term condition is derived in some way from 'to be in a certain condition',⁷ having been brought to this usage not only by the ancient philosophers but also by other Greeks. Therefore, 'condition' is a term common to all things, whether they be healthy, diseased or neither. For among the Greeks the condition of a song, or a harmony, or an argument, or a speech, is spoken of.

I.3 Disease is the opposite of health. **[VII.44K]** What is called an affection (*pathos*) or an affection (*pathema*) differs from both, just as Plato himself also distinguished when he said that should anything at all be affected,

---

¹ Reference to the two preceding books, *De morborum differentiis* and *De causis morborum*.
² Peterson (1977) takes *logos*, here rendered as 'discussion', to refer to the four treatises on diseases and symptoms collectively, comparing this to *Ad Glauconem de medendi methodo* XI.5K. This does, however, involve reading *pason* in the text as *pathon* as in the *Ad Glauconem de medendi methodo*.
³ It is difficult to find a satisfactory English rendering of ἐπιγέννημα. This matter is discussed in the section on terminology (I.4a) above.
⁴ This is the same basic subdivision as appears also for example in *De methodo medendi* X.86, in this case without 'epiphenomenon'. Elsewhere in that treatise Galen does speak of different categories of symptoms.
⁵ Galen returns here to the definition offered in *De morborum differentiis* II.1 (VI.836–8K).
⁶ The issue of a third state, neither health nor disease, is not elaborated on here – see *Ars medica* I.307K; *Herophilus*, von Staden (1989), pp. 103–8.
⁷ Galen relates here the noun *diathesis* to the verb *diakeimai*.

some affection (*pathos*) must be spoken of. This is why, I think, he calls the changes of sense perceptions, affections (*pathemata*), whether those relating to sight from white, black, yellow and the other colours, or those relating to touch from heat, cold, dryness, moisture, hardness, softness and all such things. It is the same also with regard to each of the other sense perceptions. Moreover, he calls pleasure an affection (*pathema*) and, on the whole, any movement whatever which occurs in one thing due to another.[8] For movement is a function of what is active, whilst an affection (*pathema*) or affection (*pathos*) is of what is disposed in some way by this. For, in general, to be disposed in some way is the same as to be affected. And an affection (*pathema*) differs from a condition by movement, in that when the changing ceases, the change remaining in respect to what is affected is [now] a condition of what is affected so that an affection (*pathos*) has its genesis in the very act of being converted, changed, altered and moved, and the status of a condition through remaining and being preserved in the underlying body. [**VII.45K**] Now the Greeks call the remaining condition an affection (*pathos*), just as they also call what has acted, but is not still acting, a cause. Nevertheless, this is not simply a cause nor is the remaining condition simply an affection (*pathos*) but also, strictly speaking, an affection (*pathos*) is what has happened but is no longer happening.

I.4 That it was customary for the Greeks to name things in this way has been shown in the work on medical terms.[9] But we ought to be mindful of what we have consistently said about terms – that there be agreement with one another as quickly as possible [in order] to press on to the matters themselves, and employ ourselves with, and spend time on them. But the great majority of those who say they are learned act in contrary fashion, squandering their lives on the dispute about names, so as never to be able to reach the consummation of the craft. What, then, ought one who loves the truth to do? Point out the matters that are similar to the natures of others and owing to this are overlooked, and then put names to these, especially, if it be possible, those most customary among the Greeks. If one does not know these, one should fashion what is appropriate, [**VII.46K**] ensuring

---

[8] This is taken to be a reference to the *Timaeus*, although no exact quotation is identified. In *Timaeus* 86b4–5 there is the statement: πᾶν οὖν ὅτι πάσχων τις πάθος ὁπότερον αὐτῶν ἴσχει, νόσον προσρητέον, which is very similar to that given above by Galen and which makes the distinction between *pathos* and *nosos*, although the latter term does not appear in Galen's text. Elsewhere, in his discussion of sensation, Plato appears to use the terms *pathema* and *pathos* interchangeably (*Timaeus* 62–9). Translators generally use 'affection' for both, although 'condition' is also used for the former by Bury (1929) and 'impression' for the latter by Jowett, in Hamilton and Cairns (1961). The specific consideration of pleasure occurs in *Timaeus* 64.

[9] This is taken to be a reference to *De nominibus medicis*, not included in Kühn – see Meyerhof and Schacht (1931).

above all that there is one name for each matter, so that neither any lack of clarity occurs through an identity of names, nor sophistries exist in relation to the argument, nor that some matter is left aside. Whether the name is given rightly or wrongly, in a proper sense or otherwise, is to be considered at greater leisure when we already begin to have an understanding of the matters. What is successful lies in the knowledge of these matters, not in their names. We are, then, as I said, setting down the names customary among the Greeks, and distinguishing the matters that are closely related to each other. We allow others to name as they would wish, although we do not allow [them] to pass over any matter undefined.[10]

I.5 At any rate, in these very things that we have set out, since what happens to a body by change, alteration or becoming different in any way is other than what has already happened and remains, and since what has happened is either productive of a function that accords with nature, or damaging to it, we term what has gained its existence in the process to be a function or an affection (*pathos*), whereas we term what has done so by remaining over a certain time [VII.47K] health or disease.[11] An affection (*pathos*) is distinct from a function, as what acts is distinct from what is acted upon, and disease is distinct from health, as the one being contrary to nature and the other in accord with nature. Therefore, having stated again all the definitions of these things, let us hold to them subsequently. Health is then a condition productive of function in accord with nature. It doesn't matter, as we said, whether we speak of constitution or condition,[12] or productive of function or causative of function. Likewise also it will make no difference if we do away with 'in accord with nature'. This is made evident in the remaining discussion. In this way too disease is either a constitution of the body contrary to nature, or a cause of damage to function. Or to put it more succinctly, disease is a condition contrary to nature which impedes function. An affection (*pathos*) is a movement involving matter brought about by the agent. This movement of the agent is a function.[13]

---

[10] For Galen's attitude to definitions see also *De methodo medendi* X.459K and 772K as well as Barnes in Kudlien and Durling (1991), pp. 72–6.

[11] In this rather convoluted statement, Galen attempts to clarify terminology and add to his definition of disease. The essential difference in the two pairs of terms function/health and affection/disease is that the former in each case is in progress and the latter established, as he elaborates in the following sentence.

[12] See, for example, *De methodo medendi* X.52K.

[13] I am indebted to Vivian Nutton for his comment on these two sentences (per litt. 2002). He points out that what Galen is trying to do is '. . . to distinguish process from result, and immediate from long-term results' and that this is important '. . . if one begins to think of illness as in some way the result of *functio laesa*'. He notes also the importance of recognizing that *kinesis* 'encompasses far more than spatial movement'.

I.6 That which from its own nature contributes some part of the genesis [of something] by its occurrence is called its cause. There are a number [of causes] according to class: the material, the useful, the objective, the instrumental and that from which there is the origin of movement.[14] Each of these contributes some **[VII.48K]** joint action to what happens, whereas those which contribute nothing, yet are not separate from those that do, hold the relation of 'those not without'.[15] These things being so, it is often possible when causes succeed one another for a certain series to occur, as when many small stones are placed next to each other and someone moves the first one, this [moves] the second, and that the third, and so on in order, each [moving] the one adjacent to it. In all such things, unless one distinguishes that which is said to act *per se* from that which acts *per accidens*,[16] many very absurd errors will occur in the arguments. Moreover, *per se* signifies the same as 'primary', even if some Atticizers avoid the term, whereas *per accidens* specifies the same as 'secondary'. Therefore, the one applying a finger to the first stone moves this 'primarily', whereas [he moves] the one following it *per accidens* or 'secondarily', and in the same way then also all the others. In this way too the first stone moves the second *per se*, whilst [it moves] the third and others in turn *per accidens*. And by the same argument the second [stone] 'primarily' **[VII.49K]** moves the third, whereas 'secondarily' the fourth, fifth and so on. Should one wish to make a still more precise distinction, on the basis that precision of matters is so much more useful, each of the stones 'primarily' moves the one next to it, 'secondarily' the one next to that, 'tertiarily' the one next again and 'quaternarily' the one next to that.

I.7 These things being thus and having been defined, since a disease is some condition contrary to nature and harming function, it is possible that some other condition precedes the disease itself that is contrary to nature yet not, in fact, harmful to function by reason of itself, but through the mediate

---

[14] This enumeration of causes corresponds rather closely to the basic Aristotelian account (for example in the *Physics* II.3,7). I am grateful to Hankinson for the following comment: 'Three out of the five causes are Aristotelian, but there are two types of final cause (including that translated . . . as "objective"), no formal cause, and the non-Aristotelian instrumental cause. . . . Elsewhere Galen further explores the instrumental cause (*De causis pulsuum* IX.1–9K) but the most interesting fact about him is that he standardly has nothing to do with the formal cause (mentioned in only one passage in the genuine works, and then off-handedly – *De usu partium* III.464–5K).' This is discussed in detail in the introductory section on terminology (I.4b) above.

[15] This is taken to be a technical term. Linacre has '*sine qua non*' which might correspond to the category of 'necessary but not sufficient'. See Plato, *Phaedo* 98b and also Galen's *De causis procatarcticis* VII.84.

[16] The traditional Latin terms are retained here and elsewhere for *kath' hauto* and *kata sumbebekos* despite the objections of some (e.g. Urmson 1990, pp. 85–6). Galen makes his own meaning clear in what follows.

disease. We shall not call such a condition a disease but a cause antecedent
to a disease, and here we shall give careful consideration to those who assert
that that condition is a cause of damage to function. For not *per se* and
primarily, but *per accidens* and secondarily, shall we say function is hindered
and harmed by this, whereas primarily and by reason of itself by the actual
disease. From which also, saying that a condition of the body impeding
function is [**VII.50K**] a disease is sufficient definition for those who accept
unreservedly that it is primary and *per se*. Should there be those who lis-
ten either more carelessly or more captiously, one must also add for them
'primarily', so that the definition is thus: 'A disease is a condition of a body
primarily impeding function.' Accordingly, those conditions preceding this
are not yet diseases. And even if some other conditions were to coincide
with them like some accompanying shadows, these too we shall not call
diseases, but symptoms. And for us in the same way not everything in the
body that would be contrary to nature will be what one must immediately
call a disease, but [only] what is primarily harmful to function [is called] a
disease and what precedes this [is called] a cause of disease, but not yet a
disease. If some other condition involving the body follows the disease, this
will be termed a symptom. Furthermore, the injury of function itself is a
symptom of the animal. For anything contrary to nature which could happen to the animal is a symptom. Such is the use of terms among the Greeks.
It is possible for someone to wish to change [the terms] while the matters
remain as they were, as has been said. [**VII.51K**] For instance, someone
may not wish to call [something] immediately a symptom but an epiphenomenon (*epigennema*). For a symptom is anything contrary to nature
that might befall the animal, whereas an epiphenomenon (*epigennema*) is
not anything, but what necessarily follows diseases alone. But, as I said, we
certainly shall term every change that is still occurring, an affection (*pathos*),
and everything contrary to nature that exists in bodies, a symptom.[17]

I.8 And it will sometimes happen that the same thing is called both an
affection (*pathos*) and a symptom when the signs of each are manifest in
it according to one or other definition. For example, to tremble is to be
affected, in that both change and movement occur that are not in accord
with proper function, so a tremor is both an affection (*pathema*) and an
affection (*pathos*), in that such a movement is a change as well. But it is
also a symptom, for the movement is contrary to nature. If, in fact, it were
only a change, such as might happen in seeing, hearing, smelling, tasting

---

[17] It becomes clear with these definitions that 'after-symptom' (as in LSJ) is not a suitable rendering
for *epigennema*. I have used 'epiphenomenon' but perhaps 'disease symptom' would be better. See
section I.4a above.

and touching, it should be called an affection (*pathos*) alone and not yet a symptom. For the specific characteristic of a symptom is this: it is contrary to nature. Hence, [symptoms] exist as well in all differences **[VII.52K]** where there is a change from what accords with nature. They occur, then, when there is destruction of shapes, colours, magnitudes, functions and affections (*pathemata*) that accord with nature. And this is the most specific definition of it – a change of what accords with nature. What then? Is not a disease also a change of what accords with nature? Or is it not simply a change but a certain kind of change, simply a change being a symptom? For a disease occurs in those conditions where there is both a change of what accords with nature and damage to function, and these two are necessarily required for there to be a disease. That is, it is in the class of a condition, and there is harm to function, whereas neither of these is necessarily present in a symptom. For if it is not a condition, and if it does not harm any function, at least by its being contrary to nature alone there will be enough to differentiate it. It differs from a disease in this respect, whereas it differs from an affection (*pathema*) by virtue of the fact that an affection (*pathema*) is evidently in movement and sometimes in accord with nature, whilst a symptom is not only in movement but also in relation to some permanent condition[18] and evidently contrary to nature. An affection (*pathos*) will be a change or movement still occurring with respect to material substance, and a condition what remains, **[VII.53K]** whereas a symptom is anything that should befall the animal which is contrary to nature. Consequently, a disease will be referred to under the designation of the class 'symptom', for it is in a way itself also a symptom. Furthermore, the internal antecedent (*proegoumenic*)[19] causes of diseases which exist in the actual body of the animal are subsumed under the notion of the class 'symptom'.

II.1 Therefore, now these matters have been spoken of, it is proposed in this treatise to go over specific symptoms. There is of these also a threefold differentiation. There are those that are conditions of the body itself, those that are injuries of functions, and those that follow both these, involving excess of excretions and retentions, and noises existing in the animal itself, as well as all other perceptible *differentiae*. Now let damage and privation be heard of. For not only are disordered movement (*dyskinesia*) and disordered sensation (*dysaesthesia*) damages of functions, but also absence of movement

---

[18] 'Permanent condition' is the translation of *hexis* – see Aristotle, *Categories* 8b28–9, Lee (1997) and also section I.4a.

[19] The conclusion of the discussion of causal terminology in section I.4b was that *proegoumenic* causes were those that were antecedent and internal whilst *prokatarktic* causes were those that were antecedent and external, at least as far as Galen is concerned.

(*akinesia*) and absence of sensation (*anaesthesia*); and by the same argument, not only disordered digestion (*dyspepsia*) but also absent digestion (*apepsia*). These, then, are the classes [**VII.54K**] of symptoms in which the *differentiae* must be examined in turn.

II.2 Next it would be germane to the argument to go over each [symptom], having made mention first of what we said in [the book] on the *differentia* of diseases – that [there are] those who think that health is not a condition of the body from which we function but is the functions themselves. That teaching which we now put forward on the damage of functions in symptoms, they apply to diseases, although clearly they will differ from us in terminology alone if they do not err in the matters themselves. As has often been said, there are errors in all such teachings when some *differentia* has been omitted. If then, having gone through all these, they say they are diseases and not symptoms, they will disagree with us in name only and not in the matter. What, then, must now be spoken of are the *differentiae*, bringing the argument back to its origin, since anything that should befall the animal contrary to nature was called generically a symptom, that is [to include] both diseases and their causes that exist in the body; [**VII.55K**] for the external antecedent (*prokatarktic*) causes, at least, are not symptoms. According to another, and perhaps more appropriate concept, when diseases and their causes are taken out, all things remaining that are contrary to nature are called symptoms. This is what we now propose to speak about.

III.1 It is necessary, then, having first called to mind the threefold nature of these [symptoms], to divide them all in this way in turn, making a start from the damage of functions. This one must now divide into two primary classes because the primary *differentiae* of the functions themselves are also two in number. They are those of the soul and those of nature. And on account of this, the former are called psychical and the latter physical. In turn then, having divided the prior psychical into sensory, motor and a third, or 'authoritative'[20] (for there is no harm in naming these thus for the sake of clear teaching), we also again divide each of those spoken of into the *differentiae* within itself. Thus the sensory function of the soul has altogether five *differentiae*: [**VII.56K**] sight, smell, taste, hearing and touch, whilst the motor has one particular instrument and one mode of movement of itself (for so it was shown in the writings on the movements of muscles), although this is diversified in the various organs so as to appear

---

[20] 'Authoritative' is the translation of *hegemonikos*.

to be of many kinds.²¹ The remaining function of the soul which pertains to what directs it is divided into imagination, reason and memory. And moreover, the damages common to all the sensory functions are *anaesthesias* or *dysaesthesias* (I shall call all abnormal sensations *dysaesthesias*). [These are], of each in turn, blindness (*typhlotes*), dim-sightedness (*amblyopia*) and false vision (*parorasis*) in the eyes, and deafness (*kophotes*), hardness of hearing (*baryekoïa*) and false hearing (*parakousis*) in the ears. And it is the same with respect to the tongue, the nose and touch in that, even if no specific name has been acquired, they have what corresponds to those spoken of. For the particular senses will perceive either not at all or badly. And this 'badly' will be twofold: the one indistinctly and the other falsely.

III.2 The function pertaining to touch [VII.57K] has acquired a specific and singular symptom²² beyond the other senses – pain – which arises in the other senses from the appropriate external perceptions. In the case of touch, pain comes not only from what is external, but also far more from conditions in the body itself, and often in fact so strongly that some who are overcome by suffering may kill themselves. Thus some painful state may occur in the eyes due to bright light, or in the ears due to loud or harsh sound. What is more, with respect to tastes and smells, other such affections arise that are painful, each of the senses being painfully acted upon by specific sensations. The most severe pains happen to the sense of touch. For as much as we feel pain strongly through an inflammation (*phlegmone*) of the ears, or some other condition in these, it is not of the auditory but specifically of the tactile sense. And the same is common to all sense organs, that is, to each of the other four separately. In like manner also, severe pains often occur in the eyes when the sense of touch is distressed in them. It is similar with respect to pains involving the teeth [VII.58K] and the colon.²³ Furthermore, itching is from this class of symptoms. Do not, then, go on seeking such a specific name with respect to each part, like headache (*kephalalgia*), heartburn (*kardialgia*)²⁴ and earache (*otalgia*), for you will not find one that has been given. It is sufficient for the argument to interpret all such things by speaking of pains of the bladder, kidneys,

²¹ *De motu musculorum* (IV.367–464K) – see particularly chapter 1, pp. 367–73K.
²² These two terms (*idios* and *exairetos*) are also applied to symptoms in *De methodo medendi* X.65K – see also the introductory section on terminology (I.4c).
²³ Although both LSJ and Durling (1993) have 'limb' as the only applicable translation here both Valleriola (p. 240) and Linacre (p. 1042) identify the structure described as *kolon* as the 'thick intestine'.
²⁴ Despite the derivation *kardialgia* seems initially to have been linked with the upper gastro-intestinal tract as in Hippocrates, *Epidemics* II.2.1. Elsewhere (*Epidemics* III.17) Jones (1923) translates the Greek as 'cardialgia'. Galen himself offers a definition in *De usu partium* V.4 (I.271H) of it as '. . . being a biting of the opening of the stomach'.

spleen, knees and feet and, likewise, of other parts. So, then, of such kinds and numbers are the symptoms of the sensory functions. In addition to these, two further, singular [symptoms] exist, insomnia (*agrypnia*) and coma (*koma*), involving the primary sense itself, which is, in fact, common to all the senses.[25]

III.3 Again, the primary symptoms of the motor functions are absence of movement (*akinesia*) and disorder of movement (*dyskinesia*).[26] Of *dyskinesia*, there is diminished or weak movement, or there is abnormal movement. Of the abnormal movements, there are tremor (*tromodes*), spasm (*spasmodes*), palpitation (*palmodes*), and shaking (*klonodes*).[27] Some of the symptoms spoken of, whenever they occur in the whole body, acquire a different name, such as *emprosthotonos*, *opisthotonos* and *tetanos*.[28] If there should be not only a spasm[29] **[VII.59K]** of the whole body but a cessation of the authoritative functions, such a thing is called epilepsy, just as apoplexy is a paralysis of the whole body together with the authoritative functions. These are the damages of the motor functions. If some specific and singular name has not been acquired, like *apnoea* and *dyspnoea*, or *ischuria* and *dysuria*, or *aphonia*, *kakophonia*[30] and *dysphonia*, it ought not to be thought that people have been deceived on this account and some symptom has been left out, but that the doctor himself ought to discover all such things involving each psychical function, just as he ought also, in fact, to discover the *differentiae* relating to each of these. For example, if he were to meet with *dyspnoea*, being one of the symptoms of a psychical action, i.e. of respiration, how many *differentiae* [of this] occur *in toto* is as we showed in the work on difficulty of respiration.[31] Or, how many *differentiae* [there are] in turn of *kakophonia*, as has been distinguished in the work on the voice.[32]

---

[25] Galen in classifying sleep disorders among sensory symptoms is following Aristotle's analysis of sleep (*On Sleep* I) as Valleriola (1548), p. 245, points out.

[26] As both Greek terms remain in medical usage today they are retained. In Galen's usage, however, *dyskinesia* has a more general application as the following sentence makes clear.

[27] These abnormal movements are the subject of the Galenic treatise, *De tremore, palpitatione, convulsione et rigore* (VII.584–642K), translated into English by Sider and McVaugh (1979).

[28] Again the Greek terms have been retained although in these three instances they have suffered different fates. In brief, the first is no longer in use, the second is in common use in neurology to describe severe spasms in extension whilst the third has acquired a specific meaning in relation to the motor disturbance of a particular bacterial infection.

[29] Although *spasmos* is almost always translated as 'convulsion' there are times when 'spasm' is more appropriate. Ponze de Santa Cruz (1637) provides the following definition: *Suppono quod convulsio est contractio musculi versus suam originem praeter voluntatem, in qua definitione, constat definiri, ut symptoma, non ut morbus, siquidem dicit actione laesam.*

[30] Although not a term still in regular medical usage the Greek word has been retained.

[31] *De difficultate respirationis* (VII.753–960K).

[32] *De voce* is a work is not included in Kühn – see López Férez (1991), p. 328.

Oftentimes also someone could be confused as to what class a symptom is from, as with yawning, gaping, sneezing and coughing. [**VII.60K**] But more will be said about all such things in the discussion following this, that concerning the causes of symptoms.[33]

III.4 Next would be to go through the damages of the authoritative functions, and first those of the imagination. Of this also there is something akin to a paralysis, which is termed unconsciousness (*karos*) or catalepsy (*katalepsis*); something akin to an abnormal or defective movement, which is called delirium (*paraphrosyne*); and something akin to a deficiency or weakness, as in comas (*komata*) and lethargies (*lethargiai*). Furthermore, there is also a kind of paralysis of the rational function itself, amentia (*anoia*); a kind of deficient movement, dullness (*moria*) or dementia (*morosis*); and a kind of defective [movement], delirium (*paraphrosyne*) as it is called. Often delirium (*paraphrosyne*) exists in both at the same time, i.e. in a malfunctioning imagination and an improperly functioning reasoning. Sometimes it is in relation to one of these alone. For precisely in this way was it possible for Theophilus the physician, when ill, to converse sensibly on other things and recognize correctly those present, whereas he thought some flute-players had occupied the corner of the house in which he was lying and were playing continuously at the same time as crashing about. [**VII.61K**] And he thought he saw them, some standing on the spot, but some sitting, in this way playing unceasingly so that they neither let up during the night, nor were in the least bit silent throughout the whole day. He had cried out continuously, ordering them to be cast out of the house. And this was the form of the delirium (*paraphrosyne*) in him. And when he was restored to health completely and was free of the illness, he described in detail all the other things that had been said and done by each of those coming in and remembered the delusion (*phantasma*) concerning the flute players. In some no delusion (*phantasma*) appears. They do not reason correctly because the reasoning component of the soul is affected in them. Such was the case in the deranged person who, having closed the doors within, was holding each of the household utensils through the windows and asking those passing if they would order him to throw. He spoke the name of each of the utensils quite precisely, from which it was clear that he was neither damaged in the imagination about these things nor in the memory of their names. Why then did he wish to throw all these things from a high place and shatter them? This he was no longer able to understand, but

---

[33] *De symptomatum causis* (VII.85–272K).

by the act itself he was manifestly delirious.[34] **[VII.62K]** That symptoms occur involving the remembering component of the soul, both in those who are still ill and in those who have already recovered from the illness can be learned from Thucydides, who said that some of those saved from the plague had forgotten everything that had previously happened, so not only did they not recognize their family members, but they did not even recognize themselves.[35]

IV. 1 But since the symptoms pertaining to the authoritative component of the soul have been spoken of, it is time now to pass on to the other class of functions, which they call physical. Here too there will be symptoms relating to each of these either not occurring or occurring badly. Of this class there are, of the symptoms pertaining to appetite, loss of appetite (*anorexia*), disturbed appetite (*dysorexia*) and excessive cravings for food. In turn, in relation to digestion there are failure of digestion (*apepsia*), slow digestion (*bradypepsia*) and disturbed digestion (*dyspepsia*). Furthermore, in like manner concerning distribution, and concerning the formation of the blood either not occurring or occurring badly, there will be symptoms. And the dropsies (*hyderoi*) are also of this class of symptoms. Moreover, in relation to the function of nutrition, **[VII.63K]** the failings are certain atrophies (*atrophiai*) and wastings (*phthiseis*). Abnormal nourishings bring about the *leukai*, bald patches (*ophiaseis*), alopecias (*alopekiai*) and every such kind of symptom, however many. Stoppages and irregularities are symptoms involving the function of the pulses. Further, the symptoms which exist in relation to the separation of superfluities either not occurring altogether or occurring badly, in some instances lack a specific name, like those associated with black bile, but in others are named according to common usage, like jaundice (*icterus*).

IV.2 And here the method of discovery of all these is a knowledge of the physical (natural) capacities, which we showed in the work on these to be four in each of the parts of the body: attractive, retentive, alterative and separative.[36] In fact, there will be two symptoms in relation to each of these: one when the function occurs badly and one when it does not occur at all, so that in each physical organ there will be eight symptoms in all. If, then,

---

[34] See also *De locis affectis* VIII.226K.

[35] Thucydides' detailed account of the plague, possibly typhoid, is found in II.47–58. The particular observation recorded above is in II.49.8. There is considerable uncertainty as to what 'the plague' was. Sallares (OCD, p. 1188) writes: 'Around 30 different diseases have been suggested as the cause.'

[36] *De facultatibus naturalibus* (II.1–214K). Galen does not limit the use of the term *dunamis* to these four 'capacities' or 'faculties' which are those specifically concerned with nutrition. See *De facultatibus naturalibus* III.9 (II.177–8K), *De causis morborum* VI.5.

the number of parts of the animal is known from dissection, the number of all the symptoms will quickly be discovered from this. [**VII.64K**] For those organs that are of the physical alone will be afflicted with eight symptoms only, whereas those that are of the psychical, with these and two others in addition. It has been shown a little earlier that in relation to each of the psychical functions the form of symptom will be twofold, according to whether these do not occur at all or occur badly. And it has been said that this 'badly' is also twofold: that which is, as it were, 'deficiently', and that which one would call 'defectively'. So that again, if you say that in relation to each function or capacity there are not two symptoms but three in all, dividing into two one of the two primary symptoms, there will be twelve symptoms altogether in each of the physical organs and fifteen in the psychical [ones]. The division into two primary *differentiae* creates eight [symptoms] of the physical organs and ten of the psychical. But if on the other hand the psychical organ is by virtue of a twofold principle, both sensory and motor at the same time, there will be eighteen symptoms according to the second division, whereas there will be twelve according to the first. [**VII.65K**] Having then demonstrated what was said in the case of the first or second part,[37] what we consider ourselves to have done in all these is to make someone who wishes to enumerate the symptoms direct his attention not to names (for he will not find commonly used terms in all cases) but to focus instead on the actual nature of the matters.

IV.3 Let the stomach be the organ of digestion, drawing to itself, as we have shown, the appropriate food and separating all that is otherwise.[38] But it also retains what is drawn and changes what is retained. Thus, whenever it happens that [the stomach] either does not draw to itself at all, or does so badly, consider, as I do, that there are two symptoms involving the attractive capacity. Again, one of these, that of attracting abnormally, is divided into two, even if you cannot demonstrate this clearly with terms, since no term is established with regard to these things. At any rate, as I have attempted to explain in the argument, this particular abnormality will either be like a weakness or like a defect. 'Weakly' is scarcely, with difficulty, or over a long time. 'Defectively' is like palpitatingly (*palmodos*), tremulously (*tromodos*), spasmodically (*spasmodos*) or agitatedly (*klonodos*). [**VII.66K**] Certainly, with regard to the alterative capacity in the stomach, there is the case of

---

[37] This is taken to refer to the two possible situations – i.e. no (deficient) function and impaired (defective) function.

[38] *Allotrios* may have the meaning of what is strange or alien (e.g. Plato, *Republic* 491d), what is unsuitable for the purpose (e.g. Aristotle, *Eudemian Ethics* 1218b23), what is superfluous (e.g. Plato, *Republic* 556d) or what is abnormal (Soranus II.5, pseudo-Galen, *Introductio sive medicus* XIV.780K).

nothing occurring at all, whenever all such food as is taken in remains as it is in every quality. 'Weakly' has acquired the specific term, *bradypepsia*, just as 'defectively' is a change of the food to an unusual quality, so that all three symptoms occur with the one failed function. Digestion (*pepsis*), as this function is called, is an alteration of food to the quality appropriate for the animal. *Bradypepsia* is a change to the same quality, either over a long time or with difficulty. A change to another quality, one that is not in fact in accord with nature, they call *apepsia*. Privation of function is also spoken of in the same terms to this. But it is clearer for this to be called *apepsia* alone, the defective change, *dyspepsia*, and the weak change, *bradypepsia*.

IV.4 Certainly, as Plato said, the ancients, being ignorant of most of these matters, named some not at all and others not correctly.[39] Therefore one must not be deceived by names, but direct attention to the actual essence of the matters. [VII.67K] If we do this, then we will find in like manner also that the function of the retentive capacity accords with nature whenever the time of wrapping around[40] is equal to the time of digestion and whenever the food is compressed completely from every side. Absolute privation of function, whenever it (the capacity) does not encompass at all, occurs in the *leienteries*. Weakness, on the other hand, is whenever it does not surround properly, or not to the point of complete digestion, or both occur at the same time. Since proper functioning with regard to the peristaltic[41] capacity lies in two factors – in no empty space being left between the stomach and the food, and in the time of wrapping around being equal to the time of digestion – it will function badly, either in relation to one of these alone, or to both, and symptoms will follow: splashing (*klydon*) and inflation (*pneumatosis*) in the weak wrappings around, but rapid excretions and destruction of foods in the lower stomach in those of short duration. Here I urge you to turn your attention to this, as often one [symptom] follows another symptom. In weak wrapping around [VII.68K] splashings (*klydones*) sometimes follow, but sometimes inflations (*pneumatoseis*). Deficient digestions occur wholly through short duration, there being in this connection either swift passage of

---

[39] Linacre takes this to be a general reference to Plato's *Cratylus*. I have been unable to find anything more specific.

[40] The term 'peristalsis', which has a precise physiological meaning, is used as a translation of *peristole* but does not seem appropriate here – see Galen, *De symptomatum causis* VII.219K, *De locis affectis* VIII.440K and *De facultatibus naturalibus* II.1 (II.77K). In the last Brock (1916) translates *peristole* as 'contraction' (p. 121) although he uses 'peristalsis' elsewhere (p. 263) – see his n. 1, p. 97 and n. 2, p. 263.

[41] Here Galen uses *peristaltikos*. In *De facultatibus naturalibus* III.8 (II.168–77K) both *peristoles* and *peristaltikos* are used in the same passage as well as the verb *peristello*. It is not entirely clear what the distinction is. I have used 'wrapping around' for *peristole* and 'peristalsis' for *peristaltikos*. See VI.1 and n. 219 below.

the food out, or its destruction in the lower stomach. Moistness of excretion and deficient distribution are, then, inseparable symptoms of a rapid passage out. Foul smells of corruption are of necessity in the excretions, whereas gnawings (*dexeis*) and inflations (*pneumatoseis*) are not of necessity, but sometimes there is neither of these, sometimes one, sometimes both.

IV.5 Why it is that in these, and in those discussed previously, some follow of necessity and some not of necessity, we shall go over in detail in the work on the causes of symptoms which follows this one.[42] In the present work it is time to proceed to the remaining *differentia* of the symptoms of the retentive capacity. Whenever, then, the stomach wraps itself around the food, but with a certain palpitation (*palmos*), or some kind of spasm (*spasmos*), tremor (*tromos*) or agitation (*klonos*), such an action of wrapping around would be defective. Thus, we have a clear perception of a palpitation of the stomach, even indeed of a spasm, **[VII.69K]** for the symptom is termed 'hiccup' (*lygmos*). However, our perception of its affection (*pathema*), which is like a tremor (*tromos*), is no longer a clear one. But if you pay attention to the argument, you will realize this without difficulty. Whenever, then, neither any splashing (*klydon*) nor inflation (*pneumatosis*) troubles you after having eaten, nor is there any palpitation (*palmos*), nor hiccup (*lynx*), but there is a sense of unaccustomed discomfort involving the stomach, as if it is weighed down and distressed and desirous of passing on its burden more quickly either downwards or upwards, and to this a certain eructation is added at the same time, and possibly some difficulty of respiration which is burdensome and hard to describe follows, then consider the stomach to be enclosing the food but, as it were, tremulously. A kind of agitated movement is particularly evident in rigors (*rigos*), taking hold of all the parts of the animal. More will be said about these matters in the books following this one.[43]

IV.6 Let us now pass on to the fourth capacity of the stomach, that which is called separative and expulsive,[44] of which a kind of privation arises in certain types of intestinal obstruction. Weakness on the other hand appears continually in certain slow passages of superfluities. There is too a kind of **[VII.70K]** defective movement, whenever it has been stirred to function before digestion is complete, or when complete it slows and delays, or when it occurs along with one of the already mentioned symptoms, or is in some

---

[42] See particularly *De symptomatum causis* Book III, VII.2 (VII.268–70K).

[43] See *De symptomatum causis* Book II, and for 'shivering fits', II.7.

[44] The second term here, *prostikos* is not used again in the present treatise but see *De facultatibus naturalibus* III.3 (II.148K) where Brock (1916) uses 'propulsive' (p. 231) and *De usu partium* IV.7 (I.206H, III.281K) where May (1968) uses 'expulsive' (p. 211).

other way irregular, or when the stomach attacks the actual food violently, having an uncontrolled movement like those who run down an incline and are unable to stop. In the case of the stomach, then, as the organ of digestion, the symptoms have been spoken of.

IV.7 In the manner in which it [i.e. the stomach] needs to be nourished, and to draw the nutriment to itself, and retain it, at least until it should change it and excrete the residuum, it will acquire another equal number of symptoms, as a *homoiomeric* body. Perhaps, then, it would be as well to go over all the symptoms involving the nutritive function, those that are common to the body of the stomach and to all the other parts. In this way the discussion would become clearer to those who should meet with them, and one would teach more clearly what was said a little earlier, that a symptom is also the cause of a symptom. At all events, several symptoms precede the one symptom of atrophy, whether this occurs in the whole animal, or in some one part of it. [**VII.71K**] For whatever is going to nourish itself well needs to draw to itself the appropriate nutriment and retain it until it should assimilate the changed [nutriment], and of course also separate what is superfluous. And this superfluity itself is twofold with respect to class, for there is either what is superfluous in quantity or what is superfluous in quality, there being every necessity that the atrophic part be affected by one of the things spoken of, or by more [than one]. That is, if it draws nutriment deficiently, or not at all, or defectively, the part will atrophy. Or if what there ought to be in amount and kind irrigates it, but there is some symptom involving the retentive capacity corresponding to those mentioned for the stomach, it will also atrophy in the same way. And if, even when these capacities are functioning faultlessly, the separative capacity goes wrong, evacuating more than is appropriate, in this way the part would be made withered and atrophic. But the symptoms of the alterative capacity, like privation, which we said was called *apepsia*, clearly go straight on to cause the part to be withered. [**VII.72K**] In contrast, some kind of weakness, which we call *bradypepsia*, will, over a longer period of time, sometimes itself clearly cause a withering. With the third symptom, corresponding to *dyspepsia*, the part is not withered and atrophic, but will show a complete change in form, such as appears in the *leukai* and *elephantiases*.

IV.8 We ought here to turn our attention to [colour], and distinguish whether it is by a certain humour flowing, or by things that are themselves solid being in a certain state, that things change colour. For if it is due to a humour, the symptom is from another class, and is not a failure of the alterative capacity. If it is because the whole part is not completely as it ought to be, [the fault is] of the alterative capacity. And a complete change of the colour that accords with nature occurs in the jaundices (*ikteroi*), but this is a symptom of the separative function, unless as sometimes it is a state of the veins themselves, for under these circumstances it is of the alterative capacity. The specific lack of colour in each part, if it does not occur as a result of a certain humour flowing in from without, is like some *dyspepsia* of the alterative or digestive capacity in [the part] itself. But let us exclude [**VII.73K**] from the present discussion this atrophy which is a certain malnourishment and, returning instead to the privation of nutrition called atrophy, recollect that this itself is a symptom and sometimes follows other symptoms, whether these arise in relation to the attractive, retentive, separative or even the alterative capacity itself.

IV.9 Diseases are the causes of all these symptoms. For suppose nutriment is drawn deficiently to some part and because of this the part atrophies. Some disease necessarily precedes this deficient drawing, for it has been said that whenever the actual part draws nutriment to itself more weakly, there unquestionably is to some degree a *dyscrasia* – but a *dyscrasia* is a disease. If the part is *eucratic*, but some obstruction in the organs of distribution[45] hinders the distribution, the obstruction is a disease and the damage of distribution a symptom of this. Not only when you go over each of the symptoms, those that arise due to some damage of function, would you learn that some disease invariably precedes them, but also from the essence itself [**VII.74K**] of things, it is possible for you to draw conclusions by reasoning other than inductively. For we have established that health is the cause of function and disease is the cause of damaged function.[46] But symptoms as well, which are the topic of our present discussion, we say are damages of functions. From these premises it follows that diseases are the causes of such a class of symptoms.

V.1 We shall show a little later that diseases also precede the symptoms of the remaining two classes, having the ground of cause in relation to these, when first we have gone through the whole discussion about them, beginning again from the symptoms existing in conditions of the body. There are four primary *differentiae* of these. For, as it happens, there are those that are seen, those that are heard, those that are smelt, those that are tasted, and those that are touched.[47] Those that are seen have an origin in

---

45 There is some uncertainty about the precise process indicated by *anadosis* – see section I.4c above.
46 Galen here returns to his most simple definition from *De morborum differentiis* II.1.
47 There is some uncertainty regarding the enumeration here. In the Kühn text there are said to be four *differentiae* but five are listed, *ta akousta* (those that are heard) being added. This group is not included by either Copus or Linacre and, in fact, is treated somewhat differently by Galen at the end of section V.3.

colours which are contrary to nature, either of the whole body at once, or
of certain part or parts – of the whole [body] in the case of the jaundices
(*ikteroi*), in what is called disease of the liver and spleen, [**VII.75K**] and
in certain kinds of dropsies (*hyderoi*), whereas in one part when some
singular lack of colour⁴⁸ is often seen in the tongue alone, or in parts
that have become black or livid from abscesses (*apostemata*), and as in
pustules (*anthrakes*), *erysipelata*, *herpetes* and gangrenes (*gangrainai*), when
the colours that accord with nature change. Also of this class is *alphos*,
leuke, *elephas*, and other such [diseases]. These certainly change the colours
that accord with nature. Furthermore, it is sometimes possible to find a
coincident loss of colour⁴⁹ in many parts at the same time in many of
the diseases, particularly those involving the legs, face, or whole upper or
lower body. One must in these instances consider the *differentiae* that are
seen, whereas those that are smelt are primarily in relation to respiration
and transpiration. I term the taking in and subsequent expulsion of the
ambient air through the upper windpipe, respiration, but that in relation
to the whole body, transpiration. Accordingly, the foul unnatural smells
which arise in these are arranged in the class of symptoms, and among
these [the foul smells] in relation to the ears, nose, [**VII.76K**] axillae and
as many parts as putrefy in the course of an affection (*pathos*). Moreover,
it is possible to find this same class of symptoms in eructations, when the
eructation smells smoky, acidic, foetid or fishy, or has some other such
quality. The *differentiae* that are tasted are symptoms recognized by the
sufferer himself. In fact, sometimes they taste sweat flowing into the mouth,
or there is a change in the quality of the saliva in relation to the tongue
itself. For example, in the case of blood, in those who in some way or other
evacuate this through the mouth, some have the sensation of a pronounced
sweetness or of a certain saltiness or of bitterness. So it is too when things
are brought up from the lungs or vomited from the stomach, some are
perceived as acidic, some as salty, some as bitter, some as sweet and some
as sour. Many doctors consider it right that they themselves taste the sweat
and the discharge from the ears as well, for something is also recognized
from this. Moreover, one must number *differentiae* that are touched among
these symptoms whenever they exceed what accords with nature – for
example, skin that is hard or stretched or dry. [**VII.77K**] It is the same too

---

⁴⁸ It is not clear here whether an abnormal decoloration or pallor is indicated (see, for example, the
use of *achroia* in the pseudo-Aristotelian *Problems* 967a8–9), or an abnormal colour as is indicated
in the Latin versions by Linacre and Kühn. The subsequent remarks would certainly indicate the
latter.
⁴⁹ There seems to be no doubt that *achroia* indicates loss of colour here.

when it is moist or wrinkled or has some other such *differentia*. It is clear, then, from what has been said, that this whole class [of symptoms] arises from diseases. For we learned in the *De facultatibus naturalibus* that all the *differentiae* of solid bodies themselves, pertaining to colour, odour and taste, follow 'mixings'.⁵⁰ It is the same too with *differentiae* that are touched, and much more than all those spoken of, in that I have said these are congeners to the active qualities, as they are judged by the same sense. For softness and hardness are evaluated by touch, just as are the active qualities that are their congeners.

V.2 So that whatever among these is contrary to nature, this is in every case an 'offspring' of *dyscrasia*, just as what accords with nature is an 'offspring' of *eucrasia*. But every *dyscrasia* is a disease. Consequently such symptoms are also 'offspring' of diseases. Those that arise from the flow of a certain moisture to the parts are congeners to those symptoms spoken of, both those following obstructions or compressions, and those arising in the malfunctioning of the attractive or separative capacities. **[VII.78K]** And it is necessary that these diseases are the source, as it were, of [their own] origin. Thus, obstruction in relation to the liver, being a disease of a combined and organic body, is the cause of discoloration⁵¹ in the case of jaundice. *Dyscrasia* involving each of the parts, being itself also a disease of such bodies, hinders a different capacity of them at different times, either the attractive or the separative or some other, from which, when humours flow inconsistently and irregularly in the body, they change a different part at different times in respect to colour or odour or taste or all the *differentiae* that are touched. But inasmuch as there is a class of symptoms remaining, concerning either sounds or noises in the animal, whether in those that pass outside the body or those that are held within, this is altogether an 'offspring' of diseases, either of them directly, or through certain mediating symptoms. For the diseases involving the mouth, or throat, or trachea, or lungs and thorax bring about their symptoms in the sounds, causing certain agitated, quivering, shrill or hoarse sounds. **[VII.79K]** In certain other parts of the animal, ringing sounds (*echos*) or rumblings (*borborygmos*) or murmurings (*trusmos*) or other such things are brought about, some by a narrowing of the organs or defective movement, but others by an abundant flatulent *pneuma*. And some or all of these may be present at the same time, about which more will be said in *De symptomatum causis*.

---

⁵⁰ This is taken to be a reference to *De facultatibus naturalibus* I.2 (II.2–7K).
⁵¹ Here clearly *achroia* seems to indicate an abnormal colour rather than loss of colour.

VI.1 Things expelled from the body, or retained contrary to nature, are themselves divided into three primary *differentiae*, according to whether they depart from what accords with nature in whole substances, in qualities, or in quantities. Invariably they follow diseases, either directly from them or through other, intermediary symptoms. Thus, haemorrhage belongs to the whole class of expelled substances contrary to nature. Now this occurs when there is wounding, rupture, opening up, or erosion of a vessel. Of these, wounding, rupture and erosion are diseases specific to *homoiomeres*. Opening up is specific to an organic [part], brought about sometimes when the clasping[52] capacity **[VII.80K]** is weakened, sometimes when the separative movement is excessive, but sometimes when both have been damaged at the same time. In this way too, the menstrual flow would occur either because of the symptoms of the previously mentioned functions, or because all the blood has been made thin and serous. And this exists as a symptom, its genesis diverse. For the fault is either of the capacity which produces the blood, or of that which separates what is thin and serous, or of that which expels. And it should sometimes occur when the retentive [capacity] functions excessively, or the skin is thickened, or the kidneys constricted.

VI.2 In this way, too, the sweat is secreted excessively or retained as it ought not to be, this occurring owing to the condition of the skin, or to one of the previously mentioned capacities, or necessitated by the actual nature of the humours. And clearly, as in all such discussions, we make use of disjunctive connections.[53] For invariably in the case of each of the previously mentioned symptoms some one mode of cause exists, although this certainly does not prevent two or three or all being present at the same time. Obviously **[VII.81K]** *dysuria*, retention of urine (*ischouria*), *stranguria*, and so-called 'hydrops to the chamber pot' (which some call diabetes itself and others 'flow to the urine'),[54] are symptoms of this class.

VI.3 Furthermore, with respect to the colours and odours of expulsions that are contrary to nature, we do not still need to show that these necessarily follow diseases if, in fact, none of such things occurs apart from *dyscrasia*. It is obvious that the proposition has been clearly demonstrated. For diseases

---

[52] Here *peristaltikos* is used more generally rather than in relation to the bowel specifically – hence the different translation (see n. 41 above).

[53] The point I take Galen to be making here is that a particular symptom may have more than one cause, and although a single one of these causes can bring about the symptom, a number of the possible causes can be present at the same time. For the terms translated as 'disjunctive connection' see Galen, *De plenitudine* VII.537K and Chrysippus in SVF II.71 (line 41).

[54] The last three terms are all presumed to indicate diabetes mellitus. Nutton suggests 'pot dropsy', 'real diabetes' and 'urine diarrhoea'.

must precede every kind of symptom, as there often occurs some sequence, as it were, of symptoms following each other, the first being due to the disease itself, the second due to this (the first), the third again due to this (the second), then the fourth in turn on account of this. But here we ought to pay close attention to, and distinguish carefully, symptoms from the actions of the animal. For frequently one may seem like the other, so the symptom may be thought to be an action or the action a symptom. And if someone does not have sound judgement in this too, from those things he should be mistaken about, he would criticize the argument in a pettifogging way. For if of the expulsions that accord with nature, as they call those [VII.82K] occurring in the case of the healthy, someone proposes as an object of attention the quantity, quality or actual class of the substance, and then paying attention to this assesses the symptoms, in many instances he will be wrong. For sometimes it happens that the sweat is much more than accords with nature, or the excretion[55] of the stomach, or the urine in those who are unwell, although it is not that some function is damaged, but that this occurs along with the health and care[56] of the animal. There are some things in the whole class 'contrary to nature', like haemorrhage through the nose, vomiting, bloody excretions,[57] haemorrhoids, or some other such thing, which are nevertheless not yet contrary to nature if they occur at an appropriate time. It is clear that this is 'in an appropriate time' if what is harmful is cleared out. The accord then remains, which we agreed on at the outset, i.e. that damages of functions are symptoms, and that none of those things occurring for the purpose of benefit is of this class of symptoms. For each of these is an action of nature rather than an injury.

VI.4 But perhaps someone will subsume all such things under another class of symptoms, that of a condition contrary to nature. [VII.83K] For when some vein in whatever part of the body is altogether divided, or a hole is made in it until it pours forth what it previously retained, this is not a condition that accords with nature. And surely on this point one would not be able to show that a flux of the stomach or an abundance of urine inevitably follow conditions contrary to nature. For some say that haemorrhage and vomiting are in the overall class of things contrary to nature, whereas expulsion, whether through the stomach, bladder or uterus,

---

[55] I have rendered *diachoresis* here as 'excretion' – see Hippocrates, *Aphorisms* II.18 and V.64, the latter referring specifically to blood from the bowel.

[56] It is not clear what precisely the sense of *praenoia* is here – whether it indicates foreknowledge or something working for the benefit of the animal, as seems the more likely.

[57] Galen uses *hypochoresis* here, which may be taken as a term referring specifically to 'an evacuation of the bowels by stool' (LSJ) – see Hippocrates, *Aphorisms* IV.83 and Galen, *De alimentorum facultatibus* VI.649K.

is not in the overall class of things contrary to nature. Perhaps someone will dispute the issue of sweats, that these are not in accord with nature. Thus, even Diocles made a sustained attempt towards this.[58] This opinion seems, however, to be very hard [to accept] and contrary to what is apparent, even though it has been presented most persuasively. Concerning such things, perhaps at some time there would be the occasion for us to speak again. All in all, few things remain in dispute. Regarding the whole multitude of other symptoms enough has been shown and it is now necessary to put an end to this [**VII.84K**] book. For really when someone is practised in those things agreed upon he would proceed more easily to the judgement of what is disputed.

[58] See Galen's *Hippocratis Aphorismi et Galeni in eos commentarii* XVIIB.421K and van der Eijk (2000), vol. 1, pp. 60–1, vol. 2, pp. 58–63.

On the Causes of Symptoms *I*

SYNOPSIS

I.1 A statement of aim – to examine causes of symptoms based on previously stated classificatory divisions.

II.1 Starting with sensory functions, the eye is taken as the first example. There is a threefold division: (i) the primary organ of sensation (crystalloid); (ii) the sensory capacity passing from brain to eye via the optic nerve; (iii) other, subsidiary parts of the eye. Diseases of the eye are to be understood by applying previous classifications to these three structural components.

II.2 Predominantly about the pupil, its relationship to the sensory *pneuma* presumed to flow via the optic nerve, and variations in pupillary size dependent on this flow. The prediction of outcome in couching of cataract is also considered.

II.3 More on the pupil, together with discussion of what is presumed to be the aqueous humour and its role in protecting the eye from the adverse effects of bright light.

II.4 Mainly about diseases of the choroid, including dissolution of continuity.

II.5 Galen returns to disturbances of the aqueous humour and the symptoms produced by these.

II.6 On eye symptoms arising from disturbances elsewhere in the body.

II.7 Brief consideration of 'sympathetic' affections of vision, and also of the general correspondence of the severity of symptoms to the magnitude of disturbance.

II.8 A summary of the effects of changes in the psychic *pneuma* on vision.

II.9 Disturbances of the cornea, including penetrating injuries, and their effects on vision.

II.10 A very brief statement about disorders of the conjunctiva and the eyelids.

III.1 A short restatement of overall purpose and a reiteration of the basic distinction, made clear in the case of the eye, between the primary organ (component) effecting function, the capacity (*dunamis*), and the subsidiary parts of the particular structure, which have the role of supporting the primary organ.

III.2 A summarized account of disturbances of the ear following the same classificatory division and making explicit the correspondence of the parts of the ear with those of the eye.

IV.1 Consideration of the causes of gustatory symptoms, with a brief mention of olfaction. The recurring threefold division into loss of function, reduction of function and abnormality of function is here clearly made.

IV.2 Discussion of the disturbances causing olfactory symptoms, with mention of the close connection between olfaction and respiration.

V.1 Disturbances of touch, two aspects of which are that it is common to all perceptions, and that there is a dearth of specific terms to describe different abnormalities. *Haimodia* and numbness are specifically mentioned.

V.2 Here Galen, in discussing the passage of capacity (*dunamis*) from the *arche* to the perceiving structure, distinguishes between nerves that are hollow (i.e. have a channel) and those that are solid. He describes the different ways the passage might be hindered in the two different types of structure.

V.3 Loss of sensation due to disturbances of brain or spinal cord.

V.4 After making reference to several treatises giving details of the nerve supply to different structures, Galen speculates on the reason why sometimes both sensory and motor functions are damaged when a particular nerve is damaged, and sometimes only one or the other. Lacking an awareness of the distinction between motor and sensory nerves, he invokes variation in supply of psychic *pneuma*.

VI.1 Some introductory remarks on pleasure and pain in relation to the various senses, with reference to Plato and Hippocrates.

VI.2 On some of the causes of pain.

VI.3 Causes of pain particularly, with brief reference to pleasure, in relation to the special senses. Disruption of substance (not to be confused with division of continuity) is invoked as a mechanism, and again Plato and Hippocrates are spoken of as authorities.

VI.4 Detailed discussion of the effects of sunlight and different colours on vision, in the case of the latter both those that are harmful and those that are healing.

VI.5 Consideration of what things cause distress or bring relief in hearing, taste and smell.

VI.6 After a brief discussion of touch, particularly what brings pleasure to this sense, Galen considers two related points. The first is that the use of opposites is of fundamental importance in treatment, and the second that the magnitude of the sensation (pleasure or pain) is closely related to the rapidity of the change between what accords with nature and what is contrary to nature (or vice versa), and the magnitude of that change.

VII.1 Symptoms relating to the cardiac orifice of the stomach, including 'sympathetic' affections.

VII.2 A detailed consideration of gastric symptoms and their mechanisms.

VII.3 A general discussion about the symptoms related to appetite, five being identified in all.

VII.4 Specific consideration of excessive appetite and hunger.

VII.5 A discussion of the appetite for unusual or inappropriate foods or abnormal materials (*kitta/pica*) in pregnant women particularly, but also sometimes in men.

VII.6 A concluding section on abnormalities of appetite dealing with fluids or drinks.

VII.7 After brief mention of *kardialgia* and *boulimia*, Galen gives consideration to the two *archai* (presumably brain and heart) and 'sympathetic' affection in general.

VIII.1 On the source of capacity to the sensory structures, which Galen here terms 'the primary sensorium' and which he locates in the brain. There is also a comment on sleep in relation to the supply of capacity from the *arche*.

VIII.2 Further consideration of sleep and its role in resting and restoring the psychic structures.

VIII.3 Contrary to Aristotle, Galen locates the source of disturbances of mentation and consciousness in the head, pointing out that in practical terms, that is where therapy is directed. He comments also on the adverse effects of cooling agents in relation to these disturbances.

VIII.4 After further consideration of what he identifies as neurological disturbances, particularly of the general kind such as coma, torpor, numbness, catalepsy etc., he indicates his intention to consider 'motor' disturbances, specifically spasm, tremor, palpitation and rigor, in the next book.

ON THE CAUSES OF SYMPTOMS I

I.1 [VII.85K] Let us examine in the following books the causes of symptoms, preserving the same order in the discussion that we employed in the work on their *differentiae*. There are, then, three classes of symptoms in all. But the argument we advanced regarding this first, insofar as we said that function is damaged, we thought to understand in such a way as if some [function] is lost completely. As functions are twofold in terms of class, either physical or psychical, we began from the psychical and **[VII.86K]**

divided these into three, which we called the sensory, the motor and the authoritative. Moreover, in the sensory functions, the *differentia* of symptoms is threefold. The first is when the primary organ of sense is itself affected, the second when the sensory capacity is affected, and the third is of those [parts] created for some service to the primary organ of sensation.[1]

II.1 For example, in the eye[2] the primary organ of sensation is the crystalloid,[3] for this alone was shown to be altered by colours. Then there is the sensory capacity, which comes from the brain through the nerve passing down to it, whilst all the other parts in the eye have been created for its service. And so the animal will see either badly, or not at all, when any one of the aforementioned is damaged. The diseases of the crystalloid are then in relation to the eight *dyscrasias*, whereas those of the capacity are due to either the nerve or the brain being affected. And the classes of each of these are eight in number: those diseases that occur as in *homoiomeric* [parts] **[VII.87K]** themselves; those that occur in organic [parts]; obstructions and compressions; and those which, by a flow of humours, bring about a swelling contrary to nature. Besides all those mentioned, there is the dissolution of continuity[4] common to *homoiomeric* and organic parts, which can occur not only in the brain or in the nerve but also in the crystalloid. In this, at least, an organic disease also occurs due to an alteration or change of the proper position.[5] This change, if it is towards either the greater or lesser canthus,[6] damages nothing of note, whereas if it is upwards or downwards it makes everything seen appear double. These, then, are the

[1] This initial section makes reference to a series of classificatory divisions outlined in the *De symptomatum differentiis*: (i) a general threefold division of loss of, reduction of, or damage to, function (III.1); (ii) a basic subdivision of functions into psychical and physical (III.1); (iii) a threefold division of psychical functions as above (III.1).

[2] Galen provides a detailed account of his ideas of the structure and workings of the eye in Book X of *De usu partium* (III.759–841K). May (1968), in her translation of this work, provides informative notes on the relationship of Galen's ideas to modern concepts of eye structure (vol. 2, pp. 463–503). There is also discussion by Galen of diseases of the eye in *De locis affectis* IV (VIII.217–29K) where reference is made to the present work and to a presumably lost '. . . small book I have written, having the title *Diagnosis of Affections in the Eyes*' (VIII.228–9K). A particularly detailed account of Galen's concepts of the structure and function of the eye is given by Siegel (1970), pp. 10–126.

[3] I have throughout translated *krystalloeides* simply as 'crystalloid' and *krystalloeides hygron* as 'crystalline humour' although the latter at least is generally taken to be the crystalline lens – see Durling (1993), p. 219. See also Sarton (1927), p. 282 regarding early knowledge (or lack thereof) on the lens.

[4] Dissolution of continuity is what Galen speaks of as 'a fifth class of disease' (VI.871K) although the numbering depends on how one interprets his subdivisions. See *De morborum differentiis* XI.1.

[5] *hedras* is a somewhat unusual term here, having a wide range of meaning both general and medical. Elsewhere Galen uses it in relation to a particular type of skull injury (see *De causis morborum* XI.1). Alteration of position is the fourth subclass of diseases of morphology pertaining to organic bodies, see *De morborum differentiis* X.1.

[6] Comparatives have been used here in keeping with current terminology.

diseases of the primary organ of vision and of those things supplying the capacity to it.

II.2 There are, on the other hand, the [diseases] of the things providing some service if, in relation to the aperture of the choroid or also to what is between this and the crystalloid, so great an amount of moisture or *pneuma* exists as to obstruct the primary organ of vision with respect to the discernment of things perceived. In the same way too, the part of the cornea which is in front of the pupil **[VII.88K]** obstructs vision if, either by reason of itself or in some other way, it should depart from what accords with nature. The aperture, then, changes its nature in four ways: by being increased, decreased, distorted or ruptured. But an increase always damages vision, whether it should be from birth or happen later, whereas with a decrease, if it occurs from birth there is very sharp vision, but if it occurs subsequently there is abnormal [vision]. Neither of the others, whether occurring from birth or later, damages vision in any way worth speaking about. For we have already seen often, in small prolapses of the choroid with scarring, that the pupil is drawn aside but the person is unhindered in vision whenever, at least, the part of the cornea in front of it is faultlessly transparent. Experience certainly shows these things. The cause by which dilatation of the aperture is always harmful to keenness of vision but constriction not always, is worthy of examination.[7] It seems to me with respect to the nerve which passes down to the eye from the brain, which in fact **[VII.89K]** the followers of Herophilus term 'channel', that this alone is clearly an aperture, and is the path of the sensory *pneuma*.[8] And because of this, whenever we close one of our eyes, the pupil of the other dilates, as if the *pneuma* were going to the one alone, which previously divided to both. Certainly the determination in those with cataracts (*hypochyma*) as to whether they will see if the cataract (*hypochyma*) is couched and brought down, or not, occurs particularly through this sign.[9] In those in whom dilatation occurs to the pupil when the other of the eyes is shut, there

---

[7] Current terms applied to changes in pupillary diameter, i.e. dilatation and constriction, are used here for *eurutes* and *stegnotes* respectively, these being terms also used by Galen to describe the hypothesized abnormalities of the 'theoretical' pores of Asclepiades and the Methodists.

[8] Although Alcmaeon is traditionally credited with the discovery of the optic nerve (but on this see Lloyd (1975b)), detailed description of this and other cranial nerves awaited the work of Herophilus. For consideration of his views on the structure and function of this nerve, and some comments on who 'the followers' might be see von Staden (1989), particularly pp. 159–60 and 202–4, and also Solmsen (1961). The usage of the term *poros* and its translation as either 'pore' or 'channel' are considered in section I.4c on terminology.

[9] A detailed account of the procedure of 'couching' is given by Celsus, VII.7.14 although no mention is made there of this diagnostic test. Galen himself does, however, also speak of it in *De placitis Hippocratis et Platonis* VII.4.12–17 (V.616–17K).

is the hope that they will see after couching, whereas none of those in whom there is not dilatation ever sees, nor should they be operated on even if completely painlessly and most skilfully. From all these things, it is clear that some psychical *pneuma* flows to the eyes from the brain, both to the crystalline humour itself, and to the whole space lying in front of it which the aperture of the choroid defines. Whenever, then, the pupil becomes larger, either in its initial formation or subsequently, the whole is not properly filled by *pneuma*. [**VII.90K**] Accordingly, it is compelled to flow and is broken up and dispersed. Conversely, in the smaller pupil, the *pneuma* is gathered together, compressed and thickened. It has been shown in the [writings] on the use of the parts,[10] that a gathering together and compression brings about keenness of sensation in it, whilst a breaking up and dispersion leads to disturbed sensation.

II.3 Why then is a pupil made smaller by reason of disease, not nature, rendered much worse than one of moderate size? Is it because it follows abnormal conditions, owing to which the eye so affected necessarily sees less well, and not because of the smallness of the pupil? What, then, are these conditions? This still remains for discussion. One is of the choroid membrane itself alone. A second arises from outflow of the thin fluid (aqueous humour)[11] which is located between the crystalline humour and the choroid itself. There is also a condition of the membrane itself alone, a certain displacement and relaxation of the kind often seen in joints among outside [parts], when the ligaments are made wet by superfluous moisture. On the other hand, there is a condition which is a certain deficiency of fluids owing to which, when the internal space is emptied, the choroid falls down to it [**VII.91K**] and is contracted and wrinkled, and because of this also makes the pupil small. What happens, then, in such conditions is that one sees less well or not at all, not because of the smallness of the pupil but because of the lack of fluid. For it has been shown in the writings on vision which we prepared in the treatise on the use of the parts, and in that about the teachings of Hippocrates and Plato, that the crystalline lens always requires some barrier so that it may bear external bright light painlessly.[12] Certainly one of its barriers is this fluid, with the substance

---

[10] *De usu partium* – see particularly X.4–6 (II.69–78H) and May (1968), vol. 2, pp. 475–80.

[11] Although here Galen here uses the term 'thin fluid' (*lepte hygrotes*), this is clearly the aqueous humour. In *De usu partium* X.5 (II.71H) he writes, 'That the space between the crystalline humour and the grape-like tunic (the iris) contains a thin fluid (the aqueous humour) . . .' (translation after May (1968), vol. 2, p. 476).

[12] Copus reads this as referring to three works, the two included above plus the lost work *On Vision*, although this does not seem to accord with the grammatical structure. The relevant section in *De usu partium* is X.3 (II.62–9H) and in *De placitis Hippocratis et Platonis* V.618–20K.

of the crystalline humour also aiding to some degree. Whenever, then, this fluid becomes more deficient, the crystalline humour itself doubtless becomes more dry, as it is no longer made wet by abundant moisture, and the choroid membrane falling down on itself makes the space between it and this [the lens] narrower, so compelling the crystalline humour to be in contact through a small [space] with the brightness of the external air and suffer an affection (*pathos*) like that which occurs in those who look at the sun without blinking. Some of these, then, [**VII.92K**] are blinded, but all are damaged, so they recover vision with difficulty. For we have shown that it is not possible for the organ of vision to endure bright light without pain,[13] and that because of this also, the choroid membrane set before it is, at the same time, black and dark blue, since these particularly are the colours that relieve vision that is suffering owing to bright light. This, then, is the very reason by which the fluid around the pupil becoming less is at the same time a cause that makes the sight worse and renders the aperture of the choroid smaller. Because of this, such a disease of the eyes is very hard to cure. The other condition which, due to moistness of the choroid, makes the pupil smaller, is less troublesome than this. For it is more difficult to make moist one of the *homoiomeric* parts of the body that has been dried than to make dry one that has been made moist.

II.4 These things, then, already in some way touch on therapeutic considerations, so let us say what was put forward at the start. Smallness of the pupil contrary to nature is troublesome, although good if congenital. Dilatation that is congenital is not good, whilst that which is contrary to nature [**VII.93K**] is not itself good, although less bad than constriction. For, as one might say, the *synektic* cause[14] of its genesis is tension of the choroid membrane, just as conversely relaxation is of constriction. And since it is stretched in a twofold way when it is affected by virtue of itself, either being dried as an *homoiomeric* [part], or made moist as an organic [part], its dryness is difficult to cure but its moistness is not. For inflammations (*phlegmonai*), indurations (*skirroi*), abscesses (*apostemata*) and other such diseases are of the organic parts in the case of superfluous fluids, all of which, when they exist in the choroid, the skilled doctor should prevail over without difficulty. Sometimes a tension is also added to the choroid *per accidens*, initiated by an abundance of the underlying fluids. For when it is filled like a wineskin or bladder it is stretched and distended in all

---

[13] For a discussion of the effects of bright light on vision see *De usu partium* X and in particular X.3 (II.66–9H), where Galen provides a number of illustrative examples.

[14] This is one of the few uses of *synektikon* to qualify *aition* in these four treatises.

directions by what is accumulated between it and the crystalline lens. Since the discussion has covered not only those diseases that are of the aperture in the choroid, but also has called to mind some [diseases] of the choroid itself, and those of the thin **[VII.94K]** fluid (aqueous humour) as well, the next [thing] should be to speak of the rest of the [diseases] in these, by which vision is either impeded, or destroyed altogether. Certainly, of those existing in relation to the choroid membrane, however many actually cause damage to the eyes, there still remains one disease common to both *homoiomeric* and organic [parts], a dissolution of continuity, which in this part is either a wound (*trauma*) or an ulcer (*helkos*). Whenever, then, this is so great that it is enough to disrupt the choroid, and thin fluid is poured forth externally from the membrane, so that it now touches the cornea, in this case two abnormalities necessarily occur. On the one hand, the choroid membrane falls down onto the crystalline humour and, on the other, the *pneuma* from the brain is completely unable to get through to the pupil any longer because it flows out through the wound. That not only both of these things occurring together are injurious to vision, but also either one of them should, I think, be clear to those who have not just cursorily attended to what was previously said.

II.5 It would be appropriate for me now to pass on to the thin fluid (aqueous humour), about which this much, at least, has been said somewhat earlier – that if it is increased **[VII.95K]** or decreased, it harms vision. And that if sometimes it is made thicker in consistency or too different in colour, in this way it will bring about some symptom involving the function of vision which has not been spoken of previously. Now is the time to discuss this. If this fluid becomes thicker of itself, this will both take away precision of vision and hinder it with respect to distance, so that one does not see things at a distance, nor precisely things that are near. If it is made sufficiently thick, as occurs in those with cataracts (*hypochyma*), this will prevent vision. If the whole aperture is not shadowed over by the thickened body coming together at that spot, but some part remains without blemish, they see what is external through this, each part alone not being worse than before, but they do not see many things in the same way at one time owing to the cone of vision having become narrower than it was. If the formation of a small cataract (*hypochyma*) occurs in the centre of the pupil, while what remains in a circle is clear, to those so affected everything seems as if it has a frame. For what is in the centre is not seen and seems to be cut off.

II.6 [VII.96K] If thickened bodies which are separated and not joined with each other enter into the aforementioned fluid, this will create an appearance[15] in those so disposed as if some gnats are seen moving around externally. And often, due to the consistencies of the thickened fluids, they imagine some kind of image to appear. Such a genesis of images is very often seen after rising from sleep, particularly in children and those who have imbibed too heavily, or in some other way are made full in the head. If the fluid between the crystalloid and the choroid is changed in colour, inclining towards the more dusky, this will cause a person to see as if through cloud or smoke, whereas if it is turned to some other colour, the appearance of that will be imparted to what is seen. If it changes irregularly, either in consistency or in the colour that accords with nature, should the part of it in such a condition come to the space of the pupil, it will also provide an appearance like itself to things seen. For they seem to see its colour, consistency and form externally.

II.7 From this class [VII.97K] of symptoms are the images of those with cataracts (*hypochyma*) and of those haemorrhaging from the nose or about to vomit, written about by Hippocrates.[16] Moreover, in those in whom the vision is excellent so that not even the smallest of perceptible things escape it, when certain vapours rise up from the stomach, and particularly whenever they do not digest properly, symptoms occur like those with cataracts (*hypochyma*). For in these the crystalline humour is very pure in nature, as is the aqueous humour[17] itself, about which we shall now go into detail. The magnitude of the symptoms in these is always in proportion to the magnitude of the affection (*pathos*), not only in those things I have just finished speaking about, but also in all the things previously spoken of. For example, the *dyscrasias* of *homoiomeres* that are slight bring about little damage of function, whilst those that are greater increase correspondingly the damage to these, and those that depart very greatly from what accords with nature destroy function completely. So too with those things that have been mentioned about the quantity, consistency and colour of the watery fluid (aqueous humour)[18] which, when they depart only slightly [VII.98K] from what accords with nature, harm function slightly, whereas when they depart rather more, they increase the injury to function in proportion to

---

[15] Galen uses *phantasia* here but *phantasma* in the several subsequent examples. The translation, either as 'appearance' or 'image', is intended to convey the sense of its being illusory. For a detailed discussion of the range of meaning of the former term see Siegel (1973), pp. 150–3.

[16] I am unable to locate these observations in the Hippocratic writings. Galen himself gives a detailed description of 'sympathetic affections' of the eye in *De locis affectis* IV.4 (VIII.221–9K).

[17] Galen uses the term *hydatoeides* here (which I have translated as 'aqueous humour') rather than 'thin fluid'. Both LSJ and Durling (1993), p. 317 give this meaning for the term, citing this instance only.

[18] *Hydatodes hygrotes* is a third term which I have taken to refer to the aqueous humour. It is, of course, possible that Galen means different things by these terms, but this seems unlikely.

their own injury, and when the deviation is still greater it destroys function altogether. In like manner also, those things that have been said about ruptures of the choroid or the size of the pupil damage function either a little, or more, or destroy it altogether.

II.8 In this way too, the psychic *pneuma* is either entirely pure like a cloudless sky, or moist and turbid like a cloudy sky.[19] And in terms of the amount of substance, it is either more or less. If, then, at the same time it is much and ethereal, one not only sees things in the far distance but also makes the distinction between them with precision. If it is little but clear, one discerns what is near precisely but does not see what is distant. If it happens to be quite moist and much at the same time, one sees up to what is furthest distant but not precisely, just as if it is moist and at the same time small in amount, one sees neither precisely nor up to what is furthest. And these [observations] are enough on this matter for the present.

II.9 When the part of the cornea which is in front of the pupil [**VII.99K**] has been made thicker, more dense, or more moist, it harms vision. So too, if it is changed in colour, or if it has a significant ulcer (*helkos*), or if one of those things lying in front of it externally casts an increased shadow. Therefore, a thicker and more dense cornea brings about *amblyopia*, whereas one that is more moist and more dense, whether *homoiomerically* or organically, not only brings about these things, but also one seems to see through a mist, or fog, or some vapour, or smoke. If the fluids are not great in amount but are changed in colour, a false vision (*parorasis*)[20] involving the nature of those things occurs. It is because of this at any rate that those who are jaundiced seem to see everything as pale yellow but those who have suffered a hyphaema (*hyposphagma*) as red. A significant ulcer (*helkos*) not only harms vision by collecting excess moisture, but also by compelling the crystalloid to come into contact with the surrounding light owing to the small [space]. An ulcer (*helkos*) penetrating into the pupil also pours some of the watery fluid (aqueous humour) outwards, so in this case too there is a danger that someone so affected comes to extreme blindness. [**VII.100K**] Because of this, those with wounds to the part of the cornea which is in front of the pupil, whenever the wound penetrates inwardly, are usually blinded. It is paradoxical, however, that we do not customarily see this occurring in the case of a child who has been pierced in the pupil by a

---

[19] The contrast here is taken to be that between a cloudless and a cloudy sky, as in *Iliad* VIII.556 and XV.192, but could also be that between the ether and clouds. Hippocrates (*Prorrhetic* I.39) uses *tholeros* in relation to the *pneuma*.

[20] It is not clear whether Galen is making a distinction here between *parorasis* and *phantasma* as different types of abnormal vision, or not.

stilus. For when the watery fluid (aqueous humour) immediately flows out, not only does the pupil become smaller, but also the whole cornea appears more wrinkled, yet subsequently, when treated, [the child] sees properly, the fluid that flowed out at first having clearly regathered within a short time. But these [instances] are rare, for in the majority blindness (*typhlotes*) follows such wounds, just as in all the previously recounted causes when they are increased to the extreme. Thus, if the cornea is made excessively dense, or extremely thick, or excessively moist, it casts a shadow completely over the pupils[21] so that someone in such a condition does not see at all. Why is it surprising, then, if each of the things spoken of, when increased, takes away the sight of the animal, when also, in fact, the cornea itself being wrinkled alone sometimes gives trouble in the same way? This affection (*pathema*) occurs in those who have come to the extreme of old age. What must be considered carefully in this [**VII.101K**] is the size of the pupil. For if it becomes less, the watery fluid (aqueous humour) is also reduced in such cases, whereas if it remains equal, the affection (*pathos*) is of the cornea alone. But the present work does not now require these distinctions. The major diseases occurring in the corneal membrane completely obstruct the pupils, and particularly whenever being inflamed, or suppurating, or indurated, or suffering some other such thing, as an organic part, it suffers moist diseases. Such things, then, are the nature and number of diseases of the cornea that harm vision.

II.10 Inflammation of the conjunctiva hinders the optical function *per accidens*. In the so-called *chemoses*, and additionally in *pterygia*, it is not *per accidens*, but now also primarily that it casts a shadow over the pupil. The major inflammations of the eyelids are the same, as are any unnatural swellings on them which grow to reach such a size as to cast a shadow over the pupil. All these things, then, are causes of either not seeing at all or seeing badly.

III.1 [**VII.102K**] These [examples] are sufficient concerning the eyes. For it was more for the sake of exemplification than in order to go over everything in turn that we prepared the discussion about them. Our pursuit, now at least, is to demonstrate the method through more generic arguments by the use of which someone could discover the causes of symptoms. Since one must not only know the methods, but also be practised in them in particulars as well as diversely, which not all are prepared to do, I have

---

[21] It is not clear whether Galen is referring to the eyes generally with the use of *opsis* (as Copus assumes), or more specifically to the iris (Hippocrates, *Prorrhetic* II.19) or pupil (Rufus, *On Names* XXIII). In the following sentence *opsis* is clearly used to mean sight.

now, on this account, shown in the case of the eyes the way of practice, and what kind of implementation is appropriate. In the same way, let someone approach the other sensory capacities, considering in each its primary organ and the other things which provide a certain use to it, and let him distinguish, as has just now been said, any diseases that are of the capacity itself being affected, and any [diseases] of each of the organs through which it will come about that function is damaged.

III.2 At any rate, hardness of hearing (*baryekoïa*) or deafness (*kophotetes*) will befall an animal either due to any one of the parts in the ears, or due to the nerve which comes down from the brain, or due to the brain **[VII.103K]** being damaged in that part from which its nerve has its source. Anyway, those things involving the nerve and the brain are just like those in the eyes, whereas those in the other parts are analogous but will not bring about damage in exactly the same way. For whatever *logos* the crystalline humour has in the eye, this is, in the ears, the *logos* the internal boundary in the acoustic channel has, where it joins with the widened nerve, whilst everything that is external to the curve of this channel bears a correspondence to those things that lie in front of the crystalloid in the eye. And accordingly also, their diseases carry over here from those – [that is] those that are of the *homoiomeres* in relation to *dyscrasias* and dissolution of unity whilst, on the other hand, those that are of the channel are grouped as obstructions, either due to some unnatural swelling of the parts themselves obstructing the channel – and I speak of abscess (*apostema*), inflammation (*phlegmone*), induration (*skirros*) and swelling (*oidema*) – or due to some new growth or whole swelling entirely contrary to nature, such as often occurs in the same channel, or of some callus or fleshy excrescence growing up from those things **[VII.104K]** unnaturally obstructing the channel, of which wax is the one that customarily occurs in the ears.

IV.1 Just as, then, in these [structures], the constitution of the parts showed the causes of symptoms, so too will it show [them] in relation to the tongue and the nose, when at least we know there too both the primary sensory part and the other [parts] that go to make up the whole organ. For the tongue was shown to have two functions because it serves two capacities, sensory and purposive, and we are now considering it as sensory, although we showed the organ of sense for odours to be the actual cavities of the brain.[22] The symptoms, then, of taste perception are that flavours are not perceived at all

---

[22] See *De usu partium* IX (III.714–16K). This sentence seems somewhat out of place here considering that olfaction is dealt with in the following section. In *De usu partium* olfaction is considered in Book VIII (III.647–51K), preceding a discussion of the ethmoid bone, meninges and cerebral ventricles.

or that they are perceived defectively. And defective sensation is twofold, as was shown: faintly and, as some would say, misleadingly. 'Faintly' is analogous to *amblyopia* in vision and to hardness of hearing (*baryekoia*) in hearing.[23] 'Misleadingly' is whenever people happen to see things changed in colours, forms, [**VII.105K**] magnitudes or natures, which in hearing is called *parakousis*.[24] The diseases causative of the aforementioned symptoms involving the gustatory function and capacity are in the *homoiomeric* body of the tongue, or in the membrane around it, or in the soft nerves, or particularly in that part of the brain in relation to which these grow out. The other diseases of all the things mentioned are clear. A kind of misleading perception of flavours customarily occurs, whenever the tongue is filled with some strange fluid, or when all things would seem salty to taste, or all bitter, or seem to have some other strangeness, whether this is capable of description or otherwise. For as in the case of those with cataract (*hypochyma*), the optical capacity seems to see as external, appearances that occur in the eye, in the same way the gustatory [capacity] transfers the symptoms of the organs to those things perceived in the tongue. So in those who are jaundiced, the bitterness of the bile is assumed not to be an affection (*pathos*) of the tongue, but of those things it tastes. And in certain other conditions that are salty or acid, there is the impression that these are contained in the things eaten, [**VII.106K**] the sensation that comes from without stirring up an unwholesomeness hitherto quiescent in the tongue, although the gustatory capacity perceives not what approaches it but what is abundant in it. On some rare occasions, before something is tasted, a sensation occurs of flavours in the tongue due to a precision of taste perception. Symptoms similar to this are the illusion of a cataract (*hypochyma*) occurring in the eyes in gastric conditions,[25] sounds in the ears when there is no external noise but when the actual movement in the eardrum[26] sends the illusion, and when there are certain odours in the nose from fluids contained there.

IV.2 But since we recall that the nose serves two capacities, just as the tongue also does – for it is as if this is an objective of the olfactory and

---

[23] Amblyopia meaning dimness of vision is retained in current terminology but there is no corresponding term for hardness of hearing. For the Greek term *baryekoia* see the section on terminology (I.4d) and Hippocrates, *Aphorisms* III.17.

[24] This is a term still in use – see also *De symptomatum differentiis* VII.56K.

[25] This phenomenon is that whose description was attributed earlier to Hippocrates – see n. 16 above.

[26] *Meninx* is a general term for membrane (see Hippocrates, *Fleshes* III) which came to have specific uses, particularly in relation to the eye (Aristotle, *Generation of Animals* 781a20), the eardrum (pseudo-Aristotle, *Problems* 961a38) and the coverings of the brain where, of course, it remains in use. See particularly Galen's *De usu partium* VIII.8–9 (I.476–81H) for this last application and IV.9 (I.209–14H) for his general comments on the terminology of membranes.

respiratory organs – it would be better to go over this also, just as with those things spoken of. For if some disease occurs in it that inflicts damage on the channel, the olfactory capacity will perceive odours either worse or not at all. Thus, being severely crushed, or having a polyp or some unnatural swelling, will obstruct the path of the breath. Of this [**VII.107K**] class there is also inflammation involving its internal membrane and, certainly, also those things that obstruct one of the ethmoid bones or the meninges in contact with it, or the actual perforations of the bones, these things harming the olfactory sense.[27] Still more would this be so if it were to occur in relation to the offshoots of the brain which pass down to these parts. Certainly in the catarrhs and coryzas,[28] and generally in those cases where the anterior cavities of the brain are filled by heat, cold or moisture, not only does an obstruction of the spaces occur there, but also of the breath itself which is in the cavities. In addition, some *dyscrasia* of the surrounding brain follows. Furthermore, compressions and notable divisions of the parts of it mentioned bring about dysaesthesias and anaesthesias for odours. And some kind of misleading or defective sensation occurs here due to some local bad humour which, having been made vaporous, may make turbid the foul-smelling odours carried up towards the olfactory capacity from the neighbouring bodies. A symptom such as this [**VII.108K**] occurs in relation to this capacity, like that which is said to occur in relation to the taste [capacity] in those with jaundice.

V.1 Since enough has been said about the sense perceptions occurring in specific parts of the animal, let us now speak about what is in some way or other common in all perceptions – that which they call touch. Doubtless the symptoms of this are analogous to those in the other [senses], although it uses not specific, but common terms, like some of those spoken of. For neither in the case of gustatory, nor of the olfactory capacity do we have names like *amblyopia*, blindness (*typhlotes*) or false visions (*parorasis*) in the case of the visual [capacity], or in the case of the auditory, hardness of hearing and deafness, not to mention *parakousis, parakoe*, and *parakousma*[29] – although it doesn't matter for present purposes, at least, how someone would wish to

---

[27] For a fuller discussion of the anatomical issues here see *De usu partium* VIII.6–7 (I.461–76H) where Galen also mentions Plato's description in *Timaeus* 66e. Galen refers to the ethmoid bone both in the singular and the plural.

[28] These two terms, virtually transliterated and retaining their original meaning today, are given in their common English form.

[29] These are all terms for faulty hearing. It is not clear whether Galen takes there to be some distinction between them or not. Only the first is listed in the section on terminology (I.4d) – see also VII.56K.

use the terms. Certainly the term *haimodia*[30] refers to a remarkable symptom of the tactile capacity. But this customarily occurs in the mouth, and particularly in relation to the teeth, from acidic and sour foods. Numbness (*narke*) in the whole body, and particularly in [**VII.109K**] the limbs, which is a combination of disturbed sensation and disturbed movement, is clearly seen to occur in coolings and compressions of innervated[31] bodies, to which may also be added the numbness of those touching a marine animal. If it (i.e. numbness) happens spontaneously with no such cause being added, then an idle life or abundance of foods, either thick or viscid, or some stoppage of the customary excretions necessarily precedes it.

V.2 Therefore, the *synechic* cause, or *synektic*, or *prosechic*,[32] or however someone might wish to term it, is some such condition in the nerve as to impede the capacity being sent down to it from the *arche*. So then, it is impeded if the nerve has some channel, just as is clearly seen with respect to those in the eyes due to obstruction or compression. If it does not have [a channel], it is due to contraction, cooling or compression. So it is clear to all that if the psychic capacity has some channel like a path extending from the *arche* through the nerve, it will be impeded when this [channel] is blocked up. Furthermore, that when the nerve is compressed externally, some narrowing [**VII.110K**] of the channel follows, is not unapparent either, whereas if there is no channel, but just as the rays of the sun pass through air or water, the capacity passes from the *arche* through the actual body of the nerve in the same way, that it will be hindered in its passage when these same nerves are changed to a greater thickness also does not seem to me to require lengthy proofs for someone who recalls what happens with regard to water or air. For when vapour, smoke or cloud are present in air, and mud or slime in water, they hinder and prevent the pure beam of sunlight from being carried onwards. In the same way too, if the nerve becomes thicker and harder than normal, it will do some damage to the transit of the capacity itself. And it will, of course, be thickened in some way when it is nourished by viscid and thick humours, or contracted by severe cold. And, certainly, if there is compression by some hard body coming into contact with it externally, it will not, in the same way, provide

---

[30] This term, also left untranslated, refers to the sensation of having the teeth set on edge – see Hippocrates, *Diseases* II.16 and the pseudo-Aristotelian *Problems* 863b11 but particularly Galen's own discussion in *De locis affectis* II.6–8 (VIII.86–110K) where he associates the usage with Archigenes.

[31] The term *neurodes* was not limited in application to nerve-containing structures (e.g. Hippocrates, *Ancient Medicine* XXII, Aristotle, *History of Animals* 497a14), but this is presumably Galen's intention here.

[32] This is the second use of the term *synektic* to qualify *aition* and again refers to the state of the structures affected. It appears from Galen's remark that the three terms given are interchangeable.

an unhindered passage for the capacity. So it is, then, that with respect to such nerves as are cut off by ligatures or by hands, and such as are subject to pressure from without by some inflammation (*phlegmone*) or induration (*skirros*), **[VII.111K]** and such as are narrowed by bones displaced by dislocations (*exarthrema*) or fractures (*katagma*), a numbness first occurs, but later complete anaesthesia and immobility.

V.3 Such a disturbance[33] of these [nerves] is called *paralysis*, which is in the same class as numbness (*narke*) but differs in magnitude. And if this happens in all nerves then it immediately makes the whole body anaesthetic and immobile, or brings on a swift death due to privation of respiration. If, then, the *arche* of the spine is injured, people perceive and move in the parts in the head only, so long as they should live. But if the injury occurs to the brain, they are immediately powerless and without sensation in all parts, although each may live for such a time as they would have lived had they been strangled. Those in whom the spinal cord is affected below the outgrowth of the nerves distributed to the thorax,[34] whether some vertebra is displaced or otherwise, are immediately anaesthetic and immobile in everything below [the affected level] in major conditions, whereas in lesser conditions, they are numb. They do not, however, die because respiration is preserved **[VII.112K]** in them. Nevertheless, the sensation of the arms, in those in whom the spinal cord is affected opposite the fifth vertebra, is lost entirely along with movement. In those in whom it is affected opposite the sixth vertebra the loss is not complete, for the upper parts of the arm are preserved unaffected. And this is much more so if the spinal cord is affected opposite the seventh vertebra, whilst if opposite the eighth vertebra [the loss] is very slight. If it is after this, the arms are no longer affected at all. The voice is lost in all cases should the spinal cord be affected in the neck, which is certainly not so in all the vertebrae of the back. But this much has been distinguished with regard to each case in the writings on the voice.[35] Now I seem to have again said more than is necessary. I did not intend in this book to go through all the symptoms in turn, but to reduce them to more generic causes.

---

[33] Galen here uses the term *kakosis* which might be taken as a general term for the effects of disease. See, for example, Hippocrates, *Ancient Medicine* XVII and *Airs, Waters, Places* XIX, where translators have rendered it 'harm' (Jones) or 'mischief' (Adams) in the former and 'deterioration' (Adams, Jones) in the latter.

[34] Galen is clearly referring to the cervical enlargement although this is not, of course, the origin of the nerves to the thorax but rather the phrenic nerves (C4&5).

[35] This is, presumably, the lost work *De voce* to which Galen refers frequently in *De usu partium* – see, e.g., VI.2 (I.300H) and especially May (1968), vol. 1, p. 279, n. 2.

V.4 In general then, let me say with respect to all damaged sensation, that it is by those things with which each of the nerves is furnished, when they are strong, that they are damaged, when those same things are affected.[36] If someone is anxious to know the capacity of each nerve, those which contribute to respiration **[VII.113K]** have been described in the writings on the causes of respiration, whereas those [which contribute] to sounds have been spoken of in the treatise concerning the voice.[37] These matters, then, were investigated thoroughly by us elsewhere. The nerves which provide for the neck, and the head,[38] and the abdomen, and the arms and legs, certain others before us have written about not inadequately, and we have written about in the *De anatomicis administrationibus*.[39] This, then, is the present argument regarding the symptoms in relation to the senses. Since whatever parts move by an impulse through some nerve, these also immediately have sensation through this [nerve] so a double injury necessarily occurs in them in the case of a disease of the nerve – [that is] one of sensation and one of movement. How, then, do some parts that seem to have been paralysed with regard to the impulse of the functions of movement, have sensation? And how again do others move but not sense? There is no difficulty in relation to the tongue and the eyes, since for these there are two classes of nerves. In the limbs, however, there are only hard nerves so one must distinguish the argument as follows. If **[VII.114K]** when the skin is removed, the exposed underlying muscle seems to be immobile yet when touched displays sensation, one must suppose that the injury which has befallen it is small so it receives such a part of the psychic capacity as is sufficient for sensation, but not sufficient to move the muscle. For the sense of touch is more in being affected than in effecting so it is possible for it to be brought about by less capacity. On the other hand, the movement of muscles, which has [its] function in effecting and not in being affected (for the whole body is moved by this) requires much psychic capacity. In contrast, you would never find the occurrence of an exposed muscle that moves but is not responsive to sensation. That a muscle may move, even if the skin overlying it may have lost sensation, is not a matter for surprise. Likewise nor is it that if there are two muscles one may move and the other

---

[36] The meaning of this sentence remains somewhat obscure. Copus' (1548) version reads: '. . . that nerves which supply the force of sensation while they are healthy, by the same things they damage this [power], if they have been affected'.

[37] See n. 35, particularly the May (1968) reference.

[38] A further conjunction is supplied after *kephalen*.

[39] II.215–731K. There are several recent editions/translations of this important work, notably by Simon (1906), Duckworth (1949), Singer (1956) and Garofalo (1986). The section on spinal cord damage is of particular relevance to the present discussion (VIII. 3–9, II.661–98K).

be immobile, or one be responsive to sensation but the other not. For it is possible in those cases for the nerve of the one to be injured but that of the other to be uninjured in the same way as it is possible for the nerve distributed to the skin to be injured, but that to the muscle uninjured. On the other hand, [**VII.115K**] the nerve of the skin may be uninjured but that of the muscle not uninjured. This, then, is sufficient about the symptoms set out.

VI.1 Pleasure and pain are inherent in all the senses, although clearly not to an equal degree, being least in that of vision, and most in that of touch and that of taste, whilst next to these in smell, and after these in hearing. What, then, is the common cause of all and what is specific to each? Common is what Plato also says in the *Timaeus*, writing thus: 'An affection (*pathos*) contrary to nature occurring in us violently and intensely is pain; the return to the natural state on the other hand, when it is intense, is pleasure. What is slow and slight is not perceived.' Thus, Plato. Hippocrates, who was still more ancient, said that in those who, with respect to the natural state, are changed and corrupted, pains occur. It is their being corrupted that indicates the swiftness and, at the same time, the magnitude of the change.[40]

VI.2 And with respect to touch, there are major changes of nature from the violent visitation of cold and heat, [**VII.116K**] and such things as are disposed to crush, cut, stretch or erode. For moistness and dryness without heating or cooling are non-violent in their association, as it is possible for you to learn by perusing the work on simple remedies where cold was shown to be pleasant in a way different from heat, but also to be itself painful by disrupting substance.[41] And it seems too that crushing and stretching, which carry the danger of rupture, are causes of pain to bodies, just as, in fact, both piercing and cutting are. For it is not the sequel to cutting or rupture that inflicts pain, but all such causes of pains exist in the occurring, unless pain should follow *per accidens* in those so affected, when sometimes acrid fluids sting an ulcerated body, or when sometimes inflammation (*phlegmone*) supervenes, which itself also causes pain by stretching continuously, or often too through the heat or acridness of the fluids.

---

[40] The *Timaeus* reference is 64d – see Taylor's (1928) detailed note on this (pp. 446–62). I am unable to find the exact quotation in Hippocrates but see *De placitis Hippocratis et Platonis* VII.6.32–6 and De Lacy's (1978) note, vol. 3, p. 681.

[41] This is presumably a reference to *De simplicium medicamentorum temperamentis et facultatibus* XI.753–4K.

VI.3 And the organ of taste, insofar as it shares in touch, is disrupted by the things spoken of, whereas insofar as it is specific for taste, [**VII.117K**] by sharp, bitter, harsh and pungent things, in that each of these, as has been shown, divides continuity. And the flowing vapours of the humours spoken of are distressing to olfaction because they also disrupt continuity. In hearing, there are harsh, loud and very rapid sounds, and when these come together as one in the most fearful thunders, some become completely maimed in the auditory sense through disruption of its organ by the violence of the sound. And, of course, the extreme brightness of sunlight may at once distress and destroy vision by causing separation to the greatest extent. There is also, obviously, the separation from the class of divisions, and the distressing affection (*pathos*) appears to be common among all the senses, brought about by the separation and division of a continuous and unified body, whenever this happens overwhelmingly. I shall call 'overwhelmingly' what is at the same time great and sudden. This, I imagine, is also what Plato meant when he said that disturbed sensation is brought about from a violent and at the same time overwhelming affection (*pathema*) coming upon perceiving bodies.[42] For it will make no difference whether one speaks of a distressed, [**VII.118K**] vexed, pained, disturbed or burdened perception, just as with respect to the affection (*pathema*) itself, [whether one speaks of] distress, vexation, pain, suffering or grief. And it is clear that Plato himself uses all the terms spoken of with equal weight in this matter in the *Timaeus* and the *Philebus* and if there should be any other work by him where there is discussion about these matters. And that the teaching of Hippocrates also held to the same notion in names and matters is clear from what was said a little earlier and from what is written in all his books.[43] In the same way, an altogether distressing affection (*pathos*) occurs in all the senses, whereas the converse of this, pleasure, is due to the opposite cause. For a complete return to an accord with nature of what was in danger of being sundered brings about pleasure.

VI.4 Because of this, dark blue is the most pleasing sight to the eyes, just as what is at once bright and white is the most distressing, like the sun. Next to these in what is distressing is white, whilst in what is pleasant is grey. The former [acts] through a simultaneous separation and [**VII.119K**] dissolution

---

[42] This does not appear to be a direct quotation from Plato but rather a general reference to his theory of sensation and of pain and pleasure as outlined in the two works Galen subsequently mentions, *Philebus* and *Timaeus*. Taylor's (1928) discussion, referred to in n. 40 above, is helpful here.

[43] This seems to be a general reference to Hippocrates. As with the Plato reference in the previous note, I am unable to find this statement in Hippocrates.

of its substance, the latter through an unforced gathering together. Actually to gather together is not, in fact, enough and sufficient by itself. For if this were so, one presumes black also would be pleasant, whereas now it is not, for being opposite to the substance of vision it draws it together more violently than [allows it to] return to its nature. Extreme blackness is less distressing than extreme brightness, not because the opposite distresses less than excess with respect to its congener (for on that basis black would be more distressing than extreme brightness), but because the organ of vision is of the nature of light, every ray a very fine substance, whereas black is always thick. Invariably in Nature what is composed of fine particles is more efficacious than what is composed of thick particles. Whenever, then, with respect to the same thing, the fine-particled and the thick-particled come upon one another, the thick acts less on the fine inasmuch as it is more disposed to be affected by it. In this way also, the sun distresses vision, in that being more fine-particled it readily separates it. Therefore, through the relationship of substance, the distress is less than with opposites, whereas in the strength of action it is more violent, and in this lies the swiftness of the damage to vision. [VII.120K] For our vision is affected in the shortest time in the presence of sunlight yet, on the other hand, in the greatest time when it sees no light at all but passes the time in profound darkness. In fact, when it is brought back to the light it is not able to see, because it is in some way quenched, thickened and made dark. Naturally, then, the colour most pleasant and beneficial to vision is dark blue, except when it (vision) has been dispersed by the sun. For to that, as it would already be diseased, the opposite is the remedy. On the other hand, to what is healthy but fatigued, deep blue or grey is the healthiest sight, neither separating it as do white and brightness, nor gathering it together and quenching it, as does black. Grey, then, arises when there is a simultaneous mixing of white and black, whereas dark blue arises when white and brightness come together and are incident on deep black. And this is just as Plato taught us regarding both. So these intermediate and moderate colours arise from the mixing of opposites and extremes, escaping each extreme in relation to which vision is damaged, and correct its moderate [VII.121K] fatigues, just as black does in the diseases due to separation. The manifestation of pleasure from these things is not like that in relation to the other senses in that there is not the equality of pain. For the fineness of vision is something that is not affected strongly, either by separation, owing to the relationship of substance (for it hastens beforehand to where it is led, of its own accord), or by compounding, owing to the weakness of the change. For it was shown that what is fine is weakly gathered together by what is thick. This is how it is with pleasure and pain in relation to vision.[44]

VI.5 In the case of hearing, the most pleasant sound is the smoothest and slowest, for which reason also the roughest and quickest is most painful. But these are the pleasures and pains of an entirely healthy sense. When it is fatigued, smallness is also agreeable, in addition to smoothness and slowness, whilst when it is diseased, [it is] extreme smoothness, slowness and smallness, and even more than this, rhythm. For complete silence is somewhat analogous to darkness with respect to vision, from which the question also arises, whether darkness is the opposite to light or its privation, just like [**VII.122K**] silence in the case of sound, or rest in the case of movement. There is here a greater manifestation of pleasure because there is also a greater thickness of substance. There is a still greater manifestation of pleasure in the sense of smell in that the substance is also thicker. For to the extent that air is thicker than sunlight, so vapour is thicker than air. The sensation of sight is one of sunlight; that of hearing is one of air; that of smell is one of vapour just as that of taste is one of a moist nature, and that of touch is one of a solid body. Since the sensation of smell is cognate with that of taste, differing in one aspect alone, which is the greater fineness of its substance (for vapour is moisture made fine), both will be spoken of together, starting with taste for the sake of clarity. Accordingly, the juices most pleasant to this [sense] are naturally all those that are sweet and oily, for all these were shown to be most related to the substance of the body, whilst to a sense that has been recently afflicted by one of the things that distress it, it is the oily [juices that are most pleasant] for these particularly make smooth what has been roughened. To a sense that is diseased it is the [juices] opposite to the diseases; the fine to those that are thick, the thick to those that are fine, those that cut to those that are viscid, [**VII.123K**] those that make smooth to those that make rough and, in like manner, the cold to those that are hot, the hot to those that are cold, the moist to those that are dry, and the dry to those that moist. There has been discussion about these things in the fourth [book] on the capacity of simple remedies, a discussion that should be read through carefully there, being of benefit to both diagnosis and treatment.[45] For the stomach performs a service to the internal parts and to the veins, so that those kinds of fluids these might lack are such as it strives for. Moreover, as a judge of this, the tongue puts itself

---

[44] For detailed descriptions of theories of vision both prior to Galen and Galen's own see Beare (1906), pp. 9–92 and Siegel (1970), pp. 10–126. The reference to Plato is to the *Timaeus* 68c.

[45] *De simplicium medicamentorum temperamentis et facultatibus* IV (XI.619–703K) – see particularly p. 651 but also p. 648 and Book III, p. 584.

forward, delighting particularly in those of the fluids which the stomach might lack. The cause of the association is principally the tunic surrounding it. Thus the tongue at different times delights in one or other of the fluids coming into contact with it externally. It also, then, delights sometimes perceiving sweet [fluids] in itself (this sweet fluid is a form of phlegm), so that as many times at least as when blood pours in from the veins, the tongue takes a sensation as of sweetness, it being affected in a way corresponding to that with things falling upon it externally. Certainly, in the case of the capacity of smell, the perception from without of pleasing [**VII.124K**] or distressing things has a correspondence to taste. Of the vapours that are unpleasant to it, as has been said earlier, it sometimes has a perception. It altogether does not perceive things that are sweet or pleasant, just as neither vision nor hearing do. This is because, in respect to senses that are fine-particled in substance, they do not suffer any strong affection (*pathos*) in themselves. Touch and taste themselves [suffer] nothing strong, although sometimes they do suffer such an affection (*pathos*) indistinctly, as of course the tongue [does], as has been said, in the presence of sweet phlegm, which Praxagoras and Philotimus term more specifically a sweet humour.[46]

VI.6 Touch in itself is often sensible of movement whenever it returns to an accord with nature, at least when those things that made it rough internally have been digested, transpired, or perceptibly expelled. Furthermore, those who are wearied, whenever they are softened by gently rubbing or bathing the body and after this rest, are manifestly sensible of the pleasure. Still more do they experience pleasure in the actual movements spoken of through the fatigued parts returning to an accord with nature. Not only by bathing and gently rubbing with abundant oil [**VII.125K**] do pleasures occur in the fatigued parts but also, in the more severe pains, a soft touch, gentle and smooth, brings a certain not inconsiderable relief. Now such things are external, and one must speak about them all in order. For there is nothing we still need to cover regarding smells, these being analogous to the tastes. Thus we experience pleasure in this class of sensation, to put it simply, when we return to what accords with nature. And this invariably happens to us due to opposites – if, that is to say, someone were to take the opposite, as is fitting. It is appropriate presumably to consider in all such cases what is primary and *per se*, and not through another intermediary, the cause of the final result, not what is called *prokatarchontic* or *prokatarktic*,[47] which Hippocrates saw fit to remind us of many times in other places and

---

[46] See Steckerl (1958), pp. 59–60, fragment 22.
[47] Here the causal term *prokatarktic* and its variant clearly apply to external factors.

in saying: 'It is sometimes the case in *tetanos* without a wound (*helkos*), in a well-conditioned young man during the middle of summer, that a pouring on of copious cold brings about a restoration of heat, and heat relieves these things.'[48] For someone at least might seem more unreflective about such things when declaring that sometimes some of those things contrary to nature are to be treated by similar things, [**VII.126K**] as with reference to the treatment of *tetanos* by cold baths.[49] This is simply not true, but rather all things always return towards an accord with nature owing to opposites, just as *tetanos* does too, as the result of a recall of heat. If, then, this occurs suddenly, the treatment is accomplished with pleasure, whereas if it occurs gradually, the return to an accord with nature will be unperceived. In this way also, the path from what accords with nature to what is contrary to nature, when it occurs suddenly, is altogether violent and painful, but when gradual is not perceived. And because of this, when a condition not in accord with nature is built up gradually in the body, it is absolutely unperceived, yet the return to what accords with nature, whenever this is brought about suddenly, occurs with an awareness and, at the same time, is also pleasant. And this is particularly so in the case of things most familiar to us, like sweet things in taste, and in smell, things that have a correspondence to these and are called fragrant. And the sensation of the generative parts is affected in a specific and remarkable way in that it has also a very strong capacity, the separative [capacity] of the sperm in the male class, [**VII. 127K**] whilst in the female there is not only that which is in the testes and spermatic vessels, but also the attractive [capacity] in the whole uterus.[50] For Nature has joined powerful desire and pleasure at the same time to the emission and the gathering of the sperm. But the distress, when superfluous sperm remains within, is built up gradually over a long time, and because of this, the great distress (which we shall speak about elsewhere)[51] falls short in magnitude of the pleasure which is present in sexual intercourse. When the separation of what is distressing occurs

---

[48] Hippocrates, *Aphorisms* V.21.

[49] The translation of this sentence, at least the final phrase, is something of a paraphrase. I take Galen to be saying that some people take the opposite view to Hippocrates in his treatment of *tetanos* with cold baths, recommending rather warm baths as, for example, Asclepiades – see Caelius Aurelianus, *Acute Diseases* III.89. The point is, then, whether similars rather than opposites cure opposites.

[50] For a good summary of Galen's concept of reproduction see May (1968), vol. 1, pp. 56–60. The details are set out in Books XIV and XV of *De usu partium*. The role of the attractive capacity of the uterus is to draw semen into it – see May (1968), vol. 1, p. 49 and *De facultatibus naturalibus* III.15.

[51] I am unable to find any other reference to this 'great distress' in Galen's works in the TLG. There is, however, an interesting and somewhat personal account of the adverse effects of retention of sperm in *De locis affectis* (VIII,450–1K). Distress is not mentioned there as a symptom.

suddenly there is a correspondence in swiftness between the return to an accord with nature and the magnitude of the pleasure.

VII.1 What should remain is to go through the symptoms pertaining to the opening of the stomach, which in fact they call the cardia.[52] For these are also from the class of things to do with touch, but no part has so precise a sense, nor causes a sympathetic affection of each of the two *archai* in itself,[53] as the opening of the stomach does. It is customarily called the stomach not only by the majority, but also by doctors. At any rate, what are called **[VII.128K]** gastric syncopes[54] are symptoms of this part, just as are also the heartburns (*kardialgia*) named on the basis of its other designation.[55] What is more, it brings on *dyspnoeas*, *apnoeas*, chokings (*pnix*), epilepsies, deliriums (*parakope*) and melancholies. All these, then, pertain to 'sympathetic affection',[56] whereas losses, diminutions and abnormal appetites pertain to the stomach itself. I shall call *anorexia* whenever there is no appetite at all and *dysorexia* when it is weak, whilst the abnormal appetites are either those where there is a turning aside to an excessive intake of food and drink, or those where the turning aside is to the desire for unusual qualities. One must then speak about all these in order, starting from its [i.e. the stomach's] specific symptoms.

VII.2 These follow the functions of the part in accord with nature, owing to which it also stands in need of the largest nerves from the brain, by which this extraordinary form of sensation over all things is acquired.[57] For when each animal transpires to the surrounding air through the skin, what primarily happens is an emptying of the parts underlying it, of which

---

[52] The description of the anatomy of the stomach and related structures given in *De anatomicis administrationibus* VI.2 (II.561–9K) makes no mention of 'cardia'. In that work, Galen states that his full account of the anatomy of the stomach is in *De usu partium*. This is, in fact, in Books IV and V. In these descriptions, the term *cardia* is also not used (e.g. I.201–3H). May (1968), in her translation, does provide 'cardiac' in parentheses as a qualifying term for the upper opening of the stomach – see vol. 1, pp. 208–9.

[53] It seems clear from what follows, particularly VII.6, that Galen is referring to the brain and the heart in speaking of the two *archai*. I have left the term untranslated throughout these sections.

[54] On this, Siegel (1970) writes: 'Galen described *syncope* (collapse) as an indirect (sympathetic) effect of gastric disease on the heart, since he believed that irritation of the cardia of the stomach travelled through both humors and connecting vagal fibres to the heart, especially to the left ventricle. This sympathetic irritation seemed frequently to induce fainting and collapse by suppressing the production of the vital heat in the left chamber of the heart.' He makes reference to *De usu partium* VI.18 (I.364–5H).

[55] The term *kardialgia*.

[56] For a detailed consideration of the concept of 'sympathy' and Galen's views on this see Siegel (1968), pp. 360–82.

[57] See particularly *De usu partium* IX.11 (II.30–5H) for Galen's account of the vagus and related nerves and their distribution to the stomach.

the innate capacity, [**VII.129K**] as we showed in the writings on the physical capacities, draws nutriment from what is adjacent to them to fill up what has been emptied.[58] In turn, these parts draw from those adjacent to them, and then the third [lot of parts] from those adjacent to them, and in the same way always continuously like a rapid succession occurring as in a dance, the evacuation comes to the veins passing down to the stomach. These, at least, are at the same time accustomed and naturally disposed to draw the nutriment from the stomach, being analogous to the roots which pass down into the earth in the case of plants. For this whole action is not psychical but physical, and is accomplished alike in both plants and animals. In plants, then, the earth serves in the manner of the stomach, continually 'irrigating'[59] a readily available and bounteous nutriment so long as the seasons should be in accord with nature from Zeus. That is to say, sometimes owing to the excess of droughts, the moisture from it [the earth] is dried up and the plants wither through lack of nutriment.

VII.3 For animals, inasmuch as they are not made to grow by the earth, apart admittedly from a few instances, Nature has fashioned the stomach as a storehouse of nutriment, like the earth for plants. [**VII.130K**] And it has given a perception of lack so that animals are stimulated to fill themselves with food and drink at one time. And the desire for such filling is called appetite, but it arises from the perception of lack whenever the veins draw from the stomach itself, as if to milk or suck, although the stomach does not bear the sucking, but is, as it were, 'distracted',[60] providing itself with food as a remedy for this distress. In this way, the veins turn to the foods at hand and draw nourishment from them, not from the stomach. And after the taking of food[61] what happens is that, at the same time, the veins turn themselves to the food and the stomach draws to itself from them as much as had previously been emptied by the veins. Hunger, then, is the perception of the sucking, whereas with regard to the other two, one leads in the milking of the veins, and this is also called appetite, having the same name as the other and is a physical action, not a psychical one. An emptying precedes such an appetite so there are altogether five symptoms arranged

---

[58] I take this to be a general reference to the important section III.13 of *De facultatibus naturalibus* (II.186–204K).

[59] The verb *epardo* is used in both plant and animal biology. Galen also uses it in relation to the nutrition of plants in *De semine* IV.625K.

[60] It is not clear exactly what process is envisaged here. The three Latin versions (Copus, Linacre, Kühn) use *divello*.

[61] I have used the specific meaning of 'taking in food' given for *prosphora* in LSJ, although in the use referred to there in Aristotle's *Metaphysics* (1000a14) translators such as Tredennick (1933) and Ross in Barnes (1984) use 'application'.

in order following one another. First there is the emptying; second is the physical appetite [**VII.131K**] of the emptied parts; next is the sucking of the stomach; next is the sensation of this; last of all there is the psychical appetite of this.

VII.4 And what is more, the destruction of this function happens either through the destruction of the sensation of milking, or through the milking not occurring, or through the body not being emptied. In the same way, weaknesses of appetite follow not from the destruction of those things we spoke of, but their coming near to destruction. Abnormal appetites are excesses in terms of amount, and such are called by some 'ravenous',[62] whenever either some acidic bad humour gnaws at the stomach, or also the whole body is excessively dissipated and stands in continuous need of nourishment. For a cold bad humour produces a gnawing in proportion to the sucking, whilst it arouses an appetite through a resemblance to the physical affection (*pathema*), creating a desire for food not drink, due to the cold.[63] Yet when acidic bilious bad humours gnaw at the stomach there is a desire for drink more than food. For besides heating and drying the stomach, which are causes of thirst, there also occurs in addition the flow of humours [**VII.132K**] into it and the veins. The symptom of the flow of humours may fill the containing parts just as, I think, those of cold may empty them. Moreover, cold of the parts in the stomach contributes not a little to hunger, for it makes the bodies and their coverings empty and, bringing and pressing them together, stirs them towards appetite. Especially in these, heat is a *synektic* cause[64] of not being hungry inasmuch as it loosens solid bodies by relaxing them and makes them weaker in terms of attraction, whilst moist bodies are stretched still more by dissolving. One cause, then, of a ravenous appetite is an acidic bad humour, whilst a second, as was said, is a greater emptying throughout the body, whether brought about by the strength of the heating or by the weakness of the retentive capacity. Furthermore, what happens in the first condition is that there are many evacuations of what has been taken in, whilst in the second, as it would be brought about by the emptying of the system, distributes the nutriment. Thus excessive appetites and at the same time hungers occur due to these things.

---

[62] For *kunodes* or 'dog-like' see Aristotle, *Generation of Animals* 746a35.

[63] The creation of a strong appetite by cold is considered in the pseudo-Aristotelian *Problems* 887b35 ff.

[64] Here the heat is that within the structure, i.e. it is one of the basic elements or qualities and in no sense is external.

VII.5 Those in whom some abnormal superfluity is deposited in the coverings of the stomach desire abnormal qualities. **[VII.133K]** This customarily occurs especially in women affected by bad humours, whenever they are pregnant, and the state is called *kitta* (*pica*).[65] In this they desire particularly things that are acidic and harsh, although also sometimes things that are pungent, sometimes Cimolean earth,[66] or pieces of pot, or quenched coals, or certain foods extraordinary in this way. And the majority of them suffer this up to the second or third month, whereas in the fourth month they stop, in part because the bad humour has been evacuated by vomiting, in part because it is concocted with time, the woman eating only a little as a result of aversion to food, and in part too because of the great amount being evacuated. For during the first two months the embryo draws only a little blood to itself, as it would still be very small whenever it is not yet up to the appropriate time to be called an embryo but is still a conceptus.[67] Having become larger, it needs more nourishment and not only does it draw whatever would be most useful to it in the veins just as before but, because it lacks much, it also draws some of what is abnormal. And so the whole body at that time ceases to be still *plethoric* and becomes less **[VII.134K]** bad-humoured. Certainly the embryo itself deposits in the two membranes the superfluities of the nutriment it draws and so becomes much more bad-humoured and *dyscratic*, as it would be nourished by abnormal blood unless the pregnant woman altogether avails herself of useful nutriments in the remaining time of the pregnancy. But this, at least, has no relevance to present matters. The yearning for abnormal qualities, in describing which I have called to mind *kitta* (*pica*), occurs in men as well sometimes, whenever, at least in them, some similar bad humour also attacks the opening of the stomach. These, then, are the symptoms that occur in relation to the appetite for food.

VII.6 Concerning [the appetite] for drink, there are as many other [symptoms] closely resembling these, like privation whenever either the body does not need [drink] at all owing to excessive moisture or cold, or the stomach is not sensible of the affection (*pathos*) in itself. There is a

[65] *Kitta* (or *kissa*) is the abnormal craving for food, often inappropriate food. It occurs in (but is by no means confined to) women in early pregnancy – see Siegel (1973), pp. 111, 254–5. The Latin term *pica* remains in use.

[66] This is described in LSJ as '. . . a white clay, like fuller's earth, used in baths and barbers' shops, and as a medicine'. The name presumably reflects the island of its origin.

[67] 'Conceptus' is the translation here of *kuema*, a somewhat difficult term. Peck (1942), in his introduction to Aristotle's *Generation of Animals* (pp. lxii–lxiii) writes: 'Actually it [i.e. *kuema*] covers all stages of the living creature's development from the time when the "matter" is first "informed" . . . to the time when the creature is born or hatched.' Galen, however, clearly has a very early stage of pregnancy in mind in his usage here.

deficient appetite whenever these same things occur to a lesser degree. An abnormal appetite for drinks occurs analogous to the abnormal appetite for food, [which is] sometimes of excess drink, whenever some salty or bilious bad humour is contained in the coverings of the stomach, **[VII.135K]** or sometimes [when there is] a kind of seething innate moisture in itself. People desire abnormal drinks, just as they do foods too, in proportion to the prevailing bad humour. These things, then, befall those who have passed their lives badly over a rather long time. Among those overcome by insatiable thirsts who I actually know have died, there was one bitten by a serpent (it was a *dipsas*),[68] and there were reapers who drank wine that had been standing around, in which some such serpent had died, and one who had been intoxicated by old wine, and one who wished to starve himself to death. And there were those on a ship when the water supply failed, some of whom dared to drink sea water, being more excessively thirsty than the others. Some of these, being purged with respect to the stomach and 'stung' violently, died more quickly than the rest. And I also know someone among those suffering a burning fever who drank unrestrainedly of cold [water] when the disease was still increasing, yet was never satiated right up until he died. Such in nature and number are the defects pertaining to the appetites of the stomach.

VII.7 And, in addition to these, there is heartburn (*kardialgia*), a sensory symptom **[VII.136K]** of the opening of the stomach, distressed because of mordant humours. Apart from these, there is so-called *boulimia*,[69] which is a symptom of deficiency and at the same time weakness and cooling of the stomach here. It is no wonder that swoonings (*leipopsychia*)[70] and collapses (*kataptosis*) of the capacity follow pains of this. For when some are seen to have fallen into a swoon with a whitlow (*prospaisma*) of the finger, it is not of course surprising that they are affected at the stomach, not only by the sharpness of the sensation but also by proximity of place,

68 This is both a term for thirst and, in the feminine form, for a venomous reptile whose bite leads to intense thirst – see Nicander, *Theriaca*, lines 125, 334.
69 *Boulimia* (or *boulimos*), a term which remains in use, although in a more specific sense, could be taken here simply to mean an extreme appetite for food. As mentioned earlier, it is a term considered in the pseudo-Aristotelian *Problems* (887b39 ff.). In this situation Hett (1926) translates it simply as 'appetite' although Forster, in Barnes (1984), uses 'ravenous appetite' which is the meaning given by both LSJ and Durling (1993). Galen himself gives a definition in *Hippocratis Aphorismi et Galeni in eos commentarii* XVIIB.501K in relation to Hippocrates, *Aphorisms* II.21. The word *boulimos/ia* is not found in Hippocrates. An interesting point here is that Galen may be using the term more specifically – see the discussion by Siegel (1973), pp. 253–5.
70 This is the translation of the term *leipopsychia* – see Hippocrates, *Aphorisms* VII.8, where Jones (1931) translates it as 'fainting', and Aristotle, *On Sleep and Waking*, where Hett (Loeb, vol. VIII, 1936) renders it 'fainting fits'. It is a term considered along with *boulimia* by Siegel – see previous note.

it being able to lead the two *archai* more readily to a sympathetic affection. And it is possible to find the greatest symptoms afflicting the most sensitive stomachs, as they would also be more distressed than the others in the case of all those that are distressed, and it is possible to see them transmit the injury to both *archai*. And actually, whenever the whole class of nerves is more keenly sensitive or more readily affected in someone, particularly at that time it happens that these same *archai* are brought more readily to a sympathetic affection, whenever either in some affection (*pathos*) or by nature, they are in some way weak. And whenever, at least, the four come together, [**VII.137K**] a very great affection (*pathema*) necessarily occurs. I say four with respect to the occurrence of a strong condition distressing the stomach, and its perception being especially keen, and the class of nerves or arteries being weak, and besides these, either the brain or the heart. In this way, at any rate, epilepsy supervenes in some owing to a weak stomach, as do unconsciousness (*karos*), coma (*koma*), catalepsy (*katalepsia*), delirium (*paraphrosune*) and melancholy, when the *arche* suffers a sympathetic affection in relation to the brain and nerves. The so-called cardiac syncopes supervene when the *arche* suffers a sympathetic affection in relation to the heart and the arteries. In this way too stoppages, slowings and disturbances of the pulse [arise]. *Apnoeas* [arise] when both *archai* are brought to a major sympathetic affection. *Dyspnoeas* [occur] in a twofold manner; either by a narrowing of the praecordium, or when both *archai* suffer a sympathetic affection. The causes[71] leading the animal to such affections (*pathema*) are not few. For sometimes intense cold by itself, or sometimes in the case of extremely cold phlegm (such as is like [**VII.138K**] liquefied glass in both colour and consistency, which the followers of Praxagoras and Philotimus call green and glassy humour),[72] and not least also flatulent *pneuma* which is cold, or drink, or food, or some medicine sufficiently cold, cools the actual opening of the stomach, and with it jointly cools the brain through the nerves and the heart through the great artery, in the one case by the commonality with the class of nerves in respect to the brain, and in the other case by the proximity of position in respect to the heart. For when the greatest of the arteries, having taken its origin from the heart, comes upon the spine, it is first joined and connected with the stomach by membranes, after which it extends lengthwise under the opening [of the stomach] and the stomach itself proceeding downward. Therefore, by

---

[71] This is a further use of the term *prophasis* which I have again simply translated as 'cause' for reasons given in the section on terminology. Here the usage cannot be seen as limited to external causative factors.

[72] See Steckerl (1958), pp. 59–60, fragment 22.

this being the greatest artery and growing out of the heart itself, one of the
archai suffers together with the opening of the stomach, whilst the brain
[suffers together] through the nerves. Thus, it is not surprising that, in the
case of its diseases, the greatest and most severe symptoms befall the animal.
What, then, the mode of genesis of each is **[VII.139K]** will be spoken of in
what follows. For now it is sufficient for me to go over the causes[73] themselves. These are certain mushrooms, poisonous beetles, white lead, chalk,
curdled milk, chokings (*pnix*) from the uterus in those who are widowed
and not purged, and such things as are analogous to these occurring in
men. Something will be said separately about *apnoea* elsewhere.[74]

VIII.1 It seems to me that the discussion about all the sense organs, and
also about the capacities in relation to these, is now at an end. It is time
to come in the discussion to the actual source[75] of these which sends to
the particular parts, as if from a fount, its capacities. This is, of course,
the primary sensorium. For in the actual organs severally, for each of the
senses the change comes about from the sensibilia. The part that is altered
becomes the sensorium of this from the reception of the capacity which
comes down to it from the brain via the nerves. For the brain itself is not
by nature a perceiving organ, but the perceiver of what is perceived. And
that it always sends the sensory capacity to all parts of the animal through
the nerves **[VII.140K]** is most clear from the fact that after any one of the
nerves is cut, the part to which the nerve branches is immediately rendered
incapable of sensation. It is no less clear too that during sleep the senses
are either altogether inactive, or they function weakly. It is probable, then,
that under these circumstances some small amount of capacity flows from
the *arche* to these in turn. And to fall asleep deeply or not deeply, as is
customarily said on each occasion, is dependent on the quantity of the
flow. It is, then, probable that to the extent the flow is less, so the sleep
would be deeper.

    VIII.2 Thus it seems that in that whole time in which the psychical capac-
ity is at rest during sleep, the physical [capacity] functions more strongly.
One would make this judgement on the grounds that the fatigued capacity
regains strength after sleep, and especially whenever we sleep after moderate

[73] Galen again uses *prophasis* here.
[74] See, for example, *De locis affectis* IV.10 and VI.5 (VIII.281–2K, 413–26K), *De difficultate respirationis*
VII.943K, 959K and *In Hippocratis Epidemiarum librum tertium commentarii* 1 (XVIIA.647–51K).
[75] In *De placitis Hippocratis et Platonis* Galen also speaks speaks of the *katarchon* or 'source', specifically
of sensation and voluntary movement (VII.1.6, VIII.1.1) or sensation and volition/conation (II.3.4).
There it is equated with the *hegemenon* or authoritative/governing part of the soul.

nourishment, and still more on the grounds that food is digested optimally during sleep in the whole mass of the animal, not in the stomach alone. In another way, it is also reasonable for that part of the animal in which the *arche* of the rational soul is, to rest sometimes. **[VII.141K]** For the heart obviously does this little by little so as not to need a long period of rest. On the other hand, the brain is not like this, but in wakefulness functions continuously, whilst during sleep it is at rest. And because of this, a deeper sleep befalls those who exercise more, as there would be in them a large flow of capacity from the *arche* when they are active. Owing, then, to the emptying of the capacity which the brain sends and, in addition, to the weariness it suffers by virtue of its many functions, it needs rest and, at the same time, recovery. Just as after exercises people sleep more readily and more deeply, so too do those who have taken nourishment, and the more this should be moist in nature the more they sleep, as do those also who have partaken freely of wine, or have washed the head with copious hot baths. For all such things obviously fill the brain with moisture, which it needs, being fatigued and desiccated in like manner by its many functions.

VIII.3 But, in fact, that the head being full brings sleep was adequately demonstrated by Aristotle,[76] **[VII.142K]** so there is no need for us now to go over the argument in detail. Indeed, anyone who has read his book on sleep and waking will know this very point clearly – that when the head is full sleep comes upon animals. And in addition to this, he will understand as well what is lacking in his argument. For although he was most competent to make the attempt, and most persuasive whither he would wish to lead the argument, nevertheless he was able to discover nothing very plausible as to why, when the head was full, the primary sensorium situated in the heart rests, as he supposes. For it is, of course, far more plausible for sleep to occur in moistenings of the lung, which Nature placed in a circle around the heart for no other reason than to serve it. And who of doctors entertaining contrary opinions, or reckoning from simple experience, does not approach the head in unconsciousness (*karos*), lethargies (*letharge*), comas (*koma*) and all somnolent diseases contrary to nature, pouring water over it or putting plasters on it, or shaving it, or applying cupping-glasses, or contriving anything else whatever, as if here were the root of the disease? **[VII.143K]** In the same way also, those treating madness (*paraphrosune*) and delirium (*phrenitis*), and all insomnias (*agrupnia*) contrary to nature, apply remedies to the head. But a demonstration has been provided elsewhere at

---

[76] See particularly *On Sleep and Waking* 457b20–458a23.

greater length on these matters.[77] What is useful to the present aspects of
the discussion is that when the brain itself wishes to rest from fullness of
function, it brings to the animal a natural sleep, and especially whenever
the nutritive capacity is able to benefit from abundant moisture in itself.
But if it should be weighed down by much cold moisture, it brings sleep
by comas (*koma*) and lethargies (*letharge*), and other similar diseases. The
chief features of these are moisture and cold, either each one existing alone
or both concurrently. Such, at any rate, are medicines also, all that are really
hypnotics and those that are called in this way, that bring about not sleep,
but coma (*koma*), unconsciousness (*karos*) and numbness (*narke*) of the
whole body. Those things, then, that make moist alone are properly called
hypnotics. They would say rightly that cooling things bring neither sleep
nor freedom from pain, but instead of sleep, coma (*koma*) [**VII.144K**]
and unconsciousness (*karos*), and instead of freedom from pain, loss or
disturbance of sensation, due to the excess of cold.

   VIII.4 It has also been said before, of course, that the affection (*pathema*) numbness (*narke*) is a simultaneous disturbance of sensation and of
movement of the nervous parts, and occurs, as was said, not only in relation to other causes, but it also in relation to *dyscrasias*, as in the case of
cooling medicines. In this way, then, sleep, coma (*koma*), unconsciousness
(*karos*) and numbness (*narke*) arise. On the other hand, a more excessive
dryness or heat, as in the *phrenitides*, due to either some mordant or some
hot humour, brings about irritations (*erethrismos*) or insomnias (*agrupnia*),
those at least that do not arise from pain or some anxiety. Just as such symptoms common to the whole body occur owing to the *arche* being affected,
so too do others occur involving all the functions pertaining to appeti-
tion, when the *arche* is affected. For apoplexies and epilepsies occur due
to the brain, apoplexy certainly being such an affection (*pathos*) involving
the functions related to purpose, like deep sleep in the sensory functions.
Another such, like a wakefulness in the sensory functions, is the convulsion in epilepsies. For both these are defective [**VII.145K**] movements of
the brain and, owing to this, also of all the limbs in succession. On the
other hand, both catalepsies (*katalepsia*) and inertias (*hesuchia*) are others
of its functions. Nevertheless, with respect to spasms (convulsions) of the
whole body without delirium (*paraphrosune*) or unconsciousness (*karos*),
the disease is of the spinal cord in the neck, just as when either an arm, or
leg, or one muscle, is stretched and torn violently, the injury in each case
is of the one nerve which moves the part. What precisely the cause of the

---

[77] For a discussion of these matters with appropriate references see Siegel (1973), pp. 263–77.

disease is by which the parts spasm is difficult to say, just as, indeed, is [the cause] of tremor (*tromos*), palpitation (*palmos*) or rigor (*rigos*). Now I call a rigor not a sensation of severe coldness, but an irregular shaking and agitation of the whole body. For all these things obviously involve the muscular class, either alone, or particularly compared to other parts. We shall know this more accurately when we first distinguish the notions of these. For the present, we have named four terms; spasm (convulsion – *spasmos*), tremor (*tromos*), palpitation (*palmos*) and rigor (*rigos*). What kind of symptom each is, which [the names] signify, I found to be defined precisely by not one of my predecessors. [**VII.146K**] Rather, some of them immediately go on to the substances of the diseases which the symptoms follow, whilst others do attempt to distinguish them, but are mistaken in their interpretations, as it will be possible for anyone to learn who, after our instruction, is willing to take up their books. For it is not at all difficult to detect what has been said wrongly when one already apprehends the truth. There will then be discussion of all these things in the account that follows.[78]

---

[78] The symptoms associated with disorders of motor function are considered in the next book (*De symptomatum causis* II). Galen also wrote specifically on the disorders of movement referred to here in *De tremore, palpitatione, convulsione et rigore* (VII.584–642K). Predecessors singled out for mention include Praxagoras, Herophilus, Plato and Athenaeus.

CHAPTER II.5

On the Causes of Symptoms *II*

SYNOPSIS

I.1 A list of abnormal movements, with recognition of a basic division into those that are natural but brought on by disease, and those that are not natural.

I.2 Natural movements are those due to one of the four capacities – as the separative capacity is responsible for sneezing. Movements of the capacities may be perceptible or imperceptible.

II.1 Unnatural movements include paralysis which may involve the various organs.

II.2 Spasm (convulsion) can also affect different structures and is sometimes specifically named (e.g. trismus, strabismus, epilepsy etc.). Such movements may be seen as a conflict between disease and capacity.

II.3 On the mechanism of spasm and its causes.

II.4 On the mechanism of tremor as a succession of alternating movements due to the capacity alternately overcoming and being overcome.

II.5 More on tremor, including the roles of volition, humours, and capacities.

II.6 On palpitation seen as a dilatation due to something flowing into the dilating structure. In view of the time course, this must be 'airy' rather than a humour.

II.7 More on palpitation, the movement being seen as a shaking rather than extension/flexion, and as being related to the separative capacity.

III.1 An exhortation to study and become familiar with the functions of the separative or expulsive capacity. Reference is made to the writings of Athenaeus on fever.

III.2 Consideration of the role of the separative capacity in the function of the uterus in childbirth.

III.3 The role of the separative capacity in the stomach causing either vomiting or rapid passage downward.

III.4 The actions of the separative capacity in relation to the airways involve either coughing or sneezing. Also some consideration of the intestines and bladder as well as the uterus again.

IV.1 A discussion of the mechanism of coughing, including a distinction between structures that can contract around something they need to expel, and those, like the airways, that cannot.

IV.2 Further consideration of coughing and sneezing, the latter relating to the nose and the anterior chambers of the brain. Hoarseness may precede coughing, just as nausea may precede vomiting. Reference is again made to Athenaeus with respect to the role of *dyscrasias* in coughing.

V.1 On coughing in the 'anomalous' *dyscrasias*. Reference is made to both the Pneumatists and to Hippocrates.

V.2 On pain and a sense of unease in the 'anomalous' *dyscrasias*.

V.3 A recognition of three kinds of distress in conditions of fatigue.

V.4 Shivering and rigor, and their relationship to fatigue.

V.5 More on shivering and rigor, and the role of movement of superfluities in their genesis.

V.6 A detailed consideration of causative factors in shivering and rigor, particularly the latter. Also something on the temporal relations of rigor and fever. Reference to Hippocrates on the genesis of rigors.

V.7 Continuation of the discussion of abnormal movements in relation to the function of the separative capacity. Comment also on the fact that the same symptom can follow the most opposite causes.

V.8 Further general consideration of the movements related to the separative capacity including coughing, sneezing, shivering and rigor.

V.9 On the causes of rigors in relation to fevers and otherwise. Reference to Hippocrates on the interrelationship between fever and rigor.

V.10 A brief preliminary statement on changes in the outer parts (changes in heat and in blood content) in relation to psychical affections, with comment on the 'innate heat'.

V.11 Elaboration of these matters, with attention to fear, anger and anxiety.

V.12 On changes in heat and blood distribution in relation to pain.

VI.1 A summarizing section on the various movements, specifically coughs, sneezes, hiccups, shivering, rigors, and fatigues, with mention here also of itching and its causation.

VI.2 Some summarizing remarks on coughs, sneezes, and hiccups, and their causation.

VII.1 Symptoms of the authoritative (*hegemonical*) function with the same three-fold division into loss, reduction and abnormality. The causes are either humours (particularly cooling) or *dyscrasias*.

VII.2 A final section on the various abnormalities of the authoritative function, including delirium, phrenitis, mania, melancholia, depression, irrational fear and hypochondriasis.

THE CAUSES OF SYMPTOMS II

I.1 [VII.147K] Spasm (*spasmos*)[1] and tremor (*tromos*), palpitation (*palmos*), rigor (*rigos*), shivering (*phrike*), hiccup (*lygmos*), coughing (*bex*), belching (*eruge*), sneezing (*ptarmos*), stretching (*skordinismos*), yawning (*chasme*) and rasping (*trusmos*) all have a common class, that of disordered movement.[2] They do, however, also differ among themselves, especially in one primary way, in that some of them are actions of a nature compelled to move violently by a disease-making cause, whilst others follow disease conditions, nature contributing nothing to their genesis. Some, however, occur in which both **[VII.148K]** are operative, that is disease and nature simultaneously.

I.2 I would expect you to understand the term 'nature' in the following discussion as relating to every capacity controlling an animal, whether in accordance with our choosing, or apart from this. For we shall now distinguish[3] from every cause contrary to nature by which the animal is injured or destroyed, that whole class of capacities by which it is preserved. Actions of such a capacity are sneezing, coughing, yawning, gaping and hiccup, whereas palpitation and spasm are when disease alone is operative. When both disease and capacity come together, there are all the sluggish movements and whatever others occur in those who are enfeebled but have not yet been paralysed, and tremor in addition to

---

[1] This is a situation where 'spasm' seems better as the translation of *spasmos* than the often used 'convulsion', particularly in view of the immediate association with 'tremor'. In their translation of Galen's work, *De tremore, palpitatione, convulsione et rigore*, Sider and McVaugh (1979) use 'spasm' in the title. I have generally used 'spasm' unless some epileptic phenomenon is clearly indicated. Siegel (1973) has the following: 'The Greek term *spasmos* meant both a continued contracture by a tetanic stimulus and an alternating violent contraction and relaxation of a skeletal muscle. Both types of movement are also symptoms of epilepsy. *Spasmos* (convulsion), however, appeared to Galen as exaggeration of normal motion intensified by heat, cold or dryness of the spinal nerves' (p. 245). He also makes reference to *De locis affectis* VIII.172K, 174K.
[2] These terms are all listed in the section on terminology (I.4d). In what follows they will not be transliterated again unless there is a particular issue arising.
[3] The verb *antidiaireo* has a specific usage in relation to opposition in classification – see Aristotle, *Categories* 14b34 and *Topics* 142a36.

these.[4] These are the primary *differentiae* of the class of symptoms we now put forward. Next, there are certain distinguishing features pertaining to each, about which let us now speak, starting from the movements arising due to some innate capacity. And there is an association between these and those that are entirely in accord with nature which it is necessary to mention first for the purpose of teaching clearly what [VII.149K] the genesis of these is. There are four capacities by which all nourished bodies are controlled.[5] The first is the drawing to itself of what is useful, the second the retaining of this, the third alteration, and the fourth separation of what is superfluous. When an animal is governed by the law of nature, no movement of any one of these is a symptom. But when something contrary to nature exists in the body, whenever one of the separative capacities sets out to reject this, sometimes their movements are altogether imperceptible, whilst sometimes they are perceived. Something will be said about those that are imperceptible later.

II.1 Concerning those that are perceptible, since they are in common with what are called voluntary [functions], let the elucidation be common. An injury of voluntary function, paralysis, or spasm, or tremor, or numbness, varies in the organs severally with respect to each of those mentioned, not only in the form of the symptoms, but also in the names. For paralysis of the organs effecting respiration [VII.150K] is called *apnoea*, just as also [paralysis] of those effecting speech is called *aphonia*. On the other hand, paralysis of the tongue has acquired no specific name, yet this too does away completely with speech, to no small degree a function of volition. Conversely, retention of urine (*ischouria*) will seem no less to signify something similar to *apnoea* and *aphonia*, and yet it is not a destruction of a voluntary function but of a physical one. For to pass urine involuntarily is an injury of a voluntary function. Equally, in respect to the passing of urine, retention is an injury of a physical function, whereas involuntary excretion is an injury of a voluntary function. There has been a quite full demonstration of all such things in the writings on the movement of muscles.[6] In this way the paralyses are varied in kinds.

II.2 Spasms are of the following kinds. Gnashing the teeth (*to trizein*) is an involuntary spasm of the muscles of mastication. Squinting (*strabismus*)

---

[4] The interpretation of this sentence follows Copus (1548). *Narkodes* is read as 'sluggish' but might be taken to indicate any degree of reduced movement due to partial paralysis (see, for example, Hippocrates, *Fractures* XIX, XLVIII).

[5] *Dioikeo* is taken in the sense of 'managed' or 'governed' (see e.g. Plato, *Meno* 91a), although it may also mean 'provide' or 'furnish' (see e.g. Demosthenes, XXVII.66), or even refer specifically to the digestion of food (Diogenes Laertius VI.34). Both Latin versions (Copus, Kühn) use *guberno*.

[6] *De motu musculorum* IV.367–464K.

so-called is a distortion of the [muscles] in relation to the eyes,[7] just as [the spasm] of spermatorrhoea[8] is also another *differentia*. For if this occurs with distension of the penis it is like a spasm, whereas if it occurs without this, **[VII.151K]** it is a weakness of the retentive capacity. And hiccups seem to some [to be spasms].[9] Further, a double inspiration[10] of those inhaling sometimes exists, occurring through a spasm of the muscles effecting inspiration. There exists also what is like a convulsive form of expiration, this again occurring due to spasms of the muscles which effect expiration, which was called by Hippocrates 'the breath being checked on its passage outward'.[11] That apoplexy is a paralysis of the whole body whereas epilepsy is a spasm (convulsion), has been stated previously. And it has certainly been said before about numbness, that it is a mild paralysis. The difference of the numbed parts in terms of more or less is not slight since the symptom is somehow compounded from disease and capacity. For if disease prevails over capacity completely, the limb is unable to change at all whereas, if capacity [prevails], it is not hindered at all. If there is some sort of struggle of these, [the limbs] move, but with difficulty, so that if you order those who have extended a damaged limb to maintain the extension, they are unable to do so and it falls under its natural **[VII.152K]** weight, borne downward owing to the weakness of the capacity which sustains it. For what lifts up and supports is the capacity, whereas what bears downward is the actual 'body' of the arm or the leg. The cause has been spoken of earlier in relation to the discussion regarding sensory functions, when we showed that the nerve is either contracted by coldness, or obstructed by thick and viscid humours, or weighed down and compressed by some external cause, and so is brought to numbness and paralysis.[12]

II.3 A spasm, in fact, leads nerves and muscles to the same condition to which they are also led by the psychic capacity when in accord with nature. Voluntary movements occur either when muscles are stretched towards the *arche*, or when they are filled by an influx of *pneuma*, but in the case of spasms these will happen either when flatulent *pneuma* is able to be

---

[7] See Hippocrates, *Prorrhetic* I.69 where Potter (1995) translates *illosis* as 'strabismus' (vol. 8, p. 185). See also pseudo-Galen, *Definitiones medicae* XIX.436K.

[8] I have used 'spermatorrhoea' for the Greek *gonorroia* which is now, of course, used for a specific disease. On the issue of whether the symptom occurs with or without penile erection see Caelius Aurelianus III.178 (Drabkin (1950), p. 413) and V.79 (Drabkin (1950), pp. 957–9).

[9] Galen provides a definition and description of *lynx* in *In Hippocratis librum de acutorum victu commentarii* XV.846–7K.

[10] The term *epanaklesis*, which has the general meaning of 'recall' or 'reaction' (see Hippocrates, *Aphorisms* V.21), also has the specific meaning given above – Hippocrates, *Epidemics* II.3.7.

[11] See *Regimen in Acute Diseases* XLII which has *ano* rather than *exo*.

[12] *De symptomatum causis*, Book I, V.2 (VII.109–11K).

generated in them, or in the many conditions causing tension, such as inflammation (*phlegmone*). The chief point of these is twofold, as Hippocrates made clear: a filling or an emptying.[13] Filling [occurs] in inflammatory affections (*pathos*), [**VII.153K**] emptying in very burning or very drying fevers. That stretching occurs to a greater extent in all nerve-containing bodies that are filled or emptied, the stretched strings in musical instruments show particularly well. At any rate, they break should they be put down when stretched out, in a wet and moist or dry and arid dwelling. It is because of this also that the users slacken them before they put them down. On this account, at any rate, it was also said before that a convulsive movement occurs through disease alone, in like manner to *akinesia* in the paralyses. For this will be brought about by reason of the disease. In animals, absence of movement and movement that accords with nature, whenever having stretched out an arm we are able to maintain it immobile in the stretched out position, both occur due to the psychical capacity. If, having placed the healthy arm on some solid object, we relax all the functions of the muscles, the arm is still for that period, not owing to disease or capacity but because of the natural weight in animals. Thus there are three 'quiescences' ('inertias' – *hesuche*): (i) that in the paralyses which occurs as a result of disease, [**VII.154K**] capacity, one might say, being bound at this time; (ii) that which occurs whenever we have the limb stretched out and which is due to capacity; (iii) that which, as we were just now saying, is due to neither, but which we know from what was said in the writings on the movement of muscles in relation to the outstretched arm is, in truth, from the class of functions and movements.[14] And it was said also that we term this movement 'tonic'.[15] Such a settled condition could be said in one way to be a movement, but in another to be an absence of movement. The other two [settled conditions] in no way partake of movement, just as the other two movements, convulsive and voluntary, in no way partake of immobility.

II.4 Furthermore, as the outstretched arm was said to be compounded from two movements of equal strength, the capacity carrying it up and the natural weight drawing it downward, so too tremor is itself also brought about by two movements, that which drags the limb down by its weight, and that which the capacity carries out raising it up in opposition. Thus, in the case of an arm that is strong, the capacity is not to the least degree

---

[13] Hippocrates, *Aphorisms* VI.39.
[14] This sentence has been modified somewhat, with the addition of numbered points, in the pursuit of clarity. The reference to *De motu musculorum* is particularly chapters VII and VIII (IV.396–407K).
[15] This term is used in several places in the *De motu musculorum*, for example IV.403K and IV.423K.

overcome by the weight but, being more strongly [**VII.155K**] established than the downward counterweight of the limb, continues to raise it upwards to the same degree that the other drags it downwards, whereas, in relation to tremors, although [the capacity] itself is unwilling, the limb slips down. At any rate, it is clear to see the struggle of these in that neither does the capacity permit the limb to be borne downwards as in the paralyses, nor does the weight yield to the capacity to maintain the limb raised, as when it is strong. Alternately, then, when the capacity overcomes and is overcome, and when opposing movements continuously succeed one another, tremor occurs, which is a composite movement, like the pulse of the arteries. But in the latter, perceptible cessations of movements divide diastole from systole, unless, perhaps, a very rapid pulse occurs, as in the 'formications'.[16] For here it is possible to find no perceptible cessation between opposing movements. The alternation of movement is not brought about by one nature but there is a struggle between the capacity and the weight of the body. So should someone liken the movement particularly to some other of those in the body, the resemblance is to that of the 'formicatory' pulses. For, as the movement of the artery in those [**VII.156K**] is brought about with the shortest interval, so it is in tremors with respect to whatever part of the animal should be moved by a weak capacity. Thus the genesis of this symptom is now clear – it is brought about both in association with the impetus of the movement entirely, and in association with the weakness of the capacity.

II.5 There are some who do not think the impulse is inseparable from the tremor, seeing sometimes the whole head shaking tremulously without the movement being voluntary. What they don't know is that volition also functions in maintaining any part straight and that the muscles are extended by this in a way similar to that in which they are, in fact, extended in other functions. We have shown this in the writings on the movement of the muscles,[17] so now we should provide several proofs that volition acts in tremors, and that owing to weakness it is unable to hold the part steady. At any rate, with respect to that tremor of the head, if you lie down supine on something soft, there will no longer be a tremor. In the same way, when someone writing, or cutting, or doing anything else whatsoever has acquired a tremor, if he rests [**VII.157K**] the arms, he no longer appears tremulous. Likewise, were someone walking to become tremulous in the

---

[16] I have used the term 'formication' although it came to have a specific meaning in application to a sensory symptom particularly associated with syphilis (see Mettler (1947), p. 615). In regard to the pulse, it meant 'quick and feeble', referring to the observer's sensation rather than the patient's.

[17] *De motu musculorum* IV.367–464K – see particularly chapter V (IV.440–4K).

legs, that person would not still tremble when he stopped walking. It is often possible, then, for you to see very strong young men who have laid upon their shoulders some great burden, tremble in the legs in going forward whereas, if they stop walking, or cast off the burden, they immediately become free of tremor. For, since heaviness and lightness in something are relative, a burden could be so great as to be heavy even for the strongest. Thus the greatest burden overcomes a strong capacity whereas, when it is not so strong, not only a heavy but also a light [burden overcomes it]. If it [the capacity] is weaker still, then its own body itself weighs it down like a burden – which is why all old people, whenever they attempt more vigorous functions, immediately become tremulous in the functioning parts. So too, someone approaching a beetling cliff trembles in the legs, for fear casts out capacity. Likewise, someone fleeing from a wild beast that has just shown itself is in a tremulous state. Furthermore, someone approaching a fearsome ruler trembles in the whole body [**VII.158K**] and, if [the ruler] should order him to speak, his voice is not without tremor. As, then, a psychical affection (*pathos*) producing weakness in the motor capacity brings about tremulous functions, so too do diseases of the body that damage the capacity bring forth tremulous symptoms. Those things that primarily and particularly damage capacity are those that come together in a *dyscrasia*. Moreover, old age, in that it is a *dyscrasia* insofar as it is colder and dryer, is thereby more readily afflicted by tremulous affections (*pathos*), whilst those among young men are also afflicted who are strongly cooled, or have imbibed liberally of still unmixed wine, or have suffered much indigestion, or, having filled themselves with food, remain over a long time completely idle and inactive. There are also those who take in cold water at an inappropriate time and become tremulous. All such things bring about a cold *dyscrasia*, often in the whole body, and in relation to the actual *arche* of the nerves, but sometimes in certain parts, which are weaker in nature and happen to be more susceptible to injury than others. Furthermore, thick and viscid humours [**VII.159K**] obstructing the passages of the capacity so that it flows less, constitute causes of tremors, and especially whenever they entirely block and paralyse some parts of certain nerves. For the rest of the fibres are unable strongly to extend the muscle. Nonetheless, whenever the fluids stopping up the channels of the capacity through the nerves happen to be not yet entirely impacted, they are able to be moved on and shaken up during the more violent incursions of the capacity, such movements occurring that are the kind we previously said happen sometimes in incipient paralyses, when on occasion the limb, having been lifted up, immediately falls. For under the impact of the capacity, whenever this has been stirred up and collects itself together more violently, it thrusts aside the obstructions of the nerves and the limb is moved. In turn, when those things forced away flow into the place anew, the limb falls down and rests immobile until again, for a second time, the capacity, breaking in more compactly, should disperse the humours which have occupied the channels. But this is enough about these matters.

II.6 A palpitation is a dilatation contrary to nature [**VII.160K**] and occurs in all parts – those, at least, that are disposed by nature to be dilated.[18] For bones and cartilage never palpitate because they cannot be dilated. This [palpitation] does often occur, then, in the skin, and sometimes also in the muscles underlying it. But it is also not rare in the stomach, bladder, uterus,[19] intestines, liver, spleen and diaphragm and, in a word, all those things disposed by nature to be dilated, so that it clearly befalls both the arteries and the heart itself, this other movement occurring in these alongside the pulse.[20] The affection (*pathos*) then, like tremor and spasm, is specific to neither the voluntary capacity nor the voluntary organs but, as has been said just now, occurs in all bodies capable of being dilated. These are, of course, all those that are soft in nature, such as to be able to undergo distension and collapse. It is appropriate to seek the cause of the symptom from the most evident appearances, i.e. from those palpitations that occur in the eyelids, eyebrows, forehead and cheeks. For the skin in these is seen to be lifted up and inflated [**VII.161K**] in the same way as the arteries dilate. What, then, is to be looked for in these [structures] is whether they dilate by themselves, drawing in by the dilatation what fills them, like the bellows of blacksmiths,[21] or being filled, they dilate like wineskins, this being what you must distinguish primarily in the case of palpitating parts. It is right for the class of enquiry to be likened to that pertaining to arteries but in respect to how easy it is to investigate, they differ. For it is certainly not likely that there is also some innate capacity in parts palpitating in this way, as there is in the arteries pulsating continuously and in accord with nature. It would, then, always be in these, and particularly when they are healthy. So whenever [the palpitations] are neither continuous nor in healthy [parts],

---

[18] The Greek term *palmos* clearly has a substantially wider range of meaning than has the term 'palpitation', used here in translation. The original sense is probably 'throbbing' which is used by Jones (1923) in his translation of Hippocrates' *Regimen in Acute Diseases* XXXVII (p. 93). Galen himself clarifies the use of the term in what follows. See also the pseudo-Galenic *Definitiones medicae* XIX.403K where there is a concise definition.

[19] καί is added to the Greek text here.

[20] For a discussion of Galen's conceptions (and misconceptions) of cardiac anatomy and physiology see Siegel (1968), pp. 30–47. With respect to cardiac dilatation see particularly p. 31.

[21] Aristotle uses a similar comparison in discussing expansion of the chest in respiration – see *On Respiration* VII, 474a10–16.

clearly they do not dilate by themselves. And if it is not by themselves, then doubtless it is entirely from some substance flowing into them from within. The probability in this case is twofold; either a humour or something of an airy nature. Neither the swiftness of the genesis nor the resolution of the palpitation is in keeping with a humour in that it both occurs suddenly and also ceases suddenly. No humour [**VII.162K**] flows in or out so quickly, and especially in those parts just now spoken of in the face where the skin is stretched over almost bare bones. Thus it is necessary for the cause bringing about palpitations to be some airy substance. But if this is scanty and fine it would readily flow through the body. It is, then, probably something thick, vaporous and noteworthy in amount with respect to the place in which it might be situated in each case. It dilates then, as is probable, and both lifts up and inflates the part, until having been thrust on and constrained, it should breathe towards what is like itself. This is like what happens to the bubbles in fluids that have been boiled except, at least, that these bubbles burst whereas the palpitating body does not burst owing to its strength but is lifted up until the *pneuma* should be thrust on and passed through by it. It then falls down again to its original place whenever it is completely evacuated and passed through. And it is with good reason also that palpitations befall any part whatever in those who are chilled. For that which, when it flows under normal circumstances, is fine and has been thoroughly acted upon by the heat that is innate to animals, now when it has been weakened [**VII.163K**] owing to the cold, becomes more vaporous and thicker. Thus it does not readily disperse as it did before, but is held in the skin and, being compressed in the outlet channel, is slow during its passage. And if the skin itself is thickened, the symptoms will be made twofold, the thickness of the flowing substance being added to the narrowness of the channels. So, then, in palpitations, the skin lifts up and dilates. So too do the muscles, being sometimes dilated whenever such a superfluity collects in them, lift up the whole limb.

II.7 But such a movement differs very clearly from a spasm in that it neither completely extends nor bends the limb. For certainly in the case of palpitations, the limb is neither extended nor bent to any degree worth speaking of, but is shaken in some fashion this way and that until the palpitating muscle should come to rest. The movement is effected in the same way in which a tremor is also effected, although there is a difference in the great intervals that occur compared to the small [intervals] occurring in a tremor. Certainly, whenever the size of the palpitating muscle is noteworthy, by being dilated it often raises [**VII.164K**] the entire limb with it whereas, by being contracted, it allows itself to be borne downward as if inanimate.

Thus the whole movement is contrary to nature and not, as in the case of
a tremor, in some way mixed and compound. The kind of movement that
occurs in palpitating limbs, when it is at the same time slight, slow and
intermittent, is the same as occurs in shivering fits, when it is at the same
time great, dense and rapid. I say 'great' with respect to the actual number
of the movements, whereas 'rapid' applies to the swinging nature of the
motion and 'dense' to the short duration of the periods of rest. It is not that
this movement is altogether contrary to nature like palpitation or spasm,
but it is of another kind than even tremor. It is, then, mixed somehow from
a cause contrary to nature and from the capacity of the animal, and there
is more of capacity in this than in tremors. Indeed, if one must speak the
truth, the whole movement is of the innate capacity, which it is customary
for us to call expulsive or separative, whilst the cause compelling and forcing
the capacity to move violently is contrary to nature.

III.1 [VII.165K] Anyone, then, who is sufficiently conversant with the
functions of this capacity when the animal is perfectly healthy, and is otherwise intelligent, has no need of a longer discussion on this matter. Whoever
does not, in fact, know those [functions] and is by nature more dull-witted,
I would advise him, if he is not altogether devoted to the truth, to set aside
this work. However, if he is zealous and values the truth, I would advise
him, having first started out from the works on the physical capacities[22]
and become sufficiently practised in these, then to return to this work. For
if he does not do this, he will neither follow the demonstrations of those
things we are about to talk of, nor will he understand without demonstration those things that were previously said. I then propose in this treatise to
refute no opinion. It is possible for anyone who wishes to read the twenty-
fourth book of Athenaeus to learn the causes spoken of by his medical
and philosophical predecessors concerning rigors and the extent to which
they came to absurdities, for Athenaeus refutes all these [causes].[23] It is also
possible to examine closely the actual opinion of Athenaeus, which has a
greater credibility than any of those previously held, **[VII.166K]** although
not itself true. But when there is this concern for truth in anyone, I know
that if he is instructed in this way, he will endeavour to act in this way.

III.2 Assuming a knowledge of our writings on the physical capacities,
I shall discuss a few things, having first called to mind those things I have
demonstrated in them on the uterus, stomach, intestines and bladder. For

[22] *De facultatibus naturalibus* II.1–214K.
[23] Athenaeus' writings are no longer extant. I can find no other reference to his considerations on rigors
in the Galenic corpus.

uteri have been shown to hasten foetuses towards birth by no other means than through the action of the separative capacity.[24] At any rate, having endured for nine months the weight of the foetus and their own distension, and during this whole time having their orifice so entirely closed as not to admit the round head of a probe, when the foetuses within them have reached full development, they attend to the separation of these by putting themselves in the opposite state. For their os,[25] previously closed, opens up to such an extent that it become a favourable passage for what is being born. On the other hand, the membranes, previously stretched out to the greatest extent, contract on all sides and, in fact, thrust forth the foetus, so that it escapes as quickly as possible through the cervix of the uterus. In this way the capacity is provident for foetuses, [**VII.167K**] so [the uterus can] endure being weighed down for a time of nine months whilst taking care of the mature foetus in such a way that it is safely separated. However, when the foetus is defective,[26] it immediately casts it out around the third, fourth or any other month, now opening the os in the same way it opens whenever birth is at hand. Thus, the appointed time for it to be closed or open is not limited to some prescribed period of time but is the right time for use.

III.3   In the same way, it was shown also that the stomach closes to its lower orifice after meals,[27] and permits nothing to pass through before it has been completely digested, whenever, at least, nothing else compels it to interrupt function, like abortion of the foetus in the case of the uterus.[28] For certainly some analogous affection (*pathos*) befalls the stomach when the foods in it are corrupted or, by Jupiter, often when, at the time of their intake, they are so abnormal or excessive that it is unable to bear them. And because of this, it casts out by vomiting those situated at the top whereas those already inclined downwards, it thrusts onward through that passage. But also apart from foods, the capacity of the stomach often stirs it to vomiting, [**VII.168K**] either owing to bile, or abnormal phlegm, or some other such humour, or *ichor*. For the capacity is innate in each of the parts

---

[24] Galen deals with these matters in detail in *De facultatibus naturalibus* III.3 (II.147–53K).

[25] The two terms *stomachos* and *auchen* are taken to refer to the os uteri and cervix uteri respectively although there is some variation in their usage – see Hippocrates, *Airs, Waters, Places* IX, *Diseases of Women* 1.18, 36 and Galen, *De usu partium* XIV.3. Latin translators use *fauces* and *cervix*.

[26] The verb *diaphtheiro* has a specific application to spontaneous abortion or miscarriage – see, for example, Hippocrates, *Aphorisms* V.53.

[27] Galen's account of the stomach in *De facultatibus naturalibus* follows that of the uterus – i.e. III.4 (II.152–7K). The closure of the pylorus is specifically mentioned at II.157K.

[28] See n. 26 above. The cognate noun has application to both the stomach and the uterus – see Aretaeus, *The Treatment of Acute Diseases* I.5 for the former and Hippocrates, *Diseases of Women* I.3 for the latter.

of the animal, separating what has arisen in it contrary to nature, as has been shown in the specific discussions concerning this.[29] For the present it is enough for purposes of clarification to have called to mind the actions of such a capacity, however many others have been spoken about concerning the uterus and the stomach.

III.4 For just as there is a separative capacity in the stomach in relation to vomiting, so too there is a similar one in relation to coughing in the thorax and lung. No animal is taught to be nauseated or to vomit or to cough, but very often for a long time after birth, if perfect health is enjoyed, both many other animals and also people experience neither vomiting nor coughing. But if a distressing cause takes hold of either the orifice of the stomach or the passages of respiration, then immediately the animal vomits or coughs. The stomach moves in vomiting in the same way the uterus does in giving birth, although with coughing it is otherwise. Because it is not possible for the lung to expel the distressing agent by initiating such a movement, Nature has invented [**VII.169K**] a certain extraordinarily ingenious aid. Seeing that the external air is inhaled into the bronchial tubes,[30] which are in fact cartilaginous and hard and cannot be contracted around what is contained in them, [Nature] has contrived a certain violent passage of the breath to the outside, which they call a cough. Sneezing is also of this class, by which it pushes out things in the nostrils, which are themselves passages of respiration invented by Nature. For the breath itself clears out its own passages, carrying [things] away forcibly and vigorously, just like craftsmen[31] with respect to pipes and tubes. Whatever kind of movement there is, the argument, as it proceeds, will show that this comes about. Let us accept for now what is useful to the matters put forward – that such movements are actions of Nature, although numbered among the symptoms contrary to nature because they are causes compelling Nature to move in this way. In the case, then, of the intestines, uterus and bladder, there are similar movements of the separative capacity, which should be divided into those that accord with nature and those that are contrary to nature. And because of this, [**VII.170K**] the symptoms are not clearly distinguished, although those relating to *teinesmos*, *dysenteria* and *leienteria*

---

[29] In *De facultatibus naturalibus* (II.80K) Galen speaks of the innate capacity of each of the organs which is 'given right from the beginning by Nature'. See also *De locis affectis* VIII.66K. The specific discussions of uterus and stomach are in the former work (III.3, III.4 – II.147–58K).

[30] Durling (1993) gives 'trachea' for *tracheia arteria* but here, as the plural is used, I take Galen to be referring to the bronchial tubes (as indicated in LSJ).

[31] Lloyd suggests that these *demiourgoi* are musicians.

are separative symptoms,[32] just as, in my opinion, are those relating to *stranguria* and polyuria (*diarroia eis oura*). And if one were to be precise, there is noisy flatulence, just as [there is] gurgling (*trysmos*),[33] eructation, *borborygmus* and other such things. And there will, in fact, be discussion about these in what follows.

IV.1 At least in the case of the stomach, what relates to vomiting is now more clear, yet many also say these are not actions of Nature but symptoms. In the case of coughs and sneezes, there is here greater clarity with respect to coughs [in that] sneezes do not seem to be contrary to nature in the same way. But they, as well as coughs, vomiting, diarrhoea and all other such things are of that class of symptoms in which some cause contrary to nature incites Nature to such functions. The kind of movement in all these is not the same, nor does it occur through the same capacity. Whatever things are expelled by the uterus, intestines, stomach or bladder, the parts themselves contract around these, **[VII.171K]** thrusting out what is contained in them in the same way as hands squeeze things out. The capacity bringing about the movement of these is one of the four physical [capacities]. Whenever some body is contained in the bronchial tubes, which are cartilaginous and hard and because of this are unable to contract themselves around what is contained [in them], Nature brings about a violent impulse of the breath to the exterior, setting in motion a cough. This occurs through those same organs by which it effects the great and violent exhalations which we call 'emissions of breath',[34] since a cough is nothing other than a certain very violent emission of breath in order that the breath being borne to the greatest extent and at the same time very swiftly to the exterior may carry away and propel by the rush those things obstructing its passages. And whenever, in fact, the distressing things cannot be cast out by the first expulsion, there is no hesitation in letting fall upon them a second, or a third, or as many as bring about the objective, whenever the breath itself is borne violently and the obstructing things are found to be suitable for expulsion. These are the things that are neither watery nor viscid in substance. **[VII.172K]** For those things that are watery are, due to their fineness, particularly split up by the breath rather than borne onward, whilst those that are viscid adhere to

---

[32] Three forms of abnormal defecation. In brief, ineffectual and distressing attempts at evacuation, excessive defecation (diarrhoea), and passage of undigested material – see section I.4d on terminology.

[33] I have taken *trusmos* here to be different from *trismos/trigmos* although LSJ has them as synonymous – see section on terminology I.4d.

[34] See *De difficultate respirationis* VII.795, 812K.

the trachea,[35] being hard to get rid of. Whenever, then, the breath contends with such moist things, it very often falls upon [them] violently, and the most violent coughs and those occurring with the greatest intensity arise as a result of such causes.

IV.2 Sneezes especially remove those of the watery things that are hard to dislodge and hard to throw up in the [bronchial] tubes. They have an impulse of breath still more violent than coughs although the cause of genesis is different. It is on account of distressing things in the nose, not on account of those in the trachea, that the breath is emitted forcibly, whilst something from the anterior cavities of the brain is also emitted with it. And because of this, coughs do not aid the head at all whereas sneezes, whenever they do not occur as a result of some *catarrh*, are the best cure for a head filled with vapours. It is not, I suppose, surprising that the breath is sent forth by a single impulse from the lung or from the head. For it was shown in the accounts of the muscles that the brain provides the *arche* of movement to the thorax, **[VII.173K]** whereas the thorax expands and contracts the lung.[36] Whenever, then, it starts to expel what is distressing in the nose, it makes use of both channels of expiration at the same time, the one it itself makes through itself, and the other due to the nerves passing down to the thorax like some giant hands.[37] For by these it contracts [the thorax], whilst through the ethmoid bones it itself sends forth the vaporous *pneuma*. These, then, are symptoms of the voluntary capacity.[38] Vomiting, although being somewhat analogous to these, is of the physical [capacity]. Just as nausea precedes vomiting, in the same way hoarseness precedes coughing. And in fact also, just as some are nauseated yet do not vomit, in the same way hoarseness occurs in some people yet a cough does not follow owing to the smallness of the cause. For hoarseness sometimes happens because of a slight roughness of the throat,[39] and sometimes because of a certain fine and altogether slight moisture. For invariably where the breath is checked by something, it attempts to expel it by means of a cough. This is, in fact, either moisture borne down **[VII.174K]** from the head as in *catarrhs*, or collected in the bronchial tubes as in the inflammations of

---

[35] The terminology applied to the respiratory passages is somewhat confusing, as indicated earlier. I have taken *arteria* in the singular (with or without *tracheia*) to indicate the trachea and in the plural to mean 'bronchial tubes'. See *De usu partium*, May (1968), vol. 1, pp. 352, 355, 385–6.

[36] See *De motu musculorum* IV.442–3K.

[37] For Galen's description of the nerves to the thorax see *De usu partium* XVI.7 (II.405H) and *De causis respirationis* IV.468–9K.

[38] Galen speaks of 'the voluntary capacity' only rarely – see, for example, *De causis respirationis* IV.465K where Furley and Wilkie (1984), in a note to their text and translation, make reference to Aristotle's *Movements of Animals* II (see p. 278).

[39] There is again an issue of terminology here as considered earlier.

the lungs (*peripneumonia*), pleurisies and inflammations (*phlegmone*) of the convexities of the liver, or in the cases of roughness of the throat. Apart from these, there is what is analogous to the *catarrhs* from the head, which are those things that slip down [into the bronchial tubes][40] during drinking and eating. And there is another class of cough in the case of a *dyscrasia* of the organs of respiration with which the most notable of the men of the Pneumatic sect, including Athenaeus, were well acquainted. Nevertheless, with respect to the necessity by which a cough is a consequence of a *dyscrasia*, some of them did not attempt to say anything at all, some said that the breath strikes against itself, whilst some, articulating an even more obscure explanation, think they have said something.[41] One must not blame these men for not knowing the cause but rather praise them for discovering a good subject for investigation, and one worthy of their diligence. This cough, then, occurs when the respiratory parts are cooled, yet those coughing expel nothing with it, nor does it occur at all forcibly, but is so slight and weak that it holds back, as it were, and prevents its own genesis, [**VII.175K**] either for the most part or completely. Violent coughs, at least, are not overcome by a holding of the breath. What sort of thing holding the breath is, I have already spoken about often in other places.[42] And not only are the coughs due to *dyscrasia* immediately prevented from occurring by holding the breath, but this is also their treatment if they are not very great. For the heat in the respiratory organs is increased by the stoppage of the breath, and the breath, violently compressed by the thorax, passes through all the narrow channels. When both these things occur, everything is brought to an even temperature and comes to a uniformity of mixing.

V.1 Why then, in the case of anomalous (non-uniform) *dyscrasias* of the respiratory organs, people cough (for I said the doctors of the Pneumatic sect have not worked this out very well),[43] I shall attempt to go over in detail, starting from the substance of the matter, as befits those who intend to speak by means of demonstration. Accordingly, a *dyscrasia* sometimes occurs in relation to singular qualities, when the bodies themselves are made hotter, colder, drier or more moist, [**VII.176K**] or also when they suffer this in relation to some conjunction. Sometimes what is *dyscratic* in them [occurs] with a dispersal that is dew-like. A uniform *dyscrasia* is, then, altogether painless, as the hectic fevers and many of the conditions relating

---

[40] Kühn's Latin text adds '*nobis in arteriam*' here.
[41] No detailed account of the Pneumatists' theories on the genesis of coughing has been preserved.
[42] Particularly in *De sanitate tuenda* II (VI.168–81K).
[43] See Oribasius, *Libri ad Eunapium* IV.77.2.

to cold show, taking hold of the parts evenly. For such a mixing occurs in each of the parts so disposed as if it were some additional nature. No body is distressed by its own nature. As Hippocrates said, pains occur in those things that are being changed or destroyed in their nature, not in those that have already been changed or destroyed.⁴⁴ For in being changed, and in departing from their own nature, bodies are distressed, as was also shown in the earlier discussion.⁴⁵

V.2 Whenever, then, an anomalous (non-uniform) *dyscrasia* has come into being in any one of the perceiving bodies, the magnitude of the pain is commensurate with that of the *dyscrasia*. Thus in the sharpest and strongest of the fevers, the solid parts of the animal are distressed, being changed and altered by a heat that is contrary to nature. However, when **[VII.177K]** diseases are still beginning, the majority of people at one time perceive a certain irregularity in their whole mass before they are febrile, although this is of such a kind that they are unable to speak about it. Well, I would be astounded if anyone among those familiar with these writings [of mine] were so fortunate as not also to have been seized by the symptom himself at some time. For some deep sensation occurs in relation to the whole mass as if something alien to our nature has been dispersed in it. And that which is dispersed would seem sometimes as if it were something hot, or sometimes mordant without being hot, although there are occasions when it is affected by both or, apart from these, the whole flesh is distended slightly. Certainly, in all such symptoms, people say they sense some irregularity, or they stretch the limbs, or they extend all the parts under some physical impulse, the kind we were saying just now has been given by Nature to all the parts of the animal for the purposes of safety and preservation. Particularly do they stretch after sleep, being aware of a vaporous superfluity in the flesh, collected together owing to the processing⁴⁶ of nutriment **[VII.178K]** and owing to the rest from such movements. And this the smallest of children also have without teaching. But Nature incites animals to such a movement, contriving an outlet for the vaporous superfluities.

---

⁴⁴ There is some uncertainty about this apparent quotation. The punctuation in the Kühn Greek text which suggests that what is attributed to Hippocrates precedes 'as Hippocrates said' whereas the Latin version suggests that it follows. There is the following in *Places in Man* XLII: 'For in each thing that is altered with respect to its nature, and destroyed, pains arise' (translation after Potter (1995), vol. 8, p. 85).

⁴⁵ *De symptomatum causis* I, section VI.

⁴⁶ 'Processing' is the translation of *katergasia* for which LSJ has '*working up*, frequently of food, by digestion or by chewing'. The term is found in Aristotle, *Parts of Animals* 675b5, where Peck and Forster (1937) have 'ample treatment' and Ogle, in Barnes (1984), has 'thorough elaboration'. In the pseudo-Aristotelian *Problems* 931a32 Forster, in Barnes (1984), uses 'process'.

V.3 There is another kind of this distressing sensation, that which pertains to conditions of fatigue, whether they arise after many labours or are
spontaneous. There are three kinds of sensation in fatigue: (i) that when people seem to be bruised and beaten; (ii) that when the mass of the body seems
to be stretched in every direction; (iii) that when they seem to have something like many scattered wounds (*helkos*) whenever they move.[47] With
regard to the mass being stretched, at least whenever people suffer in this way
apart from exercise, it has the name 'spontaneous fatigue in tension'.[48] This
occurs particularly as a result of a fullness which stretches the surrounding
[parts] and is not contained by them.[49] Whenever a wound-like sensation
passes through them, this also occurs more in those who are moving than
in those at rest, unless the fatigue is not very great. They think themselves
pierced by many implanted spines, for a mordant humour has brought
about the symptom. The third fatigue, in which they say [**VII.179K**] there
is distress due to *ostokopos*,[50] does not tolerate the slightest movement. There
is in these a sensation of notable heat, and at the same time also of stretching
and gnawing, abundant bad humour having been sent forth to the whole
mass of the animal. No one who is like this attempts to stretch the limbs,
fearing every movement. In the other two types of fatigue, of which they
are accustomed to call the one 'wound-like' and the other 'stretched', such
a movement also sometimes occurs, whenever they are either altogether
small, or come into being after flatulent or vaporous superfluities. At any
rate, whenever 'wound-like' fatigue is present to too great an extent, they
do not bear any movement whatever, but are in pain as with a wound, and
shiver in the body. If the symptom increases, they come near to a shivering
condition, for in this they shiver even before they move.

V.4 Just as, whenever a 'wound-like sensation' occurs, those who move
shiver, and more if more violently, so the shivering condition, whenever
it leads to movement, brings about a rigor. For all these occur through
mordant superfluities, yet they differ [**VII.180K**] from each other in the
amount of the superfluities themselves, in the movement, and in being
sometimes more mordant and sometimes less, as well as in the nature of
the fatigued body, whether it is not easily affected or easily affected, whether
it is weak, and whether it is keenly sensitive or insensitive. For that which is

---

47 I have taken some licence in the translation of this sentence, including the numbering.
48 For this term see also *De sanitate tuenda* VI.235–7K (where there is reference to Hippocrates) and
   VI.280K, 288K.
49 It is somewhat unclear exactly what process Galen is describing here.
50 I have simply transliterated the term *ostokopos* which Durling (1993), who has *osteokopos*, describes
   as 'an inflammatory attack, which makes one feel as if one's bones were giving way'.

keenly sensitive and weak is distressed by the slightest cause, whereas that which is strong and insensitive needs a substantial cause for the genesis of such a symptom. Is it, then, in these alone, or also in being moved or not being moved with respect to the cause, or when moved, being moved either more quickly or more slowly, that there is a very great difference in the symptoms? It seems to me to be like this in that the same man when at rest is sometimes seized by an irregularity alone, whereas when moved he shivers, and when he exercises he has rigors. Therefore doctors, having been taught by experience, advise those so fatigued to abstain from all movement.

V.5 But we know also that some of those with indigestion, should they rest, are not affected, whereas, should they go to the bath or stand in the sun, they shiver, and even more so if they exercise. For the sun, **[VII.181K]** bathing and exercise excite hitherto inactive superfluities to movement just as, in fact, anger also does in the psychical affections (*pathos*). Previously inactive superfluities excite to movement of themselves by heating, attenuating and vaporizing, so it is not surprising that when these [superfluities] are inactive they distress bodies less, whereas, when they are moved, they greatly distress and agitate [bodies that] shiver, have rigors, and are feverish. And indeed, such hard bodies as fall on the eyes from without, when the eyelids are closed and at rest, distress the part either very slightly or not at all, whereas, when [the eyelids] are moving, they bring a pain that is hard to bear. But also, apart from the example, it is possible to discover from the nature of the matter itself that a cause which is moving is more distressing than one which is stationary whenever, at least, what is borne occurs through perceiving bodies, as was just now proposed in relation to the eyes. For the argument was not about the humours flowing in the veins and arteries, but about those in the flesh and the whole system of the animal. Whenever, then, something carried through these is borne forcibly to the skin, **[VII.182K]** in its passage through the flesh and the skin it necessarily stabs, pierces, divides and wounds all those things it might encounter.

V.6 That every mordant and moving cause, whether it should be hot or cold, brings the animal to shivering and rigors, it is primarily possible to know from the following things. If you suddenly sprinkle boiling water on a healthy body, or plunge it into a spark-emitting fire, it will immediately develop shivering. But also sometimes, when caustic medicaments are placed on ulcerated parts, people first shiver, next have rigors, and then some become feverish. But also the tertian fevers, which are undoubtedly the most bilious and hot of all fevers, are certainly those most attended with shivering, and to the extent that they should happen to be more pure, so the rigor in them is also the more violent. But also, in someone having a bilious remittent fever (*kausos*), there is lysis when a rigor supervenes, Hippocrates says, because the bile, which until then was caught up in the veins, is preferentially driven out by Nature through the flesh to the skin.[51] Therefore, the rigor is at once a symptom and a sign of the movement and the actual bringing forth, which is made by perceiving bodies. [**VII.183K**] In consequence, those who have rigors in this way sweat, and are henceforth freed of the fever, when the bile in them is evacuated. Sometimes it makes the impulse not to the skin but to places within, and is cleared out through vomiting and, at the same time, through the stomach downwards. Often it is carried internally and externally on the same day, so that they sweat and, at the same time, vomit and pass the bile downwards. Those who think the rigor is a cause of health in a bilious remittent fever due to the cold, in that opposites are the cures of opposites, are altogether mistaken. First and foremost, if this were true it would presumably inspire them to bring about a rigor, partly by sprinkling or pouring cold water, partly by taking the sick person naked into the cold air, or throwing them into a receptacle of cold water. Thereafter, if indeed lysis does occur in those with bilious remittent fevers (*kausos*) who have rigors due to the change to the opposite, they ought to stop being feverish after the rigor. But this is not the case. For they do not, at the same time, by having a rigor cease to be febrile. In fact, after the rigor they are seized by a much greater fever than before, [**VII.184K**] but whenever they sweat profusely, they either vomit yellow bile, or it passes out[52] of them through the intestine. For after a rather violent movement of the bile, it is fitting that a rather violent fever is stirred up. That people have rigors, then, not only due to cold causes, but also due to hot [causes], has now been shown.

V.7 For what reason the same symptom follows the most opposite causes is what we must speak of next, bearing in mind again those things we showed to be distressing for the separative capacity. For this does not, of course, separate the things in the open cavities of the organs, as was shown with respect to things in the stomach, uterus, both bladders,[53] intestines, lungs and nose, yet neglect the superfluities built up in bodies themselves. Rather, every day it also separates from these things the entire excess without

---

[51] Hippocrates, *Aphorisms* IV.53.
[52] The verb *hyperchomai* has a particular application to the passing of excretory material – see also *In Hippocratis Prognosticum commentarii* XVIIIB.147K.
[53] I have supplied a conjunction before *entera* as the Latin versions do. 'Both bladders' are the gall bladder and the urinary bladder. *De usu partium* V.6 speaks of 'the bladder at the liver' and shortly afterwards (V.7) of 'both bladders' (I.272H, I.274H).

disturbance and during a transpiration imperceptible to sense – whenever, that is, the animal is governed by the law of nature. On the other hand, whenever something mordant exists in it, and particularly when this has a strong movement, [the animal] is, in fact, distressed and hastens to separate it by that method which would best allow something to be expelled from the parts of the body itself. [VII.185K] That is to say, when the parts gather together and press to themselves, and then each expels the part of the superfluity pertaining to itself. But if you suppose that all parts set in motion this same movement at the same time, a certain shaking and agitation will take hold of the whole body, such as obviously takes hold in rigors. For it must be the case, I think, when all the muscles are agitated, that they agitate the joints with themselves and, when these are agitated, there occurs a certain involuntary stretching and bending, such movement being different from that in spasms and palpitations.

V.8 In like manner to spasms, the movements are not brought about by the capacity itself, whereas, in relation to palpitations, it is not in like manner but, as has been stated before, the limb is raised by a muscle distended by flatulent *pneuma*.[54] With rigors, as was said just now, the whole part moves when the muscle clears itself out. In relation to the movement of those [rigors], the whole muscle is shaken and concussed and agitates with it at the same time the joint into which it is inserted. Such a [VII.186K] movement also occurs in the muscles of the thorax in anomalous (non-uniform) *dyscrasias*,[55] and because of this, a shorter and rougher cough follows them. For the muscles shake violently, being incited to separate those things distressing to their own flesh through the channels of the lung, whereas, in other coughs, it was shown that these fall on the lung violently, brought about for the purpose of a great and concentrated emission of breath. They attack still more violently in sneezes, which expel the breath that has concentrated there, wishing to effect a cleansing in the nose. And knowing this, some who are weak in terms of capacity yet who need to spit out things in the thorax and lung, set in motion a sneeze in themselves by irritating the nostrils so that, through the force of the movement, they spit out what they had been unable to expel with coughs. But enough has been said previously about such coughs. The coughs in a *dyscrasia* of the respiratory organs are from the same class as rigors and shiverings but differ in that the perception of them is more rapid, the respiratory organs never being at rest. For it was shown before [VII.187K] that movement particularly puts to the test such conditions in relation to the whole body. Whenever, then,

[54] See II.6 (VII.162K). [55] These are the 'non-uniform bi-*dyscrasias* (hot and cold, dry and moist).

the distressing things are moist in nature, by this violent shaking and agitation during cough or rigor, being cast out by the separative capacity, they
are in every case borne to suitable places, some upward, some downwards
to the stomach, and some outwards to the skin, so that there is a perceptible
evacuation of them. Whenever some *pneuma*-like substance alone, apart
from moisture, whether hotter than is proper or colder, passes through
the body, people at that time certainly shiver and have rigors. Sometimes,
however, owing to the same cause, they neither vomit nor sweat, nor does
anything perceptible to such people pass downward, as would be so if the
things irritating the separative capacity were air-like.[56] In the same way, in
the case of very hot baths, particularly when we approach them suddenly
and precipitately without prior warming, we immediately develop shivering. It is the same whenever we pass suddenly into cold air, or also if not
suddenly but over a long time, we are forced to be in it, as is sometimes
accustomed to happen on journeys. **[VII.188K]** The cure for such a rigor
is heat – not sweating, or vomiting, or excretion from the stomach. When,
however, as was said, either a cold or a hot cause brings about a rigor, in
heat that is airy, cold is sufficient as a remedy, whereas, in heat that is moist,
fever necessarily supervenes, and evacuation is the remedy. In cold that is
air-like, heat is the remedy whilst in cold that is moist, sometimes digestion alone suffices, sometimes evacuation, and sometimes both occurring
together.

V.9 There is, then, this antiquated opinion that a fever invariably follows
a rigor but this is not in fact altogether true. Not, that is, should one
define it properly, just as one who accepts the opinions expounded by
the ancients ought to define these things sympathetically, not refute them
unsympathetically. Nevertheless, the argument is not in this way true. Not,
that is, if in making the definition we should say that in those rigors stirred
up apart from a cause external[57] to our body, a fever will necessarily follow
them.[58] For it has been seen not only by us, but also by many doctors before
us, that rigors already exist apart from fevers although they are, at least,
not as strong as those that precede **[VII.189K]** exact tertian or quartan
fevers, or those that bring to a crisis fevers that are ardent or hot. Such
rigors customarily follow abnormal ways of life, when people in idleness
fill themselves with food and often bathe after nourishment. Often too,

---

[56] There is a difference here in the punctuation of this rather involved sentence, and consequently in
the sense, between the Greek and Latin texts in Kühn, and between the Latin texts themselves – see,
for example, Copus (1548), p. 532. I have followed the Greek version.
[57] Here *prophasis* is clearly applied to external causes.
[58] The reading of this somewhat confusing passage follows Copus (p. 541)

whenever the qualities of the foods themselves are from a more cold or phlegmatic mixture, there is the greatest susceptibility in those so disposed to be seized by unwarmable rigors. Nor is it surprising that doctors in former times never saw such rigors as there would not have been those who erred with respect to a healthy way of life equal to those there are now, nor had the use of baths become prevalent to such a degree. But, as has been said just now, such rigors are more shivering than concussive. For the first perception in us in the case of abnormal superfluities is of irregularity, and whenever, in fact, such things are pungent, the perception is mordant. The second [perception] is of a slight shivering, then more severe, then so great as already to be associated with a rigor. Then there is the rigor itself alone, concussing and shaking the parts. This rigor, in the case of cold humours, would never occur, for such [humours] are not at first moved violently [**VII.190K**] owing to thickness. But sometimes, if they are thin, they will bring a rigor, although certainly not so strong. For it is not possible for thinned phlegm to accept the same thinning that thinned yellow bile accepts. Doctors of old did not know such a rigor at all, although they did know that [which occurs] in fatal diseases. Thus Hippocrates, in the *Aphorisms*, said: 'If in a fever without intermission a rigor attacks someone already weak, it is fatal.'[59] For in such rigors, Nature sets in motion distressing things for the purpose of expulsion but, having been overcome, it collapses and is quenched, and because of this the symptom is fatal. In quartan fevers, the rigor is mixed from hot and cold. For black bile is by nature a cold humour, whereas, when it receives in addition a certain putrefaction through which it also kindles a fever, to the extent that there is a gain of heat, so there is also of putrefaction. And we have shown that rigors follow, even in hot causes.

V.10 That in all such situations [**VII.191K**] the extreme parts of the body particularly are cooled and lacking in blood,[60] and with them the whole skin and what is superficial beneath it, and for what reason this occurs is what we must next examine. And there is from the primary and, as one might say, most authoritative movements, a movement of the innate heat[61] both inward and outward, occurring in many psychical affections (*pathos*), and with it at the same time, quite clearly both *pneuma* and blood are sometimes borne inward towards the *arche* and gathered together, but

---

[59] Hippocrates, *Aphorisms* IV.46.
[60] This is an unusual verb, found, for example, in the pseudo-Aristotelian *Problems* IV (on sexual intercourse) and also in Galen in *De compositione medicamentorum secundum locos* XII.693K.
[61] Innate heat is an important concept and a point of contention among philosophers and medical writers. It is discussed in the section on terminology (I.4c). See also Solmsen (1957).

sometimes pass outwards and pour forth. Perhaps I shall have the audacity to give an opinion about the substance of the soul itself in some other work, but for what is now at hand, apart from being audacious, this is also superfluous. It seems, then, that whatever this might be, it is one of two things: either it uses the primary organs for all functions by the *pneuma* or the blood, or the heat in one or both together, or it is in these themselves.[62]

V.11 It is possible to see clearly the movements of this in many other affections (*pathos*), and particularly in those that are psychical. For example, there are fear and anger;[63] the one [**VII.192K**] leads and draws together the *pneuma* and blood inward towards the *arche* with a cooling of what is superficial, whereas the other passes out, pours forth and heats. That which is compounded from both is called being anxious,[64] and is irregular in its movements. Accordingly, the pulses of the arteries and of the heart are very small and very weak in those who are afraid, but very large and very violent in those who are angry, and are irregular in those who are anxious. In the case of shame, the movement of the psychical capacity is primarily inward. Then, having collected together, it undertakes a return again towards the exterior. If, however, it does not return, it is fear, not shame. For shame occurs suddenly, the psychic capacity expecting nothing bad but, as one might say, owing to an innate softness or cowardice, the man does not bear the association of a far stronger man but runs away, as if there were a kind of urging on from the feet occurring. And owing to this alone, it departs towards the depths, as if fleeing away from being cooled. When reason has stirred up and excited the affective part of the soul,[65] [**VII.193K**] which is what is being afraid and ashamed, it [the psychic capacity] returns and moves towards the outside, predominantly by the same kind of movement in which a recall of heat would occur after bathing in cold water. In those afraid, at least, inasmuch as reason does not completely stir up and stimulate the affective part of the soul, invariably the heat is extinguished more, so some of them also have rigors. That which they suffer in a concentrated

---

[62] Apart from *De placitis Hippocratis et Platonis*, Galen's important surviving writings on the soul are contained in *Quod animi mores corporis temperamenta sequantur* (IV.767–822K), *De propriorum animi cuiuslibet affectuum dignotione et curatione* (V.1–57K) and *De cuiuslibet animi peccatorum dignotione et curatione* (V.58–103K). See also Singer (1992, 1997) and Hankinson (1991a).

[63] See Aristotle's *De anima* 403a4–404b20 on these two emotions and their physical correlates.

[64] On *agonia* as a mental state, see the pseudo-Aristotelian *Problems* 869b6 and Chrysippus, SVF II.248. In the former there is: 'Is it because nervousness (*agonia*) is a kind of fear connected with the beginning of an action, and fear causes a cooling of the upper part of the body . . .' (Forster, in Barnes (1984), p. 1338).

[65] This is a description used by Galen predominantly in *De placitis Hippocratis et Platonis* – see particularly V.5.23–33 and V.6.22–37, where the views of other philosophers, notably Plato and Chrysippus, are considered.

way in fears, they suffer slightly in distresses, the affections (*pathos*) differing in magnitude and strength but not in the whole class. Accordingly,
some have also died in sudden fears, whenever the soul, weak in nature
and possessed suddenly by a strong affection (*pathos*), is quenched and
smothered. For quenching occurs due to the very nature of the affection
(*pathos*) which has its genesis in the cooling, whereas smothering is due to
all the blood gathering together and being borne to the *arche*. No one who
is angry dies, as there would be neither a cooling of heat nor a dissolution of
strength. Nevertheless, some pusillanimous men have died when rejoicing
greatly, just like those who are afraid. For the psychic capacity does not
move towards the exterior because of strength and seething at the same
time [VII.194K] but quite the contrary, in that, if it previously had some
strength, this it now releases and disperses. So, for example, it is broken
up whenever, being relaxed to the greatest degree, it is borne towards the
exterior.

V.12 Pain, on the contrary, compelling the soul to move, brings symptoms like great fear. For people are pale and cold, they shiver and tremble,
they have a weak or absent pulse, and finally they die, just like those who
are panic-stricken. For also in them the innate heat, being simultaneously
released and quenched, withdraws to the *arche*. When these kinds of affections (*pathos*) bring death, it is not surprising of course that they also bring
swooning (*leipopsychia*). And so, therefore, it ought not still to be surprising that the symptoms consequent upon swooning, both others and the
involuntary separation of superfluities,[66] follow. However, it is not appropriate at the present time to tarry further over such matters. Rather we
must go on with the matter in hand. Whenever, then, a rigor occurs with
humours that are simultaneously hot and mordant, it is no wonder that
all the external parts are cooled, since the psychic capacity contracts to the
depths along with the blood. For there is a sensation [VII.195K] under
these circumstances of cold of those [parts] that are external but not of cold
of those in the depths. For, in fact, some are strongly thirsty at that time,
as if the internal heat were being preserved in them. So with good reason
such things as customarily occur with rigors can be collected together here.
For if pains that settle themselves quite strongly in some one part bring
about swooning (*leipopsychia*) and cooling simultaneously, it would not be
surprising that when they exist simultaneously in the whole body, they at
least cause cooling, even if they don't bring about swooning (*leipopsychia*)

---

[66] I have retained 'separation' for *ekkrisis* and 'superfluity' for *perissoma* in the pursuit of consistency
although it seems clear that Galen is here referring to the involuntary expulsion of excretory material.

or death. For the pains during a rigor are cognate with all other pains, although they are deficient in magnitude and duration in comparison with those that destroy. For, in fact, they are less by far and of shorter duration. Certainly colicky pain often persists for two days in succession, whereas a rigor would be more brief to the extent that it is stronger. For in this the movement of the soul does not resemble that in fears, but rather more that in shame, and bathing in cold water. At any rate, the capacity both contends with, and struggles against, those things that are distressing until it should dislodge them and force them all out. Owing, then, to the violent impacts, [**VII.196K**] and because it has been collected together in the depths, it returns again with considerable heat, and stirs up fever in the case of rigors, having the material allied to its magnitude. If sometimes during the struggle it becomes fatigued before repelling the distressing material, for this happens owing to the weakness of the capacity or the greatness of the cause, death inevitably follows, as has been said before.

VI.1 Since, then, we have brought the argument to this point, let us proceed now to its summation, encompassing all the things previously mentioned under brief headings, and adding however many remain. Coughs, sneezes, hiccups and rigors are strong and violent movements of the separative capacity whereas stretching and yawning [are movements] of it, but moderate. More moderate too are the movements in shivering. Even more moderate than these are the movements in the irregularities (*anomalia*), so that one might say that such things are scarcely movements at all but only sensations, just as there are the sensations in the 'wound-like' fatigues. And more than these still [is this so] in itching (*knesis*). [**VII.197K**] For in this symptom the sensation is of superfluities associated with itching[67] alone, in that one cannot give a name to these in any other way unless one wishes to speak of something alkaline or salty or sharp, for such is their nature. It is possible to learn about these from things that are external, like the sea anemone, the squill, brine, seawater and other such things, no less than from those very things that are in the body. For itching occurs in those who do not wash, or are filthy, or have indigestion, or who eat unwholesome foods, and far more certainly in those with *psora* or *lepra*, because the humour is more copious and thicker in such conditions. And because of this, they scratch greatly and more than all those who itch without such a condition. Nor does scratching very vigorously help them, not even should they excoriate

---

[67] I have taken Galen to be referring here to superfluities that only produce itching. For the term *knesmodes* in this sense see the pseudo-Aristotelian *Problems* VII (887a35).

themselves, owing to the distressing humour which filled them remaining
in them and, as one might say, being fixed in the skin. For this is not scanty
or fine, as in those who are merely unwashed and filthy, but very copious
and thick, and sometimes also viscid. All such symptoms are, at any rate,
born of a bad humour, differing [**VII.198K**] in the nature and magnitude
of the cause and, besides these, in quietude and movement. For it is scanty,
thin, salty and motionless in those who itch whereas in the 'wound-like'
fatigues it is scanty, thin, mordant and motionless. In those with *lepra* or
psora it is great in amount, thick, salty and motionless. In the shiverings
it is scanty, thin, mordant and has a movement that is slight. If, however,
it is moved violently, or is more copious or more mordant, it brings on a
rigor not shivering. This [the rigor] is greatest when it [the bad humour]
is very copious, very strong, very mordant and moved most violently. It
is least when a moderate increase in one of these things effects a change
from shivering to rigor. There are very many others [rigors] between the
least rigor and the greatest, differing from each other in terms of more or
less, or because the cause of the movement is more or less, or because the
mordancy is more or less, or, in addition, due to the difference in amount,
or, in addition to these again, either because the cause creating the rigor is
increased in all the differences spoken of, or in some, or in one. [**VII.199K**]
And all these symptoms customarily exist when the cause is concentrated
around the skin and the flesh underlying it.

    VI.2 [As for] coughs, sneezes and hiccups, coughs occur when the causes
exist in the lung, throat or chest; sneezes occur when [causes exist] in the
nose; hiccups occur when [they exist] in the stomach and its orifice. What is
common in all the things spoken of is the separative capacity for distressing
things stirring itself to very violent movements for the expulsion of the
distressing things, just as has been said before with respect to the other
things concerning their genesis. So that sometimes a sneeze also *per accidens*
brings about a cure of humours existing together in the lung, although it
does not occur because of them. In this way also, in the stomach and
its orifice in which hiccups arise, sneezes clear them out *per accidens* and,
by virtue of this, become the cures of the hiccups. For the abdominal
muscles, being stretched out and tightly drawn in, push on the stomach so
as to bring about an impulse that is more violent on the actual disturbing
causes, which it strives to expel. I have spoken of almost all [**VII.200K**]
the symptoms of both the psychical functions and capacities along with the
causes generating these. Nevertheless, in the first book I made mention of
none of the symptoms occurring in the physical functions and capacities,
whilst in this second book, because of the commonality of the argument,

relatively little has been said about these also. But we shall, at least, provide for them a full and specific account in the third book, which follows this one.

VII.1 Now that we have completed everything regarding the symptoms occurring in the psychical capacities in the two [books], we shall speak of those involving the authoritative functions. In these there are also three primary classes of symptoms. One is destruction of function, another is damage, the third a turning aside to a difference of form. Destruction occurs in the so-called dementias (*morosis*) and amnesias (*lethe*).[68] For one has seen not infrequently certain diseases that have come to some transition lead to dementia (*morosis*) and amnesia (*lethe*). At any rate, we have seen some who have completely forgotten both letters and skills **[VII.201K]** and have not even remembered their own names, the sort of thing that Thucydides said happened in the Plague.[69] For some of the survivors did not recognize themselves or their friends, whilst one also sees some who, owing to extreme age, are overcome by very similar symptoms. From this it is clear that dementia (*morosis*) and amnesia (*lethe*) occur as a consequence of cooling. Moreover, medicines producing such symptoms are cold in their capacities. Certainly such symptoms signify a cooling of the actual body of the brain, just as also the apoplexies and epilepsies seem to occur through an abundance of phlegmatous humour gathered together in the cavities of the brain itself. And because of this, both the genesis and resolution of these things is sudden, this in no wise being able to occur in the *dyscrasias* of bodies. The moderate damages, like the 'numbness' (*narke*) of reason and of memory, occur in response to a more slight cooling, either through one of the cold medicines being taken into the body, **[VII.202K]** or being applied to the head, or when a cold humour has been gathered in the brain.

VII.2 And all the deliria (*paraphrosune*), which are defective movements of the authoritative capacity, arise on the basis of abnormal humours or through a *dyscrasia* of these in the brain. The *phrenitides* is what they are called when accompanied by fevers, *manias* when they are without these.[70] Sometimes they follow mordant and hot humours, the kind that are of yellow bile particularly, although they often arise in a *dyscrasia* of the brain

---

[68] Both these terms are mentioned by Hippocrates in *Prorrhetic* I (32 and 64 respectively). There is some textual doubt about the former whilst 'amnesia' may be too strong for the latter with 'forgetfulness' being better. See also Siegel (1968) on *morosis* (pp. 274–5) and section I.4d above.

[69] Thucydides' description of the Plague of Athens is to be found in II.47–54. The mental disturbances are referred to in II.49(8).

[70] For descriptions of *phrenitis* and *mania* see, in particular, Siegel (1968), pp. 270–4. He, however, considers delirium without fever under the heading of '*Paraphrosyne*' – see pp. 264–9.

itself tending towards more heat. The melancholic derangements alone
have a colder humour as a cause. For *phrenitis* does not simply arise on the
basis of hot humours but is brought about after inflammation involving the
brain and the meninges. In the other fevers, deliria (*paraphrosune*) occur
when such a humour is increased in the brain. And those, in fact, that arise
during the peaks of the most acute fevers have a mordant and hot vapour
rising up to the brain. The melancholic derangements vary **[VII.203K]**
by there being several kinds of false imaginings. In all these, however, one
thing seems to be common, which has been stated by Hippocrates: 'If fear or
despair continues for a long period, such a thing is melancholia.'[71] For they
are all despairing without reason, nor, were you to ask, would they be able
to say they are distressed about anything, not a few of them fearing death or
some other thing not worthy of fear. There are also those who are strongly
desirous of death. It is, at least, not surprising that fears arise through the
black bile taking possession of the *arche* of the rational soul, or depressions
or presentiments of death either. For of those things external to the body,
we see nothing so frightening to us as the darkness. Whenever, then, some
kind of darkness envelops the rational part of the soul, of necessity a person
is always afraid, as he would always be carrying around in the body the
reason for his fear. For what happens to us from an external source at a
certain time, when the deepest darkness takes hold of the ambient air,
so the same thing is stirred up by the melancholic [humours] within and
from the body itself, **[VII.204K]** when either the black bile itself takes
hold of the brain, or when some melancholic vapour rises up, just as in the
disease called flatulence or hypochondriasis.[72]

---

[71] Hippocrates, *Aphorisms* VI.23.
[72] For a discussion of Galen's views on the 'sympathetic' affection constituting *hypochondriasis* see Siegel
(1968), pp. 192 ff.

CHAPTER II.6

On the Causes of Symptoms *III*

SYNOPSIS

I.1 Preliminary remarks on the symptoms of the physical functions and their general correspondence in type to those of the psychical, i.e. loss, reduction, abnormality. This is briefly exemplified by reference to the stomach.

I.2 Changes of digestion relate to the alterative capacity itself, or to external factors. Damage to the capacity may be due to a *dyscrasia*, or to an organic disease affecting it.

I.3 'External' factors include changes in the quality or quantity of what is ingested, changes in the times or sequences of ingestion, or to lack of sleep.

I.4 Brief reference to the three components of digestion as a whole, followed by a further statement about the threefold division of symptoms into loss, reduction and abnormality of function, *bradypepsia* being the second and 'corruptions' the third.

I.5 Consideration of the post-gastric components of digestion as seen by Galen – that is, in the veins and in the 'whole system (*hexis*)'. Privation of function results in atrophy, reduced function in emaciation, and abnormal function in *leuke* and *elephantiasis*. Causative factors come down to weakness of the capacity, problems of intake, and external factors including way of life.

I.6 A statement that the doctor must not only know what has happened but why it has happened, specifically here in relation to disturbances of digestion.

I.7 Defective function of the capacity is attributable to *dyscrasia*. The resulting 'corruptions' of food have characteristics specific to the particular food.

II.1 The same threefold division applies to the 'contracting around' due to the retentive capacity – the results are 'inflations' and 'splashings'.

II.2 Defective movements of the retentive capacity involve tremors, palpitations, agitations and spasms. Also symptoms of the alterative and retentive capacities may be mixed.

II.3 Symptoms of the separative capacity include vomiting, hiccup and rapid passage downward from the stomach leading to *leienteria*. These symptoms may occur simultaneously.

II.4 There may also be failure of the attractive capacity of the stomach, particularly related to functional or structural abnormalities involving the cardiac orifice.

II.5 Symptoms of the intestines also relate to disturbances of 'wrapping around' and 'pushing forward' – peristalsis generally. Some symptoms are due to impaction of faeces. There is a correspondence between gastric and intestinal symptoms in terms of cause – *dyscrasias*, abnormal swellings, and abnormal contained material.

III.1 Distribution of nutriment from stomach to liver, and from liver to tissues, will also be abnormal in one of three ways – absence, reduction, abnormality. Causes will also be of three kinds – *dyscrasias* of the attracting parts, organic diseases of these parts, or abnormalities in the material being distributed. The first weakens capacity, the second narrows passages, and the third involves increased thickness or viscidity.

III.2 The three superfluities of digestion occurring in the veins (bitter bile, black bile, serum) will depend, in their amount and distribution, on the nature of the abnormality of function.

III.3 Resultant symptoms will be characteristic of the causative superfluity, as for example jaundice of yellow bile.

IV.1 On nutrition generally as perhaps the most necessary of the physical functions. It involves not only alteration but also assimilation. Again the threefold division of absent, reduced and abnormal is mentioned. Different visible changes in flesh will depend on variations in distribution of the different humours.

IV.2 More on the effects of nutrition on the state and appearance of the flesh with reference to Aristotle's observations in animals. Similar considerations apply to plants. There is also brief discussion of the bi-directional nature of the interaction between the nutriment and what is nourished.

IV.3 Some further consideration of this last point, followed by the specific consideration of certain conditions – *leuke*, *leientery*, dysentery, cholera and the dropsies.

V.1 Consideration of symptoms related to 'the quantity and quality of things separated', beginning with blood from various sources, i.e. haemorrhage.

V.2 Three causes of haemorrhage are identified – the capacity opening up a vessel (as in epistaxis), changes in the blood itself, and damage to blood vessels. Factors predisposing to the last are discussed. A fourth cause, that of *diapedesis*, is mentioned, which Galen particularly identifies with the passage of a bloody serum in the urine due to hepatic or renal disease.

V.3 Vomiting, and why it occurs. Things that weigh down or irritate the stomach. These are things that are unable to nourish.

V.4 On rapid passage of material downward from the stomach. This material may be useful, or may be 'corrupted' nutriment. The cause of premature downward passage lies in the amount or nature of the material, or in a weakened capacity.

V.5 On delay or reduction of downward passage. This may be due to weakness or disturbed sensation of the intestines, or to abnormalities in quantity (paucity) or quality of material (food). Weakness of the muscles of the epigastrium may contribute.

V.6 On increase in the amount of material passed downward. This may be due to the things taken in, failure of distribution, or things flowing into the stomach. There are also 'continuous separations' due to *dyscratic* weakness of the stomach, or to 'stinging' things within it. Four causes of 'stinging' are listed. Finally, continuous involuntary separation may occur owing to paralysis of the muscles controlling outflow.

VI.1 Consideration of the vaporous *pneumas* (flatus). These are related to abnormalities of cold or heat.

VI.2 More on flatulent superfluity passed via mouth or anus. Retained flatus and the sounds it may produce are also considered. There is discussion of *borborygmos*.

VII.1 Abnormal separations due to material flowing into the stomach. Reference to Hippocrates and his description of bloody diarrhoea following loss of a member.

VII.2 Abnormal separation of partially digested food. This is attributable to liver disease.

VII.3 Other abnormal excretions from the stomach may be due to failure of distribution. Blood mixed with black bile may constitute the excreted material and will have a distinctive appearance.

VII.4 Four kinds of bloody separations: (i) blood itself (severed limbs, failure of exercise); (ii) watery blood (hepatic weakness); (iii) blood mixed with black bile; (iv) blood mixed with pus and scales. The first three are continuous and copious, the fourth is intermittent and scanty and is due to ulceration of the intestines.

VIII.1 On the failure to pass (separate) urine. Galen makes the point that this may be due to problems with the bladder or its outlets, or to failure to produce urine due to renal disease.

VIII.2 More on the urine, specifically causes of bladder outlet obstruction and weakness of the bladder itself.

VIII.3 On defective evacuation of urine due to bladder weakness or changes in the nature of the urine. The latter are related to disturbances of renal function.

IX.1 A discussion of the different kind of sweats and their causes.

X.1 A general consideration of the fact that damage to capacities can variably affect the different capacities.

X.2 On the variable effects of different qualities of materials on the different capacities.

X.3 That hot and moist bodies are nourished best and, conversely, cold and dry bodies are nourished worst. The reasons for this.

X.4 On the differences in the capacities characteristic of children, together with some general comments on the relative strengths of the different capacities.

X.5 More on the differences in the capacities in children.

X.6 Discussion of the relative merits of different qualities in foods in relation to nutrition at different ages. Also consideration of the changes in nourished bodies due to age or disease and their effects on functions.

X.7 The retentive capacity is stronger in organs that are warm and dry and weaker in those that are moist and cold. The relative effects of heat, cold, moisture and dryness on hardness, strength and tension in structures, and the relation of these factors to ease of distension or otherwise.

XI.1 Galen considers what he identifies as a further class of symptoms related to the quantity and quality of material separated from various structures, particularly nose, ears, eyes, palate, throat and uterus.

XI.2 Some comments on the distinction between *catarrh* and *coryza*.

XI.3 On changes in menstruation.

XI.4 On other materials discharged from the uterus grouped under the heading of 'flux muliebris'. This may involve different materials (i.e. differing in qualities) and reflect disturbances in the uterus itself, or elsewhere.

XI.5 A brief discussion of priapism and its relation to flatulent *pneuma*, and of spermatorrhoea.

XII.1 On a final class of symptoms – that involving perceptible (by the observer) changes of colour or odour.

XII.2 Final general considerations about causation. The distinction between symptoms that follow other symptoms of necessity, and those that do not, and between effects that have a single cause, and those that have multiple causes or multiple possible causes. These points are illustrated by consideration of indigestion.

XII.3 Further consideration of indigestion in relation to the matter of whether a particular symptom necessarily follows another symptom or not.

ON THE CAUSES OF SYMPTOMS III

I.1 [VII.205K] Inasmuch as the number of symptoms that will come about in relation to the physical functions and capacities has the same method of discovery as also pertains to those supervening in the psychical functions, it is better perhaps to train ourselves in the forms of these individually, just as we trained ourselves in those of the psychical. Indeed, the chief point of discovery of all causes which inflict harm on the capacities is the knowledge of the manner by which they function when healthy. [**VII.206K**] For if the stomach digests food by kneading,[1] when it is hindered in kneading it will bring about symptoms of digestion. When it does not knead at all, it does not digest at all. When it kneads abnormally, it digests abnormally. By the same token, if it digests by putrefaction, by not putrefying it does not digest. If, on the other hand, as we showed, digestion itself is a change in quality, and occurs owing to the stomach making the food like itself, I presume it is clear to anyone that a failure of change will result in symptoms of digestion. If [the food] is altogether unchanged, the symptom is called *apepsia*, like *akinesia* and *anaesthesia* in relation to the actions of the psyche, these signifying destruction or privation of the function of the primary part of the soul. If [the food] is changed but not properly, this too is called *apepsia*, although this signifies not privation as before, but only malfunction. This malfunction is also twofold, either due to slowing and not yet taking on the proper change, or due to being completely ruined so it is altogether unable to take on the order of nature. [**VII.207K**] The former they call *bradypepsia*, whereas the latter has not received a specific name.[2] Such, then, are the damages of digestion.

I.2 Whilst there are causes of these, what is common is a failure of the objective of the alterative capacity. This may be divided according to kind and class. The two primary classes of failure are the one where the capacity itself is affected, and the one where there is a defect from without. Each is further divided – the damage of the capacity in two ways which are: (i) due to its own substance; (ii) due to some disease of the organs. The defects from without [are divided] into three which are: (i) in the super-fluities in the stomach; (ii) in the foods; (iii) in the time of sleep. But the damages of capacity involving its specific substance are certain *dyscrasias* of the active (*drastikos*) qualities, whilst others are from organic diseases in the *erysipelata*, swellings (*oidemata*), inflammations (*phlegmonai*), indurations

---

[1] Of the several options for *tribo* I have chosen 'kneading'. Brock has 'triturate' in his translation of *De facultatibus naturalibus* II.119K – Brock (1916), p. 185. In his commentary on *De methodo medendi* Hankinson (1991), p. 182, links the terms with Erasistratus' theories of digestion. For Galen's own views on the digestive process see May (1968), vol. 1, pp. 51–4 for a summary, and also both *De facultatibus naturalibus* and *De usu partium* (particularly Books IV and V). See also *De methodo medendi* (X.97–110K) for Galen's views on other theories, particularly those of the Methodists.
[2] I have retained the Greek terms, *apepsia* and *bradypepsia*, for which Galen makes his own usage clear. Neither term remains in use in the way *dyspepsia* (not included here) does.

(*skirros*), abscesses (*apostema*) and pustules (*anthrax*), and all other such diseases, either simple or combined, that arise in relation to the stomach.[3] Owing to all these, certainly, the stomach digests badly, the actual capacity by which [**VII.208K**] it digests being damaged. In the *dyscrasias* this is in relation to its specific substance, whereas in the other diseases, in however many that are simply organic, it is only hindered, and in however many that are combined from *dyscrasias* and organic [diseases], in both ways. In the presence of these causes,[4] the stomach digests badly, even when there is no defect of other things externally.

I.3 On the other hand, when the stomach itself is not affected, the animal does not digest owing to an excessive amount of food and drink, or owing to an abnormal quality, or owing to an inappropriate time, or owing to an improper order,[5] or owing to slight superfluity, or owing to lack of sleep. But in the case of abnormal qualities of foods and in the case of superfluities, such as exist in relation to the stomach, they fail to digest in conjunction with corruption,[6] and this is sometimes because of an improper order and sometimes an inappropriate time. I say 'improper order' if it so happens that they take apples and pomegranates first, and vegetables with olive and fish oil last, whereas I say 'inappropriate time' if, in the early morning before the previous food has been properly passed on or before they have exercised a little, they take breakfast. The steaming[7] 'corruptions' occur in the case of hotter and more bilious foods, [**VII.209K**] the acidic in the case of those that are colder in nature and more phlegmatic. So too, in the case of superfluities, the acidic are those that are phlegmatic and cold, whereas the steaming are those that are hot and *picrocholic*.[8] And the stomach itself, in the case of colder diseases, brings about acidic changes, but in hotter diseases, steaming changes. Those things that are hard to break

---

[3] There is some doubt about the text here since the second part of the sentence lacks a verb. The point is, however, clear in that Galen seems to be making the division he made in *De causis morborum* – that *dyscrasias* involve *homoiomeres* and combined diseases involve organs.

[4] Galen's use of *prophasis* has been discussed generally in the section on terminology in section I.4b above, with the conclusion that it is, in effect, interchangeable with *aitia*. Here this point is borne out with no suggestion that 'alleged' or 'external' is implied.

[5] Both *akairia* ('inappropriate time') and *ataxia* ('improper order') are used here in a specific sense by Galen, as he subsequently makes clear, albeit in reverse order. The term *ataxia* is generally translated simply as 'disorder' (see, for example, Aristotle, *Parts of Animals* 641b23, Plato, *Timaeus* 30a), but here it obviously relates to the sequence in which things are eaten.

[6] It is not entirely clear what Galen means by *diaphthora*. All three Latin versions have *corruptio*; hence the translation above.

[7] *knisodes* can also mean 'fatty' or 'greasy', as for example in Aristotle, *Parts of Animals* 675b11. The Latin versions use *nidorosus* (Copus, Kühn) or *fumosus* (Linacre).

[8] The Greek term *pikrocholic* has been retained, as has *melancholic*, the former meaning full of bitter bile, the latter of black bile. See Hippocrates, *Regimen in Acute Diseases* XXXIV, LXI.

down beyond the capacity or beyond sleep bring about the *bradypepsias*. Whenever, apart from corruption, complete privation of digestion occurs, one must know by this that the stomach has been completely overcome, either by an excessive quantity, as in relation to weakness of the capacity, or by severe cold. For the stomach fails to digest in such conditions because it does not attempt to digest at all.

I.4 Let these, then, also be examples for you of failure of digestion in receptacles.[9] For you will also reduce those to the same methods in turn and, in addition to those at least, those involving the third digestion, which the nourishment of the whole mass follows, since the nutriment distributed to the veins from the stomach has the same correspondence to these, whilst that from the veins to the flesh [has the same correspondence] to those, **[VII.210K]** which the things eaten and drunk have to the stomach.[10] The previously understood manner of digestion has shown us all these things. For knowing that some such mixture from the four elements which brings about the specific nature of the body of the stomach is the cause of the change of foods, and that the element heat contributes the greatest capacity to this, we are led to the discovery of causes in the *apepsias*. And this is not only in the *apepsias*, but also in all the classes of symptoms – that which is like a destruction or privation of function (or whatever else one might wish to call it), that which is like an incomplete or deficient function, and that which is like an abnormal or defective function.[11] In the stomach then, as has been said just now, there is privation of function whenever the food is not changed to the slightest degree. Deficient digestion [exists] in the *bradypepsias*, just as there is also abnormal or defective digestion in the 'corruptions'.[12]

I.5 Regarding the veins, there is privation of function in the altogether undigested humours, whereas there is deficient function in those that are partially digested and, again, **[VII.211K]** defective [function] in those in an

---

[9] For the general use of *angeion* as a 'bodily container' see Aristotle, *History of Animals* 521b6.
[10] This is a somewhat complex sentence as it stands. What I take Galen to be saying is that in relation to the three components of digestion – stomach, veins/liver, tissues – the last being that on which ultimately the maintenance of the body depends, there are three corresponding states of nutrient material: (i) food and drink as ingested; (ii) material released via the veins to the liver after processing in the stomach; (iii) the final product of these two processes which is taken up by the tissues. The tripartite division of the process of digestion is set out by Galen in *In Hippocratis librum de alimento commentarii* XV.233K. See also May (1968), vol. 1, pp. 53–5. The 'third digestion' is then taken to be that occurring in the individual parts.
[11] This is one of the basic classificatory divisions which Galen uses in *De symtomatum differentiis* – absence/reduction/abnormality of function. Here he offers two terms for each.
[12] In I.1 (VII.206K) above Galen indicates that the term is generally applied to improper digestion which is presumably what is being discussed here.

unhealthy state.[13] Likewise, in the whole system[14] of the animal, there is, as it were, a privation with undigested humours in relation to these [animals], a deficiency, as it were, with semi-digested [humours], and an abnormality with unhealthy humours in them. From these unhealthy humours the *erysipelata*, cancers (*karkinos*) and gangrenes (*gangraina*) arise, as do cancerous sores (*phagedaina*), pustules (*anthrax*), herpetic eruptions (*herpes*) and all other such things. With respect to the function of nutrition, privation of function [equates with] atrophy, deficient nutrition [equates with] emaciation,[15] and abnormal function [is seen] in the *leukai* and in relation to what is called *elephas*. The causes of all the symptoms spoken of are the same in terms of class as those previously spoken of in the case of the stomach, some of them being referrable to a weakness of capacity, some to a defect of nutrition, and a third group to practices[16] and things that happen to animals from without. And in the same manner to those, in fact, are the weaknesses of the capacity, those that are specific to the *dyscrasias* of the *homoiomeres*, and those that are not specific, but follow organic diseases. The defects of nutrition [**VII.212K**] are divided in regard to the quantity and quality of the humours, just as also, I think, those of practices and of things coming into contact from without [are divided] into 'improper order' and 'inappropriate time'. Now I call 'practices', horse riding, fishing, sexual intercourse, bathing, walking, sailing, hunting and all things in which we simply act in some way with the body.

   I.6 Of course, it behoves a doctor to be not only at the same time a diagnostician of the symptoms themselves and a discoverer of their genesis, but also of their mode of genesis, as classified in the differentiation of effecting causes.[17] For it is appropriate not only to know if the stomach

---

[13] Galen uses *kakochumia* as a general term for an unhealthy state of the humours – see also *De symptomatum causis* I (VII.106–7K) and *De methodo medendi* X.891K. The term is also used to refer to unwholesome nutriment – cf *De alimentorum facultatibus* VI.553K and VI.641K.

[14] The relationship of *hexis* to other terms describing the state or condition of the body is considered in section I.4a.

[15] I have understood *ischnotes* to indicate a pathological state rather than simply 'leanness' – e.g. Hippocrates, *Airs, Waters, Places* XXI, Aristotle, *History of Animals* 581b26.

[16] I have followed Jones (1923) in translating *epitedeumata* as 'practices', both here and in the two following usages – see Hippocrates, *Epidemics* I.23. (Jones (1923), vol. I, p. 181). 'Ways of life/living' would also be satisfactory. As with the other two terms *ataxia* and *akairos*, Galen makes his usage clear.

[17] There are two points about the final phrase of this sentence: (i) *diaphora* is singular in the Greek but made plural in the Latin, as in the titles of the first and third treatises. Here I have opted for 'differentiation' as the translation. (ii) The use of *poietikon* as qualifying *aition* is outside the division of *prokatarktic*, *proegoumenic* and *synektic* elsewhere employed by Galen. I am indebted to Hankinson for his comment that it is a 'Stoic-tinged term for efficient cause' and drawing my attention to the relevant discussion in *De causis procatarcticis*.

has not digested at all, but also for what reason – whether it is due to an overwhelming weakness of the digestive capacity, or to some excessive quantity, or to some highly abnormal quality of the foods. For a symptom due to foods is easily put right, whereas one due to extreme failings of the capacity comes to *leienteria* or so-called tympanic dropsy (*hydrops*). And in relation to the veins likewise, one must not only examine failure of blood formation, but also why it occurs [**VII.213K**] – whether it is due to a weakness of the blood-forming capacity, for it is not hard to designate it this way, or due to an abundance of cold and undigested humours distributed from the stomach, for the one is easy to remedy whereas the other ends in *hydrops*. The same applies with the flesh. Those who are violently afflicted by diseases due to undigested humours are made flatulent and dropsical in their whole system, whereas due to weakness of the capacity there are what are called the *anasarcas* of the dropsies.[18]

I.7 All the major *dyscrasias* overthrow the capacity. But those due to strong cold have it in their nature to bring about cold affections (*pathos*). Those due to heat are the opposite. The same is also known concerning the remaining opposition and conjunction. In all these, as has been said, what is common is the greatest deviation from what accords with nature. For not to function at all in the case of moderate or customary foods indicates a very great *dyscrasia* of the stomach. But if such a thing happens owing to overwhelming heat, the food is immediately corrupted, the usual corruption tending towards [**VII.214K**] steaming although each [food] has a specific [corruption] according to its nature.[19] For some things when corrupted smell, for example, of a certain noisome odour or of filth, whereas others smell of raw fish, or of an indescribable and strange putrefaction. No food when heated strongly is able to remain unputrefied. Of course, people in such a condition are immediately excessively thirsty, and sometimes become febrile with mild or slight hectic fevers, whereas if the digestion of food is altogether destroyed by excessive cold, they are without thirst and are afebrile, and preserve the precise qualities of the foods themselves, whether they wish either to belch, or to vomit as well. And if some slight function occurs during the digestion of these, and the nature of the foods is either of indeterminate[20] mixture or of one more cold, heartburns (*oxyregmiodes*)[21]

---

[18] *Anasarca*, here given as two separate words, is retained. It is a term still, in use, albeit infrequently. Interestingly, Durling (1993) does not include it.

[19] I take Galen to mean here by this terse expression that each food has a particular form of corruption peculiar to its own nature.

[20] *Mesos* is taken in the sense of being neither good or bad (see SVF III.135) with no preponderant quality.

[21] For the term *oxyregmiodes* see Hippocrates, *Aphorisms* VI.33 and Galen, *De methodo medendi* X.579K.

are brought about. When the foods are hotter with respect to mixture, or also more flatulent in nature, the stomach is filled with vaporous *pneuma*. Certainly it is possible for it to come to such *dyscrasias* quickly, whereas the stomach would never become *dyscratic* in relation to moisture or dryness to such a degree as to destroy function without a great elapse of time. [VII.215K] And *hydrops* needs the precedence of moisture, whereas old age or wasting needs that of dryness. But distinguishing such *differentiae* is a matter for another treatise.[22]

II.1 Now one must come to the retentive capacity. In this the primary differentiation of symptoms is threefold: it may not be 'contracted around'[23] at all, or deficiently, or defectively. Through it not being contracted around at all or weakly, inflations (*pneumatosis*) and splashings (*kludon*) follow. There are inflations whenever the foods are flatulence-producing,[24] or the stomach is not altogether cold. There are splashings (*kludon*) whenever either nothing is contained in it which can be made into a vapour, or it is severely cooled, for such a condition gives rise to no vapour. It is clear that without drink, splashing (*kludon*) does not occur in the stomach. Disease is the cause of it being extremely weak, whether the stomach [is taken] as an *homoiomeric* part, or as an organic part.

   II.2 About defective movements in relation to this [capacity], that they are either tremors (*tromodes*), palpitations (*palmodes*), agitations of a sort (*klonodes*), or spasms (*spasmodes*), has been stated before in the work on [VII.216K] the *differentiae* of symptoms.[25] What kind each of the afore-mentioned movements is, and what their cause is in each case, has been made clear by the previous discussion. Now one must add this much more – that the diseases and symptoms of the retentive and separative capacities are mixed. For example, the kind of convulsive movement of the stomach that happens in hiccuping is not exactly a spasm (*spasmos*), which in fact occurs in muscles alone (the stomach is not an actual muscle nor is its opening), yet it is some kind of spasm (*spasmos*), a symptom common to both capacities: of the retentive in that the hiccuping stomach is 'contracted around' the foods abnormally and not in accord with nature, whilst of the

[22] Presumably *De temperamentis* I.509–694K.
[23] The process described by the verb *peristello* is also linked to the action of the retentive capacity in the stomach by Galen in *De usu partium* IV.7 (III.281K). It is also applied to the uterus by Hippocrates (*Diseases of Women* I.34).
[24] The term *phusodes* may apply both to what is eaten or drunk (Hippocrates, *Regimen in Acute Diseases* L) and to diseases (Aristotle, *History of Animals* 605a23).
[25] *De symptomatum differentiis* III.2 (VII.58–9K).

separative, because the defective movement is primarily of that [capacity] itself being stimulated to reject some of the things distressing it.[26]

II.3 In those who vomit and those who hiccup, the movement is not the same because the condition is not the same. For by vomiting they expel things in the open space, whereas by hiccuping they expel things in the actual body of the stomach, both the condition and the movement being similar **[VII.217K]** to the kind we showed to occur in those who cough owing to *dyscrasia*, when all parts of the stomach squeeze out what is distressing them. Because of this, such a symptom occurs with respect to the stomach in those with rigors (*rigos*), and in those who partake rather suddenly of pepper or some similarly hot medicine, then afterwards drink a hot drink. And hiccup (*lynx*), in fact, occurs much more in them, whenever the pepper is extremely fine, for such a thing passes down into the actual body of the stomach more. So too with all other [things], however many are cooling or heating, that pass down into the body of the stomach, hiccup (*lynx*) follows, being primarily a defective movement of the separative capacity, and secondarily of both the retentive and the so-called clasping [capacities].[27] In like manner also, both nausea and vomiting are defective movements of the separative capacity by means of which things distressing the body of the stomach are evacuated as quickly as possible through its upper orifice. Resembling this, there is also the symptom in the *leienteriai* that whenever the stomach is distressed by something mordant or heavy, it desires to excrete this immediately. Since there are two openings in it, **[VII.218K]** one above at the cardia and, in addition, one below at the pylorus, it may incline what is distressing to either of these, making use of it for the purpose of separation. If, on occasion, such a condition happens to the whole, it may utilize both openings simultaneously, as in the *cholerai*.

II.4 Its remaining and fourth capacity, which is the attractive, is itself overcome by three symptoms according to [the following] classification. Either it is unable to attract the food at all, and such a symptom is called paralysis of the cardiac orifice,[28] or it attracts with difficulty at the time when it is starting to be paralysed but is not yet so, or third in addition to these, [it attracts] something defectively. The defective movements have frequently been spoken of, as indeed also have the conditions from which

---

[26] This matter is also considered in *De symptomatum differentiis* – see IV.5 (VII.68–9K).

[27] Galen also speaks of the 'peristaltic capacity' in the *De facultatibus naturalibus* (II.153K), where Brock (1916) renders it 'contractile faculty', and on two occasions in *De locis affectis*, once in conjunction with the retentive capacity in relation to the stomach (VIII.369K), and once alone, in relation to urinary function (VIII.408K).

[28] I can find no other reference to this condition in Galen.

they arise. Sometimes a fleshy excrescence (*blastema*) may occur at the cardiac orifice, the kind of thing that is often seen arising externally, so as either to obstruct completely the path of the foods, or to damage it incidentally to some degree. Such diseases are called organic, and there has been discussion of these in the work on the *differentiae* of diseases.[29] A stomach that is in accord with nature attracts **[VII.219K]** to itself from above through the cardiac orifice and expels downward, whereas one that is disposed contrary to nature partakes to some extent of those things below as well. For in some people, the clyster also returns by being vomited, as do faeces in fatal intestinal obstructions. It is better to assume that in such conditions the stomach does not attract, but only receives whatever might be forcibly borne upward by the compressing intestines.

II.5 For what is in accord with nature in the intestines, and now is an appropriate time to speak of these, is a 'wrapping up', as has been shown in other [writings].[30] The use of this pushes forward the nutriment as far as the end below. In certain conditions, whenever the clasping movement begins from below, the movement of what is contained in them occurs upward. In this way too, sometimes a bitter humour carried down to the fundament is borne upward again when [people] spend time in the marketplace, or some other place or activity where it cannot be released, is forcibly retained, and then borne upward. And it stings the stomach, and being vaporous fills the head, taking hold of the *arche* of movement of the psychical organ from the sphincter, so henceforth each of the intestines **[VII.220K]** pushes it onward again from itself to what is situated above in the same way as it previously pushed it towards what was below. In the same way too, wind (flatus) that has been retained sometimes goes back again. It is not, then, surprising if some part of a clyster or of faeces is sometimes brought back to the stomach contrary to nature by such violent peristaltic actions of the intestines, and then hastens in this way towards expulsion. The other movements of these (i.e. the intestines) are from the class of those that accord with nature, or are either deficient or defective, and because of this are also symptoms. One must take these as analogous to those spoken of in the case of the stomach. In this way too a privation of their movement, when it is not very small, is a symptom. And sometimes too, *ileus* may occur owing to such a cause,

[29] I take this to be a general reference to the consideration of organic diseases in *De morborum differentiis* VI–X.

[30] *Peristole* is used as a general term which Galen also applies to various structures: stomach (e.g. in *De facultatibus naturalibus* II.62, 157, 169K), veins (e.g. in *De facultatibus naturalibus* II.77K), bladder (e.g. in *De locis affectis* VIII.16K) and the intestines as above and in *In Hippocratis Epidemiarum librum sextum commentarii* XVIIB.293K. In *De methodo medendi*, Galen speaks of *peristole* and *tripsis* together. Hankinson (1991) translates the first as 'compression' and the second as 'attrition' (p. 50).

just as swellings contrary to nature will also permit the superfluities to be carried downwards, at times not at all, and at times partially. But also hard faeces impacted in a coil of the intestines may sometimes prevent the faeces lying above it from being passed on downwards. And here too **[VII.221K]** the correspondence of all the symptoms in the intestines to those spoken of in the case of the stomach is preserved, whether they occur because of some *dyscrasia*, or because of a swelling not in accord with nature, or because of the contained superfluities themselves. It is better not to tarry further on the discussion of these. Rather, it is the right moment to go on to another class of actual symptoms.

III.1 There is, then, some physical action distributing[31] nutriment, on the one hand from the stomach to the liver, and on the other from the liver to the entire body. And it has also been shown concerning this, that it comes to fulfilment when each part draws the nutriment appropriate to itself.[32] So there will also be three symptoms involving such a function in that it sometimes comes to completion deficiently, sometimes abnormally, and sometimes not at all. There are three causes, just as in the case of those things previously [mentioned]; either *dyscrasias* of the attracting [parts], or organic diseases of these same [parts], or an abnormality of the distributed nutriment. The *dyscrasias* bring about a weakened capacity, whereas the organic diseases narrow the passages. The abnormality of the nutriment is a thickness and viscidity. It is not now the right time to speak about the diagnosis of these things but one must proceed to the separations of the superfluities. **[VII.222K]** In these there are also three causes: one an actual weakness of the parts purifying them, the second a narrowing of the passages, whilst the last is an abnormality of the superfluity itself. The cause of a weakness may happen to be a *dyscrasia*, whereas that of a narrowing may happen to be an obstruction or some swelling of the organs. But the cause of swellings is a flux of humours rushing down to the actual body of the organs, whereas that of an obstruction is either a thickness or viscidity of the humours, or *blastemata*.[33] An abnormality of the superfluities themselves is either copiousness, or thickness, or viscidity.

---

[31] For discussion of the term *anadosis* as 'distribution' see the section on terminology (I.4c). See, also, particularly *De facultatibus naturalibus* II.1 (II.74–77K) and *De usu partium* IV.17 (I.237–44H).

[32] See, for example, *De facultatibus naturalibus* III.15 (II.206–14K).

[33] The term *blastema* (or *apoblastema*) is taken here to be a non-specfic term for 'outgrowth' or 'excrescence'. It has come to have, as *blastema*, a specific embryological use but this is not what is intended here. It is a term used a number of times in the four treatises. For use in relation to *chymos* see Hippocrates, *Humours* I.

III.2 In the veins there are three superfluities of digestion: one is bitter bile, the second black bile and the third serum. The bladder on the liver (gall bladder) purifies the bitter bile, the spleen the black bile, the kidneys the serum. And further, each will be purified inefficiently either owing to some weakening of the specific organs, or when the passages are narrowed in any way whatever. And inasmuch as there are two [groups of] channels, those through which the superfluity is drawn and those through which it is expelled, **[VII.223K]** a narrowing will damage the separation in relation to both. There are, however, times when none of these is damaged, but there is an abundance of superfluity, whenever it is excessive and everything cannot be purified and is borne by the blood simultaneously in every direction of the body. Of the excess of this [superfluity], there is a twofold cause: the alterative capacity not being in a good state, and an abnormality of what is eaten. A *dyscrasia* of the parts is certainly the cause of damage to the capacity as has often been said,[34] whereas an abnormality of the things eaten is specific in relation to each of the superfluities. For some are more *melancholic* in nature, some more watery, and some more *picrocholic* in their substances, as has been distinguished in the discussions about these. Furthermore, a *dyscrasia* of the alterative capacity, when it turns towards being hotter, sometimes brings about a *picrocholic* superfluity, sometimes a melancholic. Of what sort each is has been shown in other places.[35] [When the *dyscrasia*] turns towards being colder it brings about a more phlegmatic or more watery [superfluity].

III.3 A specific kind of symptom will be consequent upon each of the superfluities: jaundices with yellow bile being in excess in the whole mass, **[VII.224K]** and *erysipelata* and *herpetes* in some one part. With black bile in the whole mass, there is *elephas*, and in some one part an eroding ulcer (*karkinos*). With phlegmatic [superfluity] in the whole mass there is so-called *leucophlegmatous* dropsy, and in one part so-called *oidema* (for they speak like this of a painless or spongy swelling), whereas when the serous superfluities are in excess, the dropsy called *ascites* follows, and besides they are the originators of blisters in those parts of the animal to which the superfluities are carried up. It is like this whenever each of these is in excess in a pure state, whereas when they are mixed with each other and with the blood, very many kinds of symptoms and diseases arise, about which it is

---

[34] In these books (*De symptomatum causis*) – for example, Book II, II.5 (VII.156–60K) and Book III, I.2 (VII.207–9K).
[35] See, for example, *De atra bile* V.135, 140K, *De sanitate tuenda* VI.70, 249K, *Hippocratis Aphorismi et Galeni in eos commentarii* XVIIIA.79K.

not necessary to dilate in what follows but to return to the matter under consideration.

IV.1 The first of the physical functions, and very nearly the most necessary of all, is nutrition, which is a form of the alterative function. For alteration is in the stomach as digestion, and it is also in the veins, and it is in each part. In addition, there is a fourth alteration, **[VII.225K]** which people term assimilation which is not the same in name as nutrition, but is not a different action. Moreover, nutrition fails in its objective when it does not occur at all, or deficiently, or defectively, and this is due to the nutritive capacity, the class of which is the alterative, or to a lack of material, or to an abnormality. A lack occurs in the *atrophiai*, both such as are called 'deficient' and such as are called 'privative', whereas they speak of abnormality in the *elephantes* and the *leukai*, and there are other such things. For this happens in an accumulation of nutriment in the flesh whenever the blood is more phlegmatic, and the flesh becomes more phlegmatic. For it is not the same to be in flesh itself as to be in phlegmatic flesh, just as it is not the same to be in flesh as to be in melancholic flesh, nor, by Zeus, in *picrocholic*, or *eucratic*, or *dyscratic*[36] [flesh], and with regard to the so-called primary qualities, in more moist, or more dry, or more hot, or more cold flesh. And you will believe the argument more strongly when you consider the flesh of animals, both blood-containing and bloodless, and in addition to these [the flesh] of snakes, both those seen being born in the spring, and particularly those that look like green plants. **[VII.226K]** Well, of these, the flesh is very like the grasses. Of others, it is white and bloodless just like that of crayfish and polyps, whilst in others it is otherwise. It is not possible to name the differences of these since they are boundless in number. Whenever, then, as we were saying, flesh is nourished over a long period by blood that is at once phlegmatic and viscid, it still remains flesh, although its *differentia* is changed and turned towards another form, and is between blood-containing and bloodless flesh. Whenever such a situation comes about, what further happens to it is that it does not still try to change the nutriment brought to it to the red form of flesh, no more than in either crayfish or polyps. Owing to this, then, it very quickly becomes completely white and phlegmatic whenever it is no longer able to change the nutriment towards redness, and what is phlegmatic flows into it. The crayfish, then, and almost all oysters, have from the beginning the kind of flesh which those afflicted by the *leukai* have as a result of change. For so they call

---

[36] The *iota* subscript is restored to *duskrato*.

the affection (*pathema*) of the flesh establishing the name from the colour, [VII.227K] just as, in fact, they establish the name of flesh that is at the same time black and tuberous[37] from the animal elephant. And that comes about in the same way as in *leuke*, when melancholic nutriment flows into the flesh over a very long time. The genesis of the *alphoi* is of the same kind as in the aforementioned affections (*pathos*), although the flesh itself is not, in fact, affected throughout. Rather the *alphoi* affix certain scales,[38] as it were, to the superficial part of the skin, which are white from phlegmatic humour, or black from melancholic humour.

IV.2 How significant nutriment can be, and particularly as it relates to alteration of flesh, has also been discussed by Aristotle when he called to mind the regions in which animals that are fed become different, changing with respect to colour and other perceptible *differentiae*.[39] Those who do not concede that the nourished are changed by the nutriment, in that the name nutriment refers to what is prevailed upon and not what prevails, are unable to say anything sound about the change in animals, and still more so about that in plants, but are altogether ignorant in matters that are clearly apparent to everyone. For on the one hand no one is ignorant of the Persian plant transported from Persia to Egypt.[40] [VII.228K] In Persia it was lethal, whereas transported to Egypt it changed its dangerous quality, just as, I think, our vines, when they change places, bring forth a different wine. On the other hand, those writing about agriculture have shown this for the other plants, just as, in fact, those who write about botanical subjects have for herbs in that when transplanted from one place to another, often with a separation of less than two *stadia*, they undergo change in many *differentiae*. Therefore it behoves those who assert that nutriment is the name of what is prevailed upon, changed and transformed, not only to know and say this, but also attempt to offer an explanation of the genesis of *leuke*. For either the flesh that is nourished is the cause of the affection (*pathema*), or an abnormality of the nutriment. But if it is not the nutriment, for that is what they wish, it is necessary to say it is the flesh. Why ever, then, does the affected flesh not still make the nutriment like itself in every respect? For in this way at least, nature will become the cause of the

---

[37] LSJ links the term 'tuberous' (*ochthodes*) with leprosy although Durling (1993) does not specifically do so. Elsewhere in Galen it is used in relation to ulcers (*De methodo medendi* X.181K) or swellings in body parts such as the lips (e.g. *De methodo medendi* X.203K).

[38] The term *lepis* is variably applied to epithelial debris (e.g. in the urine – Hippocrates, *Aphorisms* IV.81), to scales (e.g. Aristotle, *History of Animals* 486b21) or flakes (e.g. Hippocrates, *Diseases of Women* I.63).

[39] See Aristotle, *History of Animals* 519a1–19.

[40] I am unable to locate the source of Galen's information on this lethal plant.

affection (*pathos*), whereas it were far better, I think, to attribute the cause to the nutriment. Although, certainly, the action of what is nourished is to make the nutriment like itself, **[VII.229K]** whereas the affection (*pathos*) of the nutriment is to be assimilated and changed, it is not impossible because of this for what is acted upon to act against what affects it, even if only very slightly. For surely we have shown quite the opposite of this in the discussions on these matters, and not only us, but also the most able of the philosophers who have been interpreters of all the functions and affections (*pathos*) of nature. At any rate, it seems that all things, even if they happen to be far stronger than the things they associate with, suffer something clear and perceptible on account of these things, if not at the first association with them, at least with the passage of time. And presumably even the sharpest iron is dulled to some degree in cutting the softest flesh, and the hardest stone has some hollow in it if it is struck by a drip over a long time.

IV.3 All know what must still be said about things mixed together. If you pour a *kotyle* of cold water into an *amphora* of boiling water,[41] the mixture of both shows not only the overcoming of the *kotyle*, but also the affection (*pathos*) of what overcomes. If, on the contrary, someone were to pour a *kotyle* of hot water into an *amphora* of cold, the *kotyle* will be overcome, while the *amphora* will also be affected to a slight extent. **[VII.230K]** But what I have also said before is that it is not my intention in this work to dispute or to speak at length, but to provide instruction as quickly as possible. *Leuke*, then, is a major fault of the alterative capacity. There are many other small faults when the flesh is changed by moisture, dryness, cold or heat. And not only will a part atrophy because of weakness of the alterative capacity, but also because of exhaustion of the attractive [capacity], or because of the separative [capacity] being moved rather excessively. The separative capacity comes to an excess of movement, just as has also been said before,[42] whenever the retentive capacity is oppressed, either by an abundance or pungency of superfluities, or a specific weakness. For in this, what is useful is necessarily expelled along with what is superfluous, as in the *leienteriai*, *dysenteriai* and *cholerai*. Owing to a weakness of the separative capacity there will necessarily be a more moist or more superfluity-filled[43]

---

[41] I have simply transliterated the two measures. LSJ gives the *amphoreus* as approximately 9 gallons and the *kotyle* as a little less than half a pint.
[42] See *De causis morborum* VII.4 (VII.32K). See also *De methodo medendi* X.847K for excessive movement of the separative capacity in relation to blood.
[43] *Perittomatikos* is a term used by Aristotle in *Generation of Animals* 766b36 where Peck (1942) translates it as 'more abundant in residue'. It is also found in the pseudo-Aristotelian *Problems* (873a18) where it is applied to people who don't exercise – 'Those who do not exercise are moist and full of superfluities.'

flesh. The greater generation of the superfluities themselves is brought about by a weakness of the alterative capacity. Whenever, then, it comes about at the same time [VII.231K] that the attractive capacity draws in much humour, but the alterative capacity is not able to act effectively on all [the humour] attracted, and because of this many superfluities arise, the separative capacity is moved less well at this time and more weakly than usual, so that an abundance of superfluities necessarily exists in the flesh. Because of this, in relation to the kind and amount of the superfluity, the flesh becomes different at different times – sometimes oedematous, sometimes flatulent, sometimes dropsical. And certainly the dropsy that is called *anasarca*[44] is of this class. But I do not think it is necessary to dilate further on such matters, for I did not set out in this discussion to go through all the symptoms in order, but to exercise those desirous of learning in the majority [of them].

V.1 So it is time for me now to pass on to some other class of symptoms akin to that pertaining to damaged functions. This, then, is the very class that lies in the quantity and quality of the things separated. It occurs either through some damage of the capacity, or an untimely irritation, or a defective movement exciting [VII.232K] the capacity, or through the opening up, rupture or erosion of an organ, just as, indeed, does the separation of blood also. One could do worse than begin from this inasmuch as so many things in the class seem to be contrary to nature. For, apart from those women who haemorrhage through the uterus, all other evacuations of blood are in the whole class of things contrary to nature, whereas the former are in amount alone. So, then, the ruptures that are of vessels occur either because of some external blows, or when someone kicks or beats [a person], or when the person is struck strongly in any other way whatsoever. And they occur to those leaping far, or falling to the earth from a high place, or as the result of a scream that is harsh and very loud, since in this the vocal parts of the organs are stretched to the greatest extent. Further, those [parts] damaged when people leap are ruptured by reason of the stretching, whilst those when people fall from a height are in the class of blows. For there is no difference when some part is bruised by a stone falling on it from without, or when a person falling lands heavily on the ground.[45] These, then, are the

---

44 This is again written as two separate words in the Greek but as a single word in the Latin.
45 The point which Galen seems to be making here is that there are two mechanisms of vessel rupture – direct trauma and excessive stretching.

visible causes[46] of rupture of a vessel **[VII.233K]** and no one is unaware of them. However, there are those [causes] stirred up from conditions of the body, when someone haemorrhages spontaneously from the nose, or when with vomiting, coughing, spitting, defecation or micturition, blood may be present. These, then, are in the whole class contrary to nature. On the other hand, in women who haemorrhage through the uterus, as has been said, the evacuation is not in the whole class contrary to nature, but only in the amount.

V.2 All such things happen from three causes: either when the capacity opens up a vessel as in haemorrhages from the nose, or by the blood itself being adversely affected, or one of the vessels [being adversely affected]. I say the blood is adversely affected when it becomes unwholesome[47] to such a degree as to erode what surrounds it, or when it is so abundant as not to be contained, for this too is sufficient to burst or open up a vessel. The abnormality of the vessels themselves lies in excessive softening, hardening or thinning.[48] And these occur naturally at the earliest time (i.e. at birth) in some who are formed badly in the womb. No less does softening occur in the case of excessive moisture, hardening **[VII.234K]** in the case of dryness, thinning in the case of atrophy. What, then, is excessively soft is more readily ruptured owing to weakness; what is particularly hard by being not easily further stretched. What is thinned meets readily with rupture due to both such conditions of the veins, not only by internal causes, but also by those that are external. All [vessels] are not equally susceptible to erosion in that what is hard and thick is not easily affected by erosion. So too are [vessels] easy to open up owing to inelasticity, softness or thinness, but not easy owing to elasticity, thickness and hardness. Opening up occurs through things that irritate the mouths of vessels, and by their being greatly burdened, and sometimes also as a result of Nature itself expelling distressing things. They also cite a certain *diapedesis* (transudation of blood)[49] as a fourth class in addition to the things spoken of. It is in no way a fourth class, being either an opening up of small vessels, or a form of separation not of blood, but

---

[46] This is the only use of *prodela* ('visible') in these treatises as a qualifying term for *aitia* ('causes'). 'Visible' and 'non-visible' causes are defined in the pseudo-Galenic *Definitiones medicae*.

[47] 'Unwholesome' is the translation of *kakochymon*. For use of this term in relation to the blood see also, for example, *Hippocratis Aphorismi et Galeni in eos commentarii* XVIIB.617K (re *Aphorisms* III.20) and XVIIIA.50K (re *Aphorisms* VI.31).

[48] Here and subsequently the Greek plurals are rendered in the singular for the three pathologies.

[49] I have retained the term *diapedesis* which remains in use. *The Oxford English Dictionary* has the following: 'The oozing of blood through the unruptured walls of blood vessels'. See also pseudo-Galen, *Definitiones medicae* XIX.457K.

of serum, in the kind of way particularly a bloody serum is often passed in the urine, or passed through below in the case of weakness of the liver or kidneys.

V.3 More will be said about these a little later, when first we discuss **[VII.235K]** what is cast out by vomiting. These things, then, are also separated, sometimes weighing down the stomach as a quantity just as, at times, abundance of nutriment [does], but at other times as what is distressing and biting, just as whenever the nutriment taken becomes acidic, steaming, pungent or bitter through lack of digestion. Of this class are the bilious, phlegmatic and serous superfluities, both those that are produced on the spot and those of a nature to flow into it [the stomach] from the system of the entire animal. There is also, in addition to these, a third class of causes which incite the stomach to vomit, even though they neither weigh down nor sting, but are only among those things that are contrary to nature. The distinguishing mark that is common to all the things contrary to nature is that if they have been digested they are unable to nourish. I think it is for this reason that not only acid or salty phlegm, but also sweet [phlegm], when it collects in the stomach, is often accustomed to provoke it to vomit. And, in fact, blood itself that has flowed into the stomach, in the same way compels it to vomit.

V.4 Furthermore, [the stomach] sometimes transmits downward too soon, or sometimes too slowly, or less, or more, or infrequently, **[VII.236K]** or frequently, either nutriment that is useful, or corrupted, or what flows into it from above, or what is produced[50] in it. But separation also comes about before the customary time when the stomach is either weighed down, as by a great amount taken in, or when it is irritated and goaded, as by what is stinging, or when it expels what is strange and unfamiliar. And we should remember, whenever we speak of much, that this has a threefold genesis: either by the capacity being weaker than normal, or by what is taken in exceeding what is exactly suitable, or because of both of these together. Apart from the things mentioned, the intake[51] of more moist or more viscid foods brings about a rapid excretion, these slipping through more readily, and particularly if people happen to walk about at leisure after them, so that they shake them yet do not, at least, bring about distribution before the proper time. For some such thing happens in shakings, since

---

[50] The verb *apogennao* is used here – see, for example, Hippocrates, *Diseases* I.25 in relation to sweat (although there is some textual uncertainty here).

[51] 'Intake' is the translation of *prosphora*. LSJ lists 'taking (of food)' as a particular meaning, citing Aristotle's *On Sleep* 458a22 and *Metaphysics* 1000a14. It is of interest to note that in the latter instance both Tredennick (1933) and Ross, in Barnes (1984), retain the primary meaning of 'application'.

there are very many coils of the intestines.[52] It is necessary, of course, that in each of these the food is borne from those that are higher to those that are lower, it being not still possible to remain there further owing to weight. [VII.237K] So those things plugging up are pushed onward by the function of the intestines[53] themselves, which have in the coils an innate separative capacity for things that distress them. Foods that are moist or viscid pass through easily, pushed onward either by weight, or the shaking of the body, or by the function of the intestines. So, the causes of a swift passage have been discussed.

V.5 The stomach separates downward later than is customary owing either to weakness or to disturbed sensation of the intestines, or owing to paucity of food, or owing to [its] quality. For the weaknesses lack the strength to propel forward, whereas the disturbed sensations perceive distressing things indistinctly, although separation of what distresses would be a cure for them. Moreover, less actual food than is required has a residue that is slight so that it does not weigh down in the same way. All those things that are thick and astringent are slow of passage in contrast to those that are viscid and moist. Excretion slows, not only because of weakness of the intestines, but also of the muscles in the epigastrium, and particularly whenever the superfluities happen to be harder. For, under these circumstances, [VII.238K] there is a need not only for strongly functioning muscles in the epigastrium, but also in the thorax. The superfluity becomes less than corresponds to the quantity of the foods whenever more of them come to distribution.

V.6 Conversely, more is excreted than corresponds to what is taken in, sometimes owing to lack of distribution, but sometimes owing to certain things flowing from above into the spaces in the stomach. Continuous separations occur owing to weakness or stinging. Thus a weakness of the organs in the stomach, as has been said often already, occurs as a result of *dyscrasia*, whereas stinging occurs as a result of the things contained in them. There are four causes of the genesis of stinging in this way: either a certain poisonous capacity[54] taken in with foods, or taken in by itself, or corruptions of the foods themselves and, in addition to these, those stinging

---

[52] There is some uncertainty about the text here, particularly regarding *atrema*, which Latin translators take to be an adverb, and the punctuation, in which I have followed the Greek rather than the Latin versions.

[53] Galen provides a detailed account of the anatomy and function of the intestines (which is relevant to what follows) in *De usu partium* IV.17–19 (I.237–47H) and V.3–5 (I.253–65H).

[54] The term *pharmakodes* is used in the sense of 'poisonous' in Soranus III.29 and III.44. In both these instances Temkin (1956) renders it 'toxic'. It can also, of course, mean 'medicinal' – see, for example, the pseudo-Aristotelian *Problems* 863b32.

superfluities that flow from the body into the [organs] in the stomach and such things as are generated in it, just as in the *dysenteriai* in the case of a malignant ulcer.[55] One would also be able to add to these at the same time a fifth cause of such symptoms, an excessive sensation **[VII.239K]** of bodies, whether this is from nature, or due to an ulcer (*helkos*). There is another kind of continuous separation, the cause of which is distinguished by class from all previously mentioned causes: that in the case of a paralysis of the muscles situated in the margin of the outlet of the superfluities. For the separation in these cases is involuntary, and because of to this untimely, uncontrolled and continuous. But this is enough about excretions.[56]

VI.1 Next one must speak about the vaporous *pneumas* which, in fact, they also call flatus. And the genesis of these is in the actual spaces in the stomach, certain phlegmatic humours or foods being dissolved to vapours right there by deficient heat. For complete cold does not entirely bring about vapour because it does not entirely thin, nor prevail upon, nor dissolve the nutriment. A strong heat, overcoming much of what it surrounds, already thins the food more than accords with the genesis of vapour, unless it is vaporous by nature. Under these circumstances, a certain turbid or, as one might say, mist-like *pneuma* is generated, and this in a brief **[VII.240K]** and very short time, as from one or a second eructation, is evacuated. The heat acting around the foods dissolves these to some degree more inadequately, but does not prevail entirely, and here is the genesis of the flatulent *pneuma*.

VI.2 In a word, just as out in the open, very cold weather conditions[57] and clear skies occur naturally in the season of north winds particularly, and the very hot weather conditions existing in the season of summer make the ambient air pure, and the [weather conditions] that are between these are those that generate cloudiness so, in the same way in animals, it is neither in the extreme weaknesses of heat, nor whenever it is strongly robust, but in the [states] between these, that flatulent superfluity is generated. And this being separated (expelled) through the mouth brings about an eructation, whilst

---

[55] In using 'malignant' for *kakoethes* I have followed LSJ but the application here should not be confused with the more specific current usage in relation to a neoplastic ulcer. The term is used in a more general sense by Galen – see, for example, *De facultatibus naturalibus* (II.131K) where Brock (1916) translates it as 'pernicious' in relation to a humour, and *De usu partium* V (III.382K, 388K) where May (1968) on both occasions translates it as 'injurious' in relation to moisture (*hugron*).

[56] It is, perhaps, appropriate to reiterate here that both *ekkrisis* and *apokrisis* (and related verb forms) are translated as 'separation' and *apochoresis* and *diachoresis* (and related verb forms) as 'excretion'.

[57] 'Weather conditions' is used for *katastasis* to distinguish this term from *diathesis* which is consistently translated as 'condition' in relation to the body.

through the limit below[58] either noisy or silent flatus. When, however, it is not brought forth by either, it creates so-called flatulence, a symptom of the stomach being too weak to expel the superfluous and cloudy *pneuma*. And in one or other of the parts of the intestines, whenever such a *pneuma* exists and moves, it creates sounds of many kinds, **[VII.241K]** not all of which have names, but are able to indicate to one who is perspicacious, of what sort and how much the superfluity is, and at which place particularly it is being rolled around. For if it sounds sharp and thin, such a *pneuma* is being borne through an empty and altogether narrow intestine, and is itself more pure and more air-like, yet when it has become more windy, it likewise makes the sound small, being enclosed in the fine intestines, but is not entirely sharp, nor thin. All such sounds arise particularly in the spaces in the jejunum. To the extent that they should pass down as far as the other fine intestines, so they are made less sonorous. There are other intestinal noises, like those from very broad clarionets of the sort the so-called funeral musicians have, which are not able to sound purely owing to the material from which they are made, and which are low-pitched owing to the width of the channel of the breath. All such [sounds] arise in the thick intestines that have become empty of superfluities. If some moisture is enclosed in them, a certain form also comes to the intestinal rumbling **[VII.242K]** from this, and people call such a sound *borborygmos*,[59] signifying the separation of moist superfluity. For the kind of sound indicates both these things in advance, signifying separation because it occurs in the case of a natural movement, but moisture in that it occurs along with *borborygmos*. And the sound of these same 'winds'[60] being borne to the outside, which is a kind of *borborygmos*, makes it clear that the separation is such that it will not yet occur, whilst a pure [sound] and, as one might say, one that is euphonious and air-like, demonstrates either that the intestine is empty, or that it has some very hard superfluity somewhere above it. Furthermore, there is also another [sound] in the middle of these like *borborygmos*, occurring in a certain intermediate condition between those spoken of. There is what is like a *trusmos* or *trismos*, for people name it in both ways, some making the chief element of the first syllable from *upsilon* whereas others make it from

---

[58] *Peratos kato* here would clearly seem to indicate the anus. It is not clear why the usual tem *hedras* is not used. Elsewhere *peras kato* is applied, for example, to the heart (*De usu partium* III.433K), to the bones of the leg (*De anatomicis administrationibus* II.409K) and to the scapula (*De anatomicis administrationibus* II.493K).

[59] I have retained the term *borborygmus* here and below, which is still used, for 'intestinal rumbling'. See Hippocrates, *Prognostic* XI for example, where Jones (1923), vol. 2, p. 25, renders it 'rumbling'.

[60] This is the translation of *phusa* as used for intestinal gas – see, for example, Hippocrates, *Aphorisms* IV.73.

iota. This occurs in the case of a simultaneous narrowing of the organs and flatulent *pneuma* along with scanty moisture.

VII.1 Since enough has been said about these matters for our present purposes at least, let us return to those things that flow into the stomach from above. **[VII.243K]** For it was certainly said as well that these constitute the causes of the moisture and magnitude of the excretions. Accordingly, the superfluity is often carried from above to the stomach by the strength of the natural separation, although sometimes owing to weakness it is not even able to bear what is useful. The superfluity is then separated in crises[61] and sometimes in a time of health, as it is, of course, in women each month. Hippocrates, too, said that such bloody diarrhoeas occur in those in whom some member had been cut off.[62] And we see this happen not only in these people, but also in certain others from some defined period.[63] All those we saw who evacuated in this way had changed from a former life of exercise to one of complete idleness. Certainly such a superfluity is abnormal only in quantity, whereas another [may be abnormal] in quality, being many times separated critically in acute diseases, sometimes by reason of colliquescence.[64]

VII.2 Between this altogether useless and abnormal superfluity and that previously spoken of as useful, **[VII.244K]** there is another, third class of superfluity, a kind which is, in fact, partially digested food in the stomach. This is separated in hepatic conditions particularly. In this way, people refer to those for whom the disease is a weakness of the liver, even if no inflammation (*phlegmone*) is associated. For under these circumstances, the affection (*pathema*) happens to the viscus somewhat like those occurring in relation to a weak stomach, when the stomach is desirous yet, should it not digest the foods it takes to itself, is weighed down and sends forth what is partially digested to the intestines. And so it itself hastens to vomit, whilst the liver is affected somewhat analogously to vomiting in that the nutriment which it has drawn to itself, as through the mouths of the vessels in the mesentery, it again sends off semi-digested through them. There is a form of such separation, just as my predecessors also portrayed it, akin

---

[61] These are, presumably, the crises of fevers, on which see, for example, Celsus, *De medicina* III.5.

[62] See Hippocrates, *On Joints* LXIX.

[63] *Periodos* may be taken as relating to a fever (see Hippocrates, *Aphorisms* IV.59), but judging by the following sentence it may here relate to a way of life (see Plato, *Republic* 407e).

[64] *Suntexis* is a term used, for example, by Aristotle, *Generation of Animals* 726a21–2, where he writes (in discussing semen), 'Colliquescence is always disease-related whereas removal of superfluity is beneficial.'

particularly to the water left over after the washing of flesh.[65] It is better, perhaps, not to speak so simply, but to add to the precision of the portrayal with the wording 'blood-containing' and 'newly slaughtered'. Furthermore, if someone calls what is separated in this way 'watery blood', he also seems to me to interpret it clearly.

VII.3 [VII.245K] This particular symptom is analogous to the vomiting of semi-digested foods. But the other, which I am about to speak of, is like the moist excretions of the stomach which have come to the most complete digestion but have failed in distribution. For as also with respect to these, of course, a stomach completely weighed down by them desires to separate them. So the liver too, in the same way, once it has sufficient benefit from the nutriment distributed to it, no longer suffers it still to remain present. Therefore, whenever this is not able to be carried onward for whatever reason, it is necessary for it to rush back to the stomach and, under these circumstances, the excreted blood appears blacker than is natural, and glistening since it is mixed from blood and black bile. Blood by itself is made black by being cooled, in addition to which it acquires no glistening, and loses even that which it had initially. Black bile, however, is more glistening than blood itself, just like the asphalt from the Dead Sea which people call Jewish.[66] For blood that has been cooled does not generate black bile, as in the case of a clot, **[VII.246K]** but when overheated has, on this account also, a preserved brightness. For black bile also has a genesis in this way, not like a clot, which is blood that has been cooled. On the contrary, black bile like ash arises entirely from overheating and boiling. It is cold in that it is earth-like, but partakes of heat just as do ash and vinegar. The humour distributed from the stomach comes to the condition spoken of, when it remains longer in the liver, by not having distribution from that source. Such a kind of separation is called by some *dysenteria*, for they are also often stinging like the *dysenteriai*, inasmuch as, I think, the yellow bile becomes bitter in them by the blood being overheated. Therefore, let each call it what he will.

VII.4 There are, in all, four *differentiae* of the bloody separations consequent upon four conditions. One is of blood itself, brought about for a

---

[65] Galen also uses the description watery and bloody in relation to diarrhoea in *De locis affectis* I.5 (VIII.46K) and in relation to dislocation of the hip in *In Hippocratis De articulis librum commentarii* XVIII.730K (re *On Joints* LXX).

[66] Galen speaks of the asphalt from the Dead Sea in *De simplicium medicamentorum temperamentis et facultatibus* XX (XVIIa.689–91K) and of its description as Jewish in *De compositione medicamentorum per genera* (XIII.536K, 560K, 781K).

certain period either when limbs are severed or when exercises are neglected. The second is due to a weakness of the liver when there is a casting out of watery blood, which people liken to the water left after the washing of flesh. The third, [VII.247K] now spoken of, is of melancholic and glistening [blood]. These three, then, bring about a separation that is both continuous and copious, whereas the fourth is a separation that occurs little by little and over a short time, sometimes of pure blood and sometimes of clot. In this there is often also concomitant expulsion of a small amount of pus, or of what are called scales, or certain membranous bodies which are parts of the intestines themselves. But as well as these, compact faeces having drops of blood in them are often separated. The conditions of the first three have been spoken of a little earlier whilst the condition of the fourth now spoken of is an ulceration of the intestines. Some think this alone merits the name *dysenteria*. But, as I have often said, in the need to give great attention to not neglecting the matter, one must give scant attention to terms. There is from the same class, in the previously mentioned *dysenteria*, also what is called *teinesmos*, which is an ulcer (*helkos*) in the rectum, bringing other similar symptoms, although the strainings are far more violent compared to the *dysenteriai*.

VIII.1 [VII.248K] The stoppages and abnormal evacuations of urine have a correspondence to the stoppages of the superfluities in the stomach and the separations contrary to nature. For [the urine] is retained either when the bladder is unable to expel, or when its orifice is closed. Both these diseases of the bladder have, then, one common symptom, retention of urine (*ischouria*), for the urine is retained in it. No less do many doctors call that symptom 'retention of urine', although it is not retention, whenever the urine does not come to the bladder at all because the function of the kidneys has been destroyed. And one must, at least, agree with them in calling it thus, since they lack a specific term, although it is certainly not appropriate to be ignorant of the difference between the conditions. For it is one condition whenever the bladder is full yet expels nothing, whereas it is another whenever it is empty since it contains absolutely nothing within it. At any rate, in respect to such a condition in which the bladder is full, either its orifice is closed, or when this is in its natural state, [the bladder] is too weak to contract and expel the urine to the outside. [VII.249K] The stoppages of the orifice are, then, brought about by obstruction, or by closure.[67]

---

[67] Galen here indicates the derivation of the specific terms *ischouria* and the verb *ischoureo* from *ischo* ('to retain') and makes two important clinical distinctions. The first is between the failure to pass

VIII.2 An obstruction also occurs due to a clot, or thick pus, or a stone, or a calculus, or due to some new growth (*blastema*) growing up in the channel itself, such as is seen occurring in all other external parts in relation to the ears, the nostrils, the genitals and the anus. A closure occurs either due to some unnatural mass (*onkos*), or due to extreme dryness. A mass (*onkos*) comes about as a result of inflammations (*phlegmone*), indurations (*skirros*) and other swellings (*oidema*), and things which, having lifted up the neck of the bladder, extend the mass (*onkos*) to the internal channel.[68] Dryness comes about in very burning or very dry fevers, in which often we see those afflicted being unable to utter a sound without wetting the mouth. I do not need to say anything more about the causes of weakness in the bladder for I have already spoken frequently [of these] in the case of many parts, either as they happen to *homoiomeres* themselves, or to organic [parts]. This is something that seems to happen to a greater degree in a bladder that is overfull, which not only we ourselves have seen happen, but have also learned of from others.[69] **[VII.250K]** For when people are ashamed to depart from a feast to urinate although the bladder is full, it comes about that they destroy the function and are no longer able to pass (separate) urine, even if they happen to exert sufficient force. It seems that such a thing also occurs in relation to the stomach and the intestines, but escapes the notice of many in the case of those who suffer this in the stomach itself, when they are overtaken by choking. In the case of those who have collected together the superfluity in all the intestines, the doctors are distracted to other things by the accompanying symptoms. Such a thing customarily occurs by purgatives alone being collected in the intestines, or remaining in them. These same conditions bring on a privation, as it were, of the separation of urine, whilst the congeners of these, when they are lacking in magnitude, bring about, for example, weak and sluggish functions.

VIII.3 In other conditions, a third class of symptoms is disposed by nature to supervene, consisting of defective evacuations. There are many forms of these. The first is so-called *stranguria*,[70] brought about by a

---

urine due to bladder and outlet tract pathology (true *ischouria*), and that due to renal failure (anuria). The second is between an atonic bladder unable to expel urine, presumably neurogenic in origin, and some outlet obstruction, mechanical or neurogenic. See his more complete description in *De locis affectis* VI.4 (VIII.402–14K).

[68] Whilst both the Greek and the Latin version in Kühn, as well as Linacre, have 'internal channel', Copus has 'external channel'.

[69] It is not clear who these others are but in his account in *De locis affectis*, Galen does mention some specific cases – see VIII.407K.

[70] This is Galen's term for difficulty of micturition which embraces disturbance of the passing of urine and pain on its passage (modern 'dysuria'). A clear explanation of the range of the term is given in

weakness of the bladder or a sharpness of the urine. The second [**VII.251K**] is like the fluxions involving the stomach, about which it is better to say more here and now. Certainly something like a dissolution, or colliquescence, or releasing, or whatever one should wish to call it, occurs, sometimes of the whole body, but sometimes of the humours alone in the veins. And the waste material of this sometimes flows to the stomach, sometimes to the urine, and sometimes rids itself to the sweat. Thus, when the humours in the veins are dissolved to serous fluids, the kidneys are disposed by nature to draw such[71] superfluity, and particularly whenever they happen to be healthy. So, on the one hand, they purify the serous fluid of the veins and, on the other hand, they carry the flux continuously to the bladder. Whenever, also, the kidneys happen to be unable to draw, the veins either send down such a serum to the stomach, or they distribute it to the whole body, bringing on sudden watery states. If the waste material is thicker and of a kind that the kidneys are not disposed by nature to draw, it all, of necessity, flows to the stomach. When the class of flesh has been liquefied thus, either the stomach receives the flux whenever it is thicker, or many sweats supervene, [**VII.252K**] whereas when it has been dissolved into vapour, there are sweats. This is enough for the moment at any rate on the colliquescence involving the flesh and the blood. In respect to the other symptoms of the urine, some demonstrate a certain condition of either the bladder or the kidneys, about which Hippocrates wrote in the *Aphorisms*,[72] whereas others provide information on the degree of failure of digestion or of indigestion in the blood itself. There has been writing about these in the *Prognostic*.[73]

IX.1 Now is, then, an appropriate time to proceed to sweats, about which there has been discussion, I suppose, at least to the extent that sometimes they occur when the system is released, and the affection (*pathema*) is called *syncope*.[74] The opposite state to this is that in the critical sweats[75] which

---

De locis affectis VI.4 as follows: 'The occurrence of strangury in cases of stinging urine is a symptom of the bladder and not an affection. That which occurs due to ulceration or atonia is as a result of an affection of the bladder, just as that due to stinging sometimes is a result of an affection of the kidneys and sometimes a result of some other of those things able to send a bad humour to the urine, or pus when someone is afflicted by an abscess' (VIII.402K).

[71] I am indebted to Greg Horsley who pointed out to me (per litt.) that the addition of ν to τοιοῦτο is post-classical, representing a failure of Galen to maintain his usual Atticizing policy.

[72] Hippocrates, *Aphorisms* IV.69–83.   [73] Hippocrates, *Prognostic* XI.

[74] The application of the term 'syncope' is considered in detail by Siegel (1968), pp. 347–52. The term is also defined in the pseudo-Galenic *Definitiones medicae* XIX.420–1K. Durling (1993) gives 'a sudden loss of strength' as the meaning of the Greek term *syncope*.

[75] Although dating from Hippocrates at least (see, for example, *Prorrhetic* I.149), it is of interest to note that this concept persisted until at least the eighteenth century – see Mettler (1947), p. 417.

indicate a strong rather than a dissolved nature. Certainly such sweats purify the body. Resembling these, there are those associated with moderate exercise, or baths, or the summer heat. In excessive exercises already something of what is useful departs as well. Moreover, they have a smell and colour like evacuated superfluity. The abundance [of sweat] is either due to the thinness **[VII.253K]** of the body, or due to the amount of superfluity, or due to the fineness of what is evacuated. Owing to the opposites of these, on the other hand, they are disposed by nature to be held back whenever the superfluity happens to be small in amount, or viscid, or thick, or when the channels are stopped up. They suffer this as a result of obstruction or closure. They are obstructed by thick or viscid humours, whereas they are closed by atrophy, or cold, or softening. There also occurs, owing to weakness of the capacity involving the flesh, a retention or separation of sweat, just as of other superfluities too. For truly, both the bladder and the stomach sometimes retain more of the contained superfluities within themselves, delaying to separate [them], but often, on the other hand, they do not bear them for the shortest time, but are weighed down and cast them out forthwith.

X.1 I have reserved this discussion of what is common to all the parts to go over finally, all cases at the same time. For it seems to be a difficulty, when a body is damaged, that it is not concomitantly damaged equally with respect to all its capacities, but **[VII.254K]** some more, some less, and others not at all. It is clear to everyone that unless the substance of each of the existing things is harmed somewhat, it is not possible for its function to be impaired. Often, when each of the parts functions, sometimes one and sometimes another of the functions is damaged, for there does not need to be a like condition of the alterative and effective functions. Alteration occurs to all things that come into association with one another, and requires nothing else, neither transfer from place to place, nor the laying hold of something, nor to retain, nor to press against, whereas, when something is about to draw (attract),[76] retain or separate, it is necessary that the function occur with a movement in place.

X.2 On this basis, what is so soft as to be moist, or liquid, or unstable,[77] is equally unable to draw (attract), retain or separate. For in all such actions

---

[76] I have given both 'draw' and 'attract' here because, although the relevant capacity is termed 'attractive', 'drawing' seemed the more appropriate translation in this context and in what immediately follows.

[77] Galen also uses the term *asteriktos* in *De usu partium* II.15 in relation to the movements of the arm (I.108H).

there must be a point of stability and tension for functions,[78] although it is able to change what comes into association if it is very moist, and particularly whenever it is also very hot at the same time, for none of the active qualities seems so quickly to effect change in what comes near [VII.255K] as heat. From these things it is clear that a very hot and very moist body will most rapidly bring about change. That is, it will digest and at the same time assimilate to itself the appropriate nutriment. Something that is hard to the extent that it is not difficult to bend, yet is securely fixed, will be able to draw (attract) vigorously whatever it should wish, or expel forcibly, or retain strongly. For it does not slacken in tension, as do things that are exceedingly soft, yet there is no danger of it being ruptured by being stretched more violently. And those things it once takes hold of, it retains having enveloped them, in a way which neither those things that are difficult to bend owing to hardness, nor those that are soft through being moist, are able to do. For some things it does not encompass securely, whereas others of the things it lays hold of make use of the attachments being weak to slip away easily.[79]

X.3 Thus, bodies that are moist and hot are nourished best, for they most rapidly both change and also receive the nutriment into themselves, and they assimilate and adapt [it]. Cold and dry bodies, on the other hand, are nourished worst, being able neither to change nor receive [the nutriment] into themselves, nor assimilate, nor adapt [it]. So, then, [VII.256K] what is hottest changes most rapidly, as was said before. This is what digestion is. However, that what is most moist and most soft readily receives into itself what has been changed, stands more in need of recall than proof, just as does the fact that what is dry and hard permits nothing to enter into it before it is broken up in some part, as if ulcerated. Furthermore, no one is unaware that things which are more moist adhere and coalesce more readily and rapidly, whilst those that are harder do so not at all, or only with difficulty. So that, at any rate, if someone were to disregard copper, iron, gold and stone, and direct the discussion to lead, it is obvious that this does not at all coalesce with other lead without being made liquid by heating.

X.4 In children then, and in such other bodies as are hotter and moister in their mixtures, there are those that are best in matters of digestion and

---

[78] Hippocrates speaks of an *aposterixis* in *Instruments of Reduction* 42, where Withington (1928) renders the term 'fulcrum'.
[79] Galen discusses the role of 'adhesion' in nutrition in *De facultatibus naturalibus* I.11 (II.24–7K).

administration of food, and of adhesion, and of nourishing.[80] For digestion and nutrition are changes, whereas administration of food occurs when what is nourished receives the nutriment into itself in a dew-like fashion.[81] Adhesion is a binding together and unifying in all instances, of which [VII.257K] moisture of the body being nourished is of no small benefit to assimilation, being like what is doing the nourishing with respect to consistency. The organs of distribution in children, even if they are not very strong in their functions, are, nevertheless, at least sufficient, and in no way lacking. For the veins already have an exactly suitable hardness and tension.[82] The retentive capacities are, however, weaker in them, and because of this they separate more quickly, if they are sometimes burdened by something, or if they are otherwise distressed. Similar to these, the separative [capacities] are moderate in weakness. And yet not in children alone, but also in all others, the retentive capacities seem weaker than the separative, even if they are alike, owing to the long period of function. For the retentive capacities function to the greatest extent in order to do the work of retaining, whereas the separative capacities have a short duration of function, being able to force onward and cast out what is distressing at a single stroke. As, then, in the case of these, the same man who is most adequate to cast out the burden externally, being unable to bear it through the whole day, is also able to thrust away into the organs internally what is distressing [VII.258K] more readily than retain it longer.

X.5 At any rate children, who are the subject of the discussion, have a stronger alterative capacity than those in their prime, but a weaker attractive capacity than those in their prime, although the latter is not, in fact, deficient, at least in terms of its own need. With respect to the remaining two [capacities], they are weaker compared to those in their prime. But the weakness of the separative [capacity] is not put to the test owing to the short duration of its service. For they vomit and defecate more frequently than those in their prime, not by the strength of the separative, but by the

---

[80] In this sentence I have translated *prosthesis* as 'administration' (see Hippocrates, *Aphorisms* I.19) and *prophysis* as 'adhesion', i.e. adhesion of food to tissues – see X.2 and the previous note. Brock (1916), in his translation of *De facultatibus naturalibus*, has the following note: 'One is almost tempted to retain the terms *prosthesis* and *prophysis* in translation, as they obviously correspond much more closely to Galen's physiological conceptions than any English or semi-English words can' (p. 39, n. 6). In his translation of the pseudo-Aristotelian *Problems* (866b21), Hett (1926) renders *prophysis* (in relation to nutriment) as 'transmission'.

[81] Elsewhere Galen uses the term *drosoeides* in relation to semen – see *De facultatibus naturalibus* II.3 (II.86K).

[82] The tension (*tonos*) of veins (and also arteries and nerves) is also spoken of by Galen in *De methodo medendi* X.881K.

weakness of the retentive [capacity]. In digestions in the stomach, those things that are moist and soft, they digest about equally to those in their prime, whereas those that are hard, they digest worse. For in children the heat is more vaporous, but in those in their prime more dry. Furthermore, in the former the body is more moist [so] there is need for more moist nutriments, whereas in the latter it is more dry so there is need for more dry [nutriments].

X.6 If, then, digestion is a change to a suitable quality to those nourished, the softer and moister of foods are more suitable to children, whereas **[VII.259K]** the harder are more suitable to those in their prime. In the aged, however, the body is in a bad condition with respect to almost all functions, for it is very much drier than in those in their prime, and cold in the aged alone. They do not, therefore, digest well owing to a lack of heat, nor are they nourished owing to a concurrent dryness and weakness of the alterative capacity. In them, distribution is brought about slowly and weakly, as if by organs already become numb as a result of cold. In the case of separations, those of short duration do not reveal the weakness of the capacity, whereas those of longer duration, they perform badly. In terms of the active functions, an organ that is dry and hot is the more suitable, whereas one that is moist and cold is the more weak. Between both of these stand the remaining two conjunctions. Among the ages, then, you would not find a body that is moist and cold, for that of the aged was shown to be cold and dry. In abnormal mixings there are those that accord with nature in respect to form in each case, and there are those that occur in acquired conditions. *Phrenitis*, for example, **[VII.260K]** is a dry and hot disease and because of this is very strong in the active functions. *Lethargos*, on the other hand, is weak, soaking the parts with abundant moisture and cold. Such also is the class of the dropsies (*hydrops*), especially of the *leucophlegmatasias* and the *anasarcas*. And cold is always weaker and torpid, whether it be associated with dryness, or with moisture.

X.7 In the same way, the retentive of the physical capacities is stronger in the case of drier and warmer organs, but weaker in those that are more moist and colder, whether this is from birth, or comes about later in some other way. One should direct one's attention to the magnitude of the excess in the case of each part. For example, nerves, tendons, muscles and ligaments, to the extent that they are drier, are necessarily stronger up to that excess at which they become difficult to bend through hardness and, as if brittle, through dryness. For in this way they are seized with spasms. Again, the physical organs, to the extent **[VII.261K]** that they are more moist, are nourished better, even if they are exceedingly moist in their mixtures. In terms of digestions, they are neither better than they are themselves, nor than those that are more dry, if they are also in like manner hot. Unless, that is, you give dry nourishment to a dry and parched organ, and do not mix abundant moisture with it. Bodies that are very hard are abnormal in regard to distributions and separations, for they both dilate and contract with greater difficulty, of which the one brings about attraction and the other expulsion. So that one may give attention to few points, I shall divide the whole under headings. Increases of heat effect change quite adequately until they should come to such a strength as not yet to melt, for then, in the first place, they are altogether useless. Coldness is useful to no function. Dryness is useful to strength and tension up to the point of not yet making things difficult to move or easy to break. Moisture is most suitable to nutrition, although very opposing to other functions apart from growth, for which it is more useful than in nutrition. **[VII.262K]** For what is going to be properly increased needs to be very readily extended and distended in every direction.

XI.1 Perhaps this is now enough to put an end to the treatise here, for as I said in what has gone before, it was not to go over everything in turn, but for the sake of exercising those eager for knowledge with more examples that I directed the discussion towards the many kinds and classes of symptoms. In extending the size of the book still further, something will also be said about the [symptoms] which have been omitted. For if something separates from the nose, or the ears, or the palate, or the eyes, or the throat, or the uterus, or any one of all the other [parts], it is appropriate to consider both the quantity and quality in these, and [thirdly] the manner of separation, referring to the causes already spoken of. For all symptoms will be found to have arisen owing to *dyscrasias* of the *homoiomeres* and diseases of the organic [parts], besides the quality and quantity of the material itself.

XI.2 For example, **[VII.263K]** the brain is the cause of both *catarrh* and *coryza*, as a *homoiomere* being brought to a *dyscrasia* by cooling and likewise by sun-stroke (*ekkausis*), and being heated as an organ.[83] Diarrhoea is the sort of affection (*pathos*) that occurs in the stomach in disordered digestion, like each kind of the things spoken of in the brain. We use the term *catarrh* whenever the superfluity flows to the mouth, but *coryza* whenever it flows to the nose. Hoarseness occurs in the case of the *catarrhs* when

[83] The term *ekkausis* is taken to indicate sun-stroke specifically here as the Kühn Latin translation assumes. See, for example, Galen's *De instrumento odoratus* II.884K.

the throat is soaked in fluids. If the flux falls down to the uvula it either generates in it what is called uvulitis (*staphyle*) or otherwise provokes it to a swelling (*onkos*), whilst if to the glands situated opposite each other on both sides in the boundary of the mouth, tonsillitis (*antias*), and if to what is adjacent to these, adenitis (*paristhmion*). If the flux from the head is also carried down to the stomach and to the trachea, it is greatly distressing to both. But others prior to us have discussed more carefully the damages from such fluxes and we shall say more about them in the writings on therapeutics.[84] Regarding things expectorated from the lung and chest, **[VII.264K]** we have already spoken beforehand in the writings on crises.[85]

XI.3 Neither will those things pertaining to stoppage of the monthly periods, nor abnormal separation of all the things from the uterus, still be difficult to discover, if we refer to similar objectives. For, in fact, the body of the uterus itself when thick and hard will be a cause of stoppage, being such in nature as never to be entirely evacuated unless someone modifies it for the better with medications, and over a long time, or for a certain time after that condition which might happen on each occasion to take hold of uteri.[86] And narrowing of the veins comes into existence immediately from the beginning when the female is abnormally formed in this [the uterus]. Corresponding to this also there is a pressure in the vessels from the surrounding structures whenever the body [of the uterus] is excessively thickened. A *dyscrasia* of the uterus occurs both naturally and in certain conditions, just like a thickening. There will be sometimes also a stoppage of the monthly period due to the material itself whenever what is being evacuated becomes thick or viscid. **[VII.265K]** But even if it should be good, when some obstruction from humours of this sort has occurred beforehand in the vessels passing down to the uterus, in this way also the monthly flow will be obstructed. But because of the whole body, sometimes the uterus will be not at all purged, or sometimes less, or more, or abnormally. 'Not at all' is due to much exercise or a meagre way of life, or to the redirection of humours to other parts, whereas 'less' is due to these same things occurring more moderately than is natural. 'More', however, is due to great idleness or a sumptuous[87] way of life.

---

[84] Fluxes (*reumata*) are considered extensively in both *De methodo medendi* – see, for example, IV.4 and VII.11 (X.250–75K), and in *Ad Glauconem de medendi methodo* – see, for example, I.15 and II.1–2 (X.510–18K).

[85] *De crisibus* IX.686K – see also *De sanitate tuenda* VI.421K and *De locis affectis* VIII.289K.

[86] Galen presumably means pregnancy here.

[87] *Hadros* I have rendered as 'sumptuous' following Copus' *opiparus*.

XI.4 But there are also abnormal fluxes through the uterus, the symptom being called 'flux muliebris' (*rous gynaikeios*),[88] when a purging of the whole body occurs through this part. What is evacuated in each case is such that in form it is also like what is in excess in the animal. One is red, a liquor of the blood, another white from phlegm, another yellow which is *picrocholic*, another watery, and another again serous. Apart from these, there is abnormal evacuation of those things from the uterus **[VII.266K]** due to some affection (*pathos*) arising in the uterus itself. Besides, [there is] also such a suppression of the menstrual flow when due neither to lack of blood, as has been spoken in the case of excessive exercises and a meagre way of life, nor to an affection (*pathos*) having arisen in the uterus, but sometimes due to vigour, when the blood flows down into other parts, the purifications in the uterus are kept back. But, as I said just now, it is not, I think, difficult for each person trained in the many matters addressed in these treatises to discover such things himself. And it is, I presume, clear to anyone that through the individual diseases in the uterus, whether existing in the horns, or in the neck, or in the whole cavity, that sometimes the menstrual flow is carried more than before, sometimes less, and sometimes not at all, or abnormally. Moreover, imperforate women are also to be subsumed under this class in the division of the argument.

XI.5 In like manner also, what is called *priapism* is an involuntary swelling and distension of the penis of males, a symptom generated by flatulent *pneuma*. **[VII.267K]** Furthermore, the spermatorrhoeas (*gonorroia*), other than when the penis is being put on the stretch, are due to a weakness of the retentive capacity in the spermatic vessels, whereas when it is stretched in any way, they bring about something akin to a spasm of those things affected.[89]

XII.1 There is, then, no need to go over such things any further. Rather, we shall pass on to the remaining class of symptoms, which itself does not require much discussion because of what has already been said about symptoms following other [symptoms]. So we may now put an end to the work here. Colours, then, will be changed, to speak briefly, as a result of humours departing from their natural form, or sinking down to the depths, or overflowing, as it were, the skin, but in specific cases as a result of causes compelling the humours to come to such movements and conditions. There

---

[88] I have kept this term in its Latin form. Galen clearly has more in mind here than the normal menstrual flow, for which the term *katamenia* is more common – although compare Hippocrates, *Aphorisms* V.56 and V.57 in Jones' (1931) translation. See also Aristotle, *History of Animals* 521a28.

[89] Galen provides a detailed account of these and related matters in *De locis affectis* VI.6 (VIII.437–52K).

are, of course, the psychical affections (*pathos*) and the changes of the air surrounding us towards hot or cold. And there are conditions of the body itself, which has its blood hotter, or colder, or less or more, or pushed to the exterior, or drawn to the interior. [**VII.268K**] Of this class also is every bad humour which changes the colour of the whole body according to its own form, in jaundice (*ikteros*), dropsy (*hydrops*), *elephas* and weaknesses of the spleen and liver. Analogous too are the decolorations which will arise in relation to any part whatever. And the natural forms will be changed when the parts are filled or evacuated more excessively, or removed from their particular place, or forcibly drawn aside. The causes of these are obviously in each case numerous, but to discover them is no longer difficult for anyone by whom the foregoing has not been read superficially. In like manner, it will no longer be difficult to discover too the causes of bad odours, or of softening, or of hardening, or of such other things as correspond to these, starting from what has previously been said. But, in fact, I have already said something about this at the end of the book written on *differentiae* of symptoms.[90]

XII.2 It is not, therefore, necessary to elaborate further on these matters, but rather to let the work on causes in symptoms have an end at this point when I have added this alone, which I deferred demonstrating there in the work on the *differentiae* of symptoms.[91] [**VII.269K**] That is, that some symptoms follow others of necessity, but some not of necessity, a matter which it seems to me does not itself require protracted discussion. It will be enough to have demonstrated its method by one example for one to be excused from the majority of them in turn. Above all, I urge you to consider whether it is by one cause that an effect is brought about, or by many. If it is by one, then it will necessarily follow its acting, whereas if it requires many for genesis, it is not of necessity. This same method, then, is common in all matters. And in the case of symptoms, you ought to look at it in this same way. If one [effect] occurs from one [cause], it has consequent necessity. On the other hand, when some other causes are also added to the genesis of a second symptom, it will no longer necessarily follow what is prior. For if there is indigestion, flatulence (*empneumatosis*) does not necessarily follow, just as gnawing (*dexis*) does not, nor watery or copious excretion, nor nausea (*nautia*), nor an intense appetite, nor a sluggishness with regard to actions, nor a torpor of mentation,[92] nor a heaviness of the head (*karebaria*), nor insomnia (*agrypnia*), [**VII.270K**] nor heartburn

---

90 *De symptomatum differentiis* V and VI (VII.74–84K).
91 Galen discusses this in general terms in *De symptomatum differentiis* I.6 (VII.47–9K).
92 Galen does not employ a specific term for any of the three preceding symptoms.

(*kardialgia*), and still more not epilepsy, nor derangement (*paranoia*), nor distraction (*ekstasis*), nor coma (*koma*), just as there is not necessarily despair (*dysthymia*), nor other distress, nor, far more, melancholy, nor altogether any pain of the colon, kidneys, liver, spleen, thorax or joints, just as there is not malaise (*anomalia*), shivering (*phrike*), rigor (*rigos*) or fever (*puretos*). And yet with each of these and almost all other symptoms, it is not possible to find that which does not at some time appear in those with indigestion, but depending on the magnitude of the indigestion and the *differentia*, and the strong or reduced sensibility of the nature of the person, and the strength or weakness of each of the parts in the body, different symptoms will arise at different times.

XII.3 For severe indigestion (*apepsia*) brings greater and more numerous symptoms. Mild indigestion, on the other hand, brings lesser and fewer. Accordingly also, the *differentiae* of those suffering indigestion, when they tend towards the cold and phlegmatic, are generators of one sort of symptoms, and when they tend towards the steaming and hot, of another. So it is too with respect to gnawing and not gnawing, and with dissolving to vaporous *pneuma* and not dissolving. Also the nature, [**VII.271K**] as has been said, of the person acts with or acts against the generation of symptoms. For example, in those in whom the stomach is of reduced sensibility, there is not severe gnawing, nor do they experience pain, nor do they separate much. In the same way, they neither suffer heartburn (*kardialgia*) nor are they easily troubled in the head. In those with strong sensation, all the symptoms readily follow these because the *arche* has sent them down from above. Why must one say that in each of those suffering indigestion that part is most perceptive of damage which should be weakest? And because of this, it is not possible to say that any symptom of necessity follows indigestion. However, either privation of the nutriment distributed to the body, or weakness of the function, necessarily brings atrophy (*atrophia*), just as, in fact, damage of the alterative capacity in each part also does, or failure of the separation of the superfluities of the blood, being itself a symptom of the separative function, necessarily brings the symptoms of discoloration. And one of these is called jaundice (*ikteros*), whereas another is without a name in the case of melancholic superfluity. In the same way, [**VII.272K**] in every class of symptom you will find those that invariably follow others, and those that do not. Eschewing elaboration, I shall end the work here.

PART III

Conclusion

CHAPTER III.I

Conclusions

These four translated treatises constitute an important component of Galen's considerable oeuvre, signified by their incorporation into the core material of the medical training curriculum well into the second millennium. Like others of Galen's major works, they have a well-defined purpose which might be summarized as the systematic examination of the nature and causation of disease and related phenomena. Unlike many of his works, they are singularly devoid of *ad hominem* arguments and the often quite virulent abuse heaped upon those with opposing views. Indeed, a strikingly even-handed, if somewhat cursory, treatment is given to one particular theory, the *anarmoi/poroi* theory of Asclepiades and its subsequent developments, which is elsewhere shown to be a particular Galenic *bête noire*. These treatises are, however, disappointingly lacking in any detailed consideration of earlier and other views and are, as a consequence, a poor source of information on such views, unlike a number of other Galenic works. This is especially unfortunate with respect to nosology.

In summarizing the content of these works, three aspects of diseases and their symptoms are considered: definition, classification and causation. Based on the sequence of the argument, and on the relative space devoted to these three matters, the impression is that the first two, definition and classification, are primarily to be seen as instruments for the analysis of the third – causation. Nonetheless, all three are obviously independently important despite their close interrelationship.

Taking each of these three subjects in turn, Galen's concern for accurate and comprehensive definition is obvious and is reflected in the content of the opening sections of the first and third treatises, *De morborum differentiis* and *De symptomatum differentiis*. The key definitions are those of health and disease but also important are other terms, specifically symptom and affection. He also attempts a definition of 'cause', although this is somewhat *en passant* (*De symptomatum differentiis* I.6). In fact, one must look to the other works discussed in chapter I.6 for a full understanding of Galen's ideas on what a cause is and how causation operates. However, in the key definitions, foundational as they are to his taxonomic project, he is consistent, both within these treatises and across other treatises. The definitions of health and disease themselves depend on three key terms: 'condition'/'constitution' (*diathesis/kataskeue*), 'function' (*energeia*), and 'in accord with/contrary to nature' (*kata/para phusin*). As he describes it, the body is always in some particular 'condition' or of some particular 'constitution', these terms, according to Galen, being interchangeable for the purpose of definition. They apply, moreover, to the individual components or parts (*moria*) of the body identified as either *homoiomeric* or organic structures. Each part is charged with the performance of a certain function or else has the role of aiding a functioning part to carry out its function. 'Function' (*energeia*) is, then, the second key component of the definitions. Both 'condition'/'constitution' and 'function' must be either in accord with or contrary to nature.

Health then, according to Galen's basic definition, is properly constituted parts carrying out their appointed functions (or presumably their subsidiary roles, although he does not make this distinction explicit) in accord with nature. Disease, conversely, is a departure from this desired state. In essence, it is a disturbance of condition/constitution damaging function such that the latter is contrary to nature. A proper condition or constitution is one that is 'in balance' (*summetros*). Balance, in turn, is to be defined in terms of the basic structural components, i.e. either *anarmoi/poroi* according to Asclepiades and those of like mind, or the four qualities (hot, cold, moist and dry) as Galen himself believes. His definitions, then, apply independently of one's position vis-à-vis basic structure. A condition or constitution not 'in balance' is identified as 'imbalanced' (*ametros*). In these four treatises the possibility of some intermediate state is once mentioned but never given detailed consideration. Degrees of health and disease are, however, recognized and their existence taken to support Galen's own continuum concept of structure.

There are two main, and interrelated, problems with these definitions which Galen only in part, and only partly in these treatises, addresses. The first, alluded to above, is to what extent the categorization of bodily states as either healthy or diseased is exhaustive. Galen clearly recognizes this problem. There are, at least, the other states or phenomena which the terms 'symptom' and 'affection' designate. With respect to the four putative 'entities' (health, disease, symptom, affection) there are, then, problems with respect to demarcation and coexistence in theory which translate to recognition and description in practice. He does attempt to resolve these issues, particularly in section II of *De symptomatum differentiis*, but also elsewhere in these treatises, and in other treatises, most notably *De methodo medendi*. These attempts are based on variations of duration of change in altered states and their accord or otherwise with nature. Ultimately, however, he is forced to accept some degree of overlap both in the actual states themselves and in terminology. Clearly, also, disease and symptom can, and possibly must, coexist just as health and affection can coexist, especially if one accepts Plato's definition of affection as Galen does. This overlap reflects an enduring problem in clinical practice. When does some 'departure from accord with nature' become a disease rather than say a variant of health, or a symptom, or an affection? Is a symptom, say headache, invariably a manifestation of disease or can it exist independently as is generally taken to be the case, and if so is the term 'symptom' appropriate? Also, when is an affection a symptom or a disease? Galen does not satisfactorily resolve these issues and, indeed, seems to accept that they are beyond definitive resolution.

The second problem is the definition of the terms in the key definitions themselves. Neither condition/constitution, nor function, nor nature (particularly in the sense used by Galen) is beyond further definition, or even self-evident in terms of meaning. Indeed, all three are to a significant extent vague. This is especially so with the first and third terms. In fact, it is not clear whether the term condition/constitution is to be taken primarily in the physiological, or in the anatomical sense, or whether, perhaps, the two terms (*diathesis* and *kataskeue*) are intended to denote physiological and anatomical states, respectively. Even more is there a laxity in the term 'nature' in this context. These are issues which Galen does not attempt to deal with in the way he attempts to clarify the demarcation between the defined terms. It is notable that in these treatises he does not often give vent to his exasperation about perceived quibbling over terminological points, as he is wont to do in other works, although on several occasions he does express his view that the objective to be kept in mind is the achievement of accord on the matters themselves even if this comes at the expense of some terminological variation. These various difficulties notwithstanding, for the purposes of his exposition his definitions do work, at least to a significant degree.

Deficiencies in the definitions do, however, create difficulties with his classifications, although this is not explicitly acknowledged. In the first and third of the treatises, Galen advances classifications of diseases and symptoms respectively. These classifications are themselves dependent on other classifications, apart from the definitions considered. In general,

308 *Galen*

the classifications are unexceptionable. The first is basically structural and involves two levels of structural analysis. What might be termed the macroscopic is the division of bodily structures into *homoiomeric* and organic. This is not dissimilar in a general way from the modern division into tissues and organs where the basis of division is certainly similar in intent even if different in fact. Not so the microscopic structural level where, in Galen's time, there was a clear division between continuum theories (elements/qualities/humours) and atomic (particles/void) theories. In these four treatises, Galen does no more than give a very abbreviated account of disease classification on the basis of the particular development of particle theory associated with Asclepiades and the subsequent Methodic school, whilst at the same time drawing attention to some of the problems which it entails in explaining pathological processes, especially those involving degrees of change. This latter is part of the same problem more generally conceived which bedevilled such theories. On the other hand, he declares his strong support for a continuum theory of structure, and takes every opportunity to point out this theory's distinguished lineage, particularly those predecessors he most reveres: Hippocrates, Plato and Aristotle. One must, however, look to other works, such as the *De elementiis secundum Hippocratem*, for Galen's own detailed discussion of his concepts of basic structure.

The second classification, that of symptoms, has a different basis, although why this should be so is not an issue which Galen addresses. Diseases are essentially divided into those involving 'microscopic' structure (*dyscrasias*) and those involving 'macroscopic' structures (abnormalities of form, number, size and arrangement), with the additional 'rogue' category of 'dissolution of continuity'. Symptoms, however, are classified on the basis of function. Where diseases are related to *homoiomeres* and organs, symptoms are related to psychical and physical functions and the organic (instrumental) structures underlying them. For taxonomic purposes, psychical functions are subdivided into sensory, motor and authoritative (*hegemonical*). Physical functions are subdivided on the basis of the physical capacities described in detail in *De facultatibus naturalibus*. In both cases, psychical and physical, classification is based on the tripartite division of disturbed function into complete loss, partial loss, and abnormal function. Thus, Galen's classifications of diseases and symptoms were based on three foundational components. The first was the group of broadly acceptable, and indeed possibly novel, although not sharply demarcating, definitions of 'health', 'disease', 'symptom' and 'affection'. The second was a concept of macro-structure that was also generally acceptable. The third was a concept of micro-structure that was to a definite degree contentious, and has not survived, even in broad terms, as the opposing concept has.

The difficulties inherent in Galen's definitions, and the classifications based on them, essentially revolve around the inevitable imprecision of the definitions, not least the lack of clear definition of the key terms of the definitions themselves, and the failure in part to meet the basic criteria for successful classification. These imperfections notwithstanding, he does arrive at two workable classifications commensurate with the level of histological, anatomical and physiological knowledge of his time.

The third component of these treatises, causation, is at once the most important and the most problematic. It is important in that a basic tenet of rational medicine is that to know the cause or causes of a disease is to understand the disease, and so be able to identify appropriate prophylactic measures, or institute rational and effective therapy if the disease has already occurred. It is problematic insofar as the whole issue of causation was then, and is now, contentious. The purpose of the detailed discussion in the introductory chapter I.6 was to bring out the nature of this contention between those, such as the Sceptics, who downplayed the importance of causation, and others who saw causation as universal, whether conceptually or physically. The brief historical overview was aimed in part at showing that the former have had their intellectual progeny, and influential ones at that, whilst the latter, likewise, have their modern successors. It was, in essence, this division that defined the medical schools identifiable in Galen's time. Attention was also drawn, in that section, to variant views amongst which might be numbered Aristotle's account of causation and the reductionist approaches to causation in disease adopted by Erasistratus and by Asclepiades and the subsequent Methodics.

What emerges from an analysis of the four treatises, particularly the second and fourth, and from a wider examination of Galen's works, is that he clearly believed in the universality of causation. Every event is attributable to a cause or causes. Whether these causes are evident or not, they are what affect both the body and the mind, and effect the changes in underlying condition or constitution which bring about diseases, symptoms and affections. In terms of the medical schools prevalent in his time, Galen could be categorized as a Dogmatic at heart, but an Eclectic to the extent that he showed definite Empiric tendencies, and was by no means altogether at odds with the Pneumatics. That is to say, he believed, contrary to the Empirics and the Sceptics, that in every case a single cause or multiple causes could be implicated in disease states and their symptoms, and even though these causes might not be immediately identifiable, they could be speculated on and should be sought. He believed also that variation in the relation between putative cause and observed or predicted effect could be satisfactorily accounted for by variations in the magnitude, duration and means of application of the cause, and the underlying condition of the body being acted on. Contrary to the Methodics, he did not believe in a severely reductive account of disease causation, in their case based on what he considered to be an erroneous view of basic structure. He also did not accept Erasistratus' reductive account, although based on what were, to him, acceptable views on structure. Finally, he did not share the Pneumatics' view of the critical importance of *pneuma*, although *pneuma* did occupy a significant place in his concepts of physiology and pathology.

On causation, Galen's eclecticism is particularly evident in his use of different concepts and terminology. As discussed in the introductory chapter on terminology (1.4), there were available to him terms, and their underlying concepts, developed and used by various predecessors, most notably by Plato, Aristotle, the Stoics (perhaps predominantly Chrysippus) and possibly Athenaeus, together with the standard terms for cause – *aitia, aition* and *prophasis*. With respect to these three terms, throughout all four treatises he uses the first two interchangeably, whilst *prophasis* is used in *De symptomatum causis* without comment on its particular connotations. The impression is that Galen employs it to indicate an obvious, or a postulated cause which would be in keeping with its use generally. As for the specific causal terms, those for example listed in the pseudo-Galenic *Definitiones medicae*, he does endeavour to make clear the distinction between *proegoumenic* and *prokatarktic*, which is that both are antecedent but the former is internal whilst the latter is external. He does not, however, use either term to any extent in the actual description of causes in these treatises. Even less does he use the term *synektic*, and less still the other special terms. As for Aristotle's theories of causation, although Galen, in his general definition of cause in the important opening sections of *De symptomatum differentiis*, does offer a quasi-Aristotelian classification, he makes no further use of the fourfold Aristotelian division in these treatises. He does, however, pay attention to the distinction between primary (*per se*) and secondary (*per accidens*) causes.

On the issue of causation, what Galen is mainly concerned with in these four treatises is cataloguing known causes and relating them to diseases, either kinds of diseases or individual diseases. In keeping with his lack of use of specific causal terminology, he does not, in general, attempt to analyse the actual mechanism by which the cause brings about its effect apart from some superficial analogies with inanimate objects in the case of heating, cooling etc. In fact, the works have throughout a distinctly practical flavour. One further important point to emerge from an analysis of these and other works is that the application of physical concepts of causation to psychical functions presented no problem to Galen insofar as he accepted a physical basis for the normal functioning of the latter, a position altogether in keeping with the mainstream of current neurophysiological and medical thinking.

Ultimately I believe that these four works must be judged favourably for the following main reasons:

1. They represent the first systematic and coherent attempt in the Western medical tradition to deal with three of the most fundamental aspects of medical theory: the definition of key terms, the classification of diseases and symptoms on other than a simple topographic basis, and the causation of disease.

2. In doing this they are an important repository of information on what diseases were identified in the ancient world, and how they were thought of in terms of mechanism and effects.

3. Although theoretical in their basic aim, these works had an obvious and immediate relevance to then current medical practice.

4. Owing in no small part to their intrinsic merits, they endured as a substantial component of the body of material on which medical teaching was based, both in Europe and in the Arab world, for well over a millennium.

5. Finally, even today, when shorn of the obviously outmoded concepts of structure, they could be taken as a model of how such fundamental theoretical issues in medicine should be approached.

On a personal note, apart from the very considerable insight that these and related Galenic works have provided into the historical development of ideas in medicine, I found in these treatises a strong implicit argument for a greater awareness by doctors of the philosophical issues involved in such subject matter, and in medical theorizing more generally. This is, of course, an argument which Galen makes quite explicitly elsewhere. For me, studying these treatises engendered the wish that I had pursued these matters early rather than late in my own medical studies. I can only think that Galen himself would have found such a cause–effect relationship, if it were generalized and could occur early in each individual's experience, most appropriate.

Bibliography

GALEN

(1) COLLECTED EDITIONS AND TRANSLATIONS (LISTED UNDER EDITOR/TRANSLATOR)

Brain P. (1986): *Galen on Bloodletting*, Cambridge University Press, Cambridge. (*De venae sectione adversus Erasistratum, De venae sectione adversus Erasistrateos Romae degentes, De curandi ratione per venae sectionem.*)

Daremberg C. (1854–6): *Oeuvres anatomiques, physiologiques et médicales de Galien*, 2 vols., J.-B. Baillière, Paris. (*Que le bon médecin est philosophe, Exhortation à l'étude des arts, Que les moeurs de l'âme sont la conséquence des tempéraments du corps, Des habitudes, De l'utilité des parties du corps humain, Des facultés naturelles, Du mouvement des muscles, Des sectes aux étudiants, De la meilleure secte, À Thrasybule, De lieux affectés, De la méthode thérapeutique, à Glaucon.*)

Furley D. J., Wilkie J. S. (1984): *Galen on Respiration and the Arteries*, Princeton University Press, Princeton. (*De usu respirationis, An in arteriis natura sanguis contineatur, De usu pulsuum, De causis respirationis.*)

Grant M. (2000): *Galen on Food and Diet*, Routledge, London. (*On the Humours, On Black Bile, On Uneven Bad Temperament, On the Causes of Disease, On Barley Soup, On the Powers of Foods I–III.*)

Kühn K.-G. (1821–33): *Claudii Galeni Opera Omnia*, 20 vols. Georg Olms Verlag, Hildesheim, 1997 reprint, 122 titles.

Marquardt J., Müller I., Helmreich G. (1884–93): *Claudii Galeni Pergameni Scripta Minora*, 3 vols. BT, Leipzig. (Vol. 1: *De animi morbis et peccatis, De optima doctrina, De parvae pilae exercitio, Adhortatio ad artes addiscendas*; vol. 2: *Quod optimus medicus sit quoque philosophus, De consuetudinibus, Quod animi mores corporis temperamenta sequantur, De ordine librorum suorum ad Eugenianum, De libris propriis*; vol. 3: *De sectis ad tirones, Thrasybulus, De facultatibus naturalibus.*)

Singer P. N. (1997): *Galen: Selected Works*, Oxford University Press, Oxford. (*My Own Books, The Order of My Own Books, The Best Doctor is also a Philosopher, An Exhortation to Study the Arts, To Thrasybulos, The Affections and Errors of the Soul, The Soul's Dependence on the Body, The Construction of the Embryo, Mixtures, The Best Constitution of our Bodies, Good Condition, The Exercise with the Small Ball, The Thinning Diet, The Pulse for Beginners, The Art of Medicine.*)

Walzer R., Frede M. (1985): *Three Treatises on the Nature of Science*, Hackett Publishing Company, Indianapolis. (*On Sects for Beginners, An Outline of Empiricism, On Medical Experience.*)

(II)   INDIVIDUAL EDITIONS AND TRANSLATIONS
(LISTED UNDER LATIN TITLE)

De alimentorum facultatibus

Powell O. (2003): *Galen on the Properties of Foodstuffs*, Cambridge University Press, Cambridge.

De anatomicis administrationibus

Duckworth W. H. L., Lyons M. C., Towers B. (1962): *Galen on Anatomical Procedures. The Later Books*: IX.6–XV, Cambridge University Press, Cambridge.

Garofalo I. (1986): *Anatomicarum administrationum libri qui supersunt novem. Earundem interpretatio arabica Hunaino Isaaci filio ascripta*, vol. 1, libri I–IV, Naples.

Simon M. (1906): *Sieben Bücher Anatomie des Galen*, ed., trans. and comm., 2 vols., Leipzig.

Singer C. (1956): *Galen on Anatomical Procedures*, Clarendon Press, Oxford.

De captionibus

Edlow R. B. (1977): *Galen on Language and Ambiguity*, E. J. Brill, Leiden.

De causis contentivis

Lyons M. (1969): *Galen on the Parts of Medicine, On Cohesive Causes, On Regimen in Acute Diseases in Accordance with the Theories of Hippocrates*, CMG, Suppl. O.II, Akademie-Verlag, Berlin.

De causis procatarcticis

Bardong K. (1937): *Galeni De causis procatarcticis libellus a Nicolao Regino in sermonem Latinum translatus ad codicum fidem recensuit in Graecum sermonem retro vertit*, CMG suppl. II, Teubner, Leipzig and Berlin.

Hankinson R. J. (1998): *Galen on Antecedent Causes*, Cambridge University Press, Cambridge.

De elementis secundum Hippocratem

Helmreich G. (1878): *Galeni de elementis ex Hippocratis sententia*, Deicherti, Erlangen.

Bibliography

De Lacy P. (1996): *Galen on the Elements According to Hippocrates*, CMG, V.I.2, Akademie-Verlag, Berlin.

De facultatibus naturalibus

Brock A. J. (1916): *Galen on the Natural Faculties*, Loeb Classical Library, Harvard University Press, Cambridge, MA (1963 reprint).

De homoeomereis corporibus differentia

Strohmaier G. (1970): *Galeni De partium homoeomerium differentia libelli*, CMG, Suppl. O.III, Akademie-Verlag, Berlin.

De locis affectis

Siegel R. E. (1976): *Galen on the Affected Parts: Translation from the Greek Text with Explanatory Notes*, S. Karger, Basle.

De methodo medendi

Hankinson R. J. (1991): *Galen on the Therapeutic Method: Books 1 and 2*, Oxford University Press, Oxford.

De nominibus medicis

Meyerhof M., Schacht J. (1931): *Galen, über die medizinischen Namen* (Arab text, German translation), Abh. Akad. Wiss., Berlin.

De placitis Hippocratis et Platonis

De Lacy P. (1978): *Galen on the Doctrines of Hippocrates and Plato* (Books I–V), CMG, V.4,1,2, Akademie-Verlag, Berlin.

De praecognitione

Nutton V. (1979): *Galen On Prognosis*, CMG, V.8.1, Akademie-Verlag, Berlin.

De propriis placitis

Nutton V. (1999): *Galen On My Own Opinions*, CMG, V.3.2, Akademie-Verlag, Berlin.

De sanitate tuenda

Green R. M. (1951): *A Translation of Galen's Hygiene*, Thomas, Springfield, IL.

De semine

De Lacy P. H. (1992): *Galen On Semen*, CMG, V.3.1, Akademie-Verlag, Berlin.

De tremore, palpitatione, convulsione et rigore

Sider D., McVaugh M. (1979): 'Galen on tremor, palpitation, spasm and rigor', *Transactions and Studies of the College of Physicians, Philadelphia* 1, pp. 183–210.

De usu partium

Helmreich G. (1907–9): *De usu partium libri XVII*, G. B. Teubner, Leipzig (1968 reprint).

May M. T. (1968): *Galen on the Usefulness of the Parts of the Body*, 2 vols., Cornell University Press, Ithaca.

(III)   RENAISSANCE LATIN TRANSLATIONS AND COMMENTARIES
         (LISTED UNDER TRANSLATOR)

Copus G. (1548): *Commentarii in sex Galeni libros de morbis et symptomatibus*, commentary by F. Valleriola, Venice.

Du Bois J. (1539): *Methodus sex librorum Galeni in differentiis et causis morborum et symptomatum in tabellas sex*, Paris.

Leoniceno N. (1528): *Claudii Galeni de differentiis morborum liber 1 de causis morborum liber 1*, Paris.

Linacre T. (1528): *Galeni de symptomatum differentiis liber unus. Ejusdem de symptomatum causis libri tres*, Paris.

Nuñez de Zamora, Antonio (1621): *Repetitiones super caput primum et tertium libri de differentiis symptomatum Galeni, in publicis praelectionibus, relatae etc.* Salamanca.

Ponze de Santa Cruz, Antonio (1637): *Antonii Ponze Sanctae Crucis operum libri III* (a commentary on Galen's works *De morbis and De symptomatibus*), Madrid.

Roselli J. F. (1628): *Ad sex libros Galeni de differentiis et causis morborum* (N. Leoniceno interprete) *et symptomatum* (T. Linacre interprete) *commentarii*, Barcelona.

Santorelli, Antonio (1628): *J. F. Roselli censura [of Galen's six books De differentiis et causis morborum etc.] ad censuram vocata. In qua definitio actionis depravatae ab auctore primum tradita adversus ipsorum defenditur etc.*, Naples.

Sebisch, Melchior the Younger (1630–2): *Praes. Libri sex Galeni de morborum differentiis, morborum causis, symptomatum differentiis, et causis, in theseis partum contracti, partum in epitomes redacti et ad disputandum in Academia Argentoratensi propositi a M Sebizio, Access*, Strasbourg.

Wolffius, Joannes of Frankfurt (1632): *Resp. liber Galeni de symptomatum causis tertius: in theseis contractus et ad disputandum propositus a M. Sebizio*. Strasbourg.

CLASSICAL WORKS OTHER THAN GALEN

ANONYMUS LONDINENSIS

Jones W. H. S. (1947): *The Medical Writings of Anonymus Londinensis*, Cambridge University Press, Cambridge.

ANONYMI MEDICI

Garofalo I. (1997): *De morbis acutis et chronicis*, E. J. Brill, Leiden.

ARISTOTLE

Balme D. M. (1991): *History of Animals, Books VII–X*, Loeb Classical Library (Aristotle, vol. XI), Harvard University Press, Cambridge, MA.

Balme D. M. (1992): *De partibus animalium I and De generatione animalium I*, Clarendon Press, Oxford.

Barnes J. (1984): *The Complete Works of Aristotle*, 2 vols., Princeton University Press, Princeton, NJ.

Cook, H. P., Tredennick H. (1938): *Categories, On Interpretation, Prior Analytics*, Loeb Classical Library (Aristotle, vol. I), Harvard University Press, Cambridge, MA (1983 reprint).

Freese, J. H. (1926): *Art of Rhetoric*, Loeb Classical Library (Aristotle, vol. XXII, Harvard University Press, Cambridge, MA (1994 reprint).

Hett W. S. (1926, 1937): *Problems*, Loeb Classical Library (Aristotle, vols. XV, XVI), Harvard University Press, Cambridge, MA (1970, 1983 reprints).

Hett W. S. (1936): *On the Soul. Parva naturalia. On Breath*, Loeb Classical Library (Aristotle, vol. VIII), Harvard University Press, Cambridge, MA (1986 reprint).

Lee H. D. P. (1952): *Meteorologica*, Loeb Classical Library (Aristotle, vol. VII), Harvard University Press, Cambridge, MA (1987 reprint).

Peck A. L. (1942): *Generation of Animals*, Loeb Classical Library (Aristotle, vol. XIII), Harvard University Press, Cambridge, MA (1979 reprint).

Peck A. L. (1965, 1970): *History of Animals, Books I–III, IV–VI*, Loeb Classical Library (Aristotle, vols. IX and X), Harvard University Press, Cambridge, MA (1970, 1993 reprints).

Peck, A. L., Forster E. S (1937): *Parts of Animals, Movement of Animals, Progression of Animals*, Loeb Classical Library, Harvard University Press, Cambridge, MA (1993 reprint).

Tredennick H. (1933, 1935): *Metaphysics*, Loeb Classical Library (Aristotle, vols. XVII, XVIII), Harvard University Press, Cambridge, MA (1975, 1990 reprints).

Wicksteed P. H., Cornford F. M. (1929, 1934): *Physics*, Loeb Classical Library (Aristotle, vols. III and IV), Harvard University Press, Cambridge, MA (1996, 1995 reprints).

CAELIUS AURELIANUS

Drabkin, I. E. (1950): *Caelius Aurelianus on Acute Diseases and on Chronic Diseases*, University of Chicago Press, Chicago.

CELSUS

Spencer W. G. (1935–8): *Celsus: De medicina*, 3 vols., Loeb Classical Library, Harvard University Press, Cambridge, MA (1971–94 reprints).

CICERO

Rackham H. (1942): *Cicero* (vol. IV), Loeb Classical Library, Harvard University Press, Cambridge, MA (2001 reprint).

DIOCLES OF CARYSTUS

Van Der Eijk P. J. (2000): *Diocles of Carystus. A Collection of Fragments with Translation and Commentary*, vol. I, *Text and Translation*, E. J. Brill, Leiden.
Van Der Eijk P. J. (2001): *Diocles of Carystus. A Collection of Fragments with Translation and Commentary*, vol. II, *Commentary*, E. J. Brill, Leiden.

DIOGENES LAERTIUS

Hicks R. D. (1925): *Diogenes Laertius*, Loeb Classical Library, Harvard University Press, Cambridge, MA (revised edns., vol. 1 (1972), vol. 2 (1931); 1995 reprint).

EMPEDOCLES

Wright M. R. (1981): *Empedocles. The Extant Fragments*, Yale University Press, New Haven and London.

EPICURUS

Bailey C. (1926): *Epicurus. The Extant Remains*, Clarendon Press, Oxford.
Usener H. (1887): *Epicurea*, Brown Reprint Library, Dubuque, IA (reprint of Teubner edition).

ERASISTRATUS

Garofalo I. (1988): *Erasistrati Fragmenta*, Giardini Editori e Stampatori, Pisa.

HEROPHILUS

Von Staden H. (1989): *Herophilus. The Art of Medicine in Early Alexandria*, Cambridge University Press, Cambridge.

HIPPOCRATES

Adams F. (1886): *The Genuine Works of Hippocrates*, 2 vols., William Wood and Co., New York.
Jones W. H. S. (1923–31): *Hippocrates*, Loeb Classical Library (Hippocrates, vols. I, II, IV), Harvard University Press, Cambridge, MA (1984, 1992 reprints).
Littré E. (1839–61): *Oeuvres complètes d'Hippocrate*, 10 vols., J.-B. Baillière, Paris.
Lonie I. M. (1981): *The Hippocratic Treatises 'On Generation', 'On the Nature of the Child', 'Diseases IV'*, Walter de Gruyter, Berlin and New York.
Potter P. (1988–95): *Hippocrates*, Loeb Classical Library (Hippocrates, vols. (V, VI, VIII), Harvard University Press, Cambridge, MA.
Smith W. D. (1994): *Hippocrates*, Loeb Classical Library (Hippocrates, vol. VII) Harvard University Press, Cambridge, MA.
Withington, E. T. (1928): *Hippocrates*, Loeb Classical Library (Hippocrates, vol. III), Harvard University Press, Cambridge, MA.

ORIBASIUS

Raeder J. (1926–33): *Collectiones Medicae, Synopsis ad Eustathium filium*, CMG, VI.1–5, Teubner, Leipzig.

PLATO

Archer-Hynd R. D. (1883): *The Phaedo of Plato*, Macmillan & Co., London.
Burnet J. (1911): *Plato's Phaedo*, Clarendon Press, Oxford (1989 reprint).
Bury R. G. (1929): *Timaeus, Critias, Cleitophon, Menexenus, Epistles*, Loeb Classical Library (Plato, vol. IX), Harvard University Press, Cambridge, MA (1989 reprint).
Fowler H. N. (1914): *Euthyphro, Apology, Crito, Phaedo, Phaedrus*, Loeb Classical Library (Plato, vol. I), Harvard University Press, Cambridge, MA (1982 reprint).
Hamilton E., Cairns H. (1961): *Plato: The Collected Dialogues*, Princeton University Press, Princeton, NJ (1989 reprint).
Lamb, W. R. M. (1924): *Laches, Protagoras, Meno, Euthydemus*, Loeb Classical Library (Plato, vol. III), Harvard University Press, Cambridge, MA (1977 reprint).
Taylor A. E. (1928): *A Commentary on Plato's Timaeus*, Clarendon Press, Oxford.

PRAXAGORAS

Steckerl F. (1958): *The Fragments of Praxagoras of Cos and his School*, E. J. Brill, Leiden.

RUFUS OF EPHESUS

Daremberg C., Ruelle C. E. (1879): *Oeuvres de Rufus d'Éphèse*, Paris (Amsterdam reprint 1963).

SEXTUS EMPIRICUS

Annas J., Barnes J. (1994): *Sextus Empiricus. Outlines of Scepticism*, Cambridge University Press, Cambridge.
Bury R. G. (1933–49): *Sextus Empiricus*, Loeb Classical Library (Sextus Empiricus, vols. I–IV), Harvard University Press, Cambridge, MA (1983–93 reprint).

SORANUS

Temkin O. (1956): *Soranus' Gynaecology*, The Johns Hopkins University Press, Baltimore, MD.

THEOPHRASTUS

Einarson B., Link G. K. K. (1976–90): *Theophrastus. De causis plantarum*, 3 vols., Loeb Classical Library, Harvard University Press, Cambridge, MA.

THUCYDIDES

Smith C. F. (1919): *History of the Peloponnesian War, Books I and II*, Loeb Classical Library (Thucydides, vol. I), Harvard University Press, Cambridge, MA (1980 reprint).

OTHER WORKS

Ackerknecht E. H. (1982): 'Diathesis: the word and the concept in medical history', *Bulletin of the History of Medicine* 56, pp. 317–25.
Algra K., Barnes J., Mansfield J., Schofield M., eds. (1999): *The Cambridge History of Hellenistic Philosophy*, Cambridge University Press, Cambridge.
Allbutt T. C. (1921): *Greek Medicine in Rome*, Macmillan, London.
Annas J. (1996): 'Scepticism, old and new', in Frede and Striker (1996).
Annas J., Barnes J. eds. (1985): *The Modes of Scepticism*, Cambridge University Press, Cambridge.
Anscombe G. E. M. (1993): 'Causality and determination' (reprint of 1971 lecture) in Perry J., Bratman M. (1993), pp. 250–60.
Balme D. M. (1939): 'Greek science and mechanism, I: Aristotle on nature and chance', *Classical Quarterly* 33, pp. 129–38.
Balme D. M. (1941): 'Greek science and mechanism, II: the Atomists', *Classical Quarterly* 35, pp. 23–8.
Balme D. M. (1962): 'Development of biology in Aristotle and Theophrastus: theory of spontaneous generation', *Phronesis* 7, pp. 91–104.
Bardong K. (1942): 'Beiträge zur Hippokrates- und Galenforschung', *Nachrichten der Akademie der Wissenschaften in Göttingen* 7, pp. 577–640.
Barnes J. (1979): *The Presocratic Philosophers*, Routledge & Kegan Paul Ltd, London (1996 reprint).
Barnes J. (1993): 'Galen and the utility of logic', in Kollesch and Nickel (1993), pp. 33–52.

Beare J. L. (1906): *Greek Theories of Elementary Cognition*, Clarendon Press, Oxford.

Bobzien S. (1999): 'Chrysippus' theory of causes', in Ierodiakonou (1999).

Botros S. (1985): 'Freedom, causality, fatalism and early Stoic philosophy', *Phronesis* 30, pp. 274–304.

Boudon V. (1994): 'Les Définitions tripartites de la médecine chez Galien', *Aufstieg und Niedergang der römischen Welt* II.37.2, pp. 1468–90.

Burnyeat M., ed. (1983): *The Skeptical Tradition*, University of California Press, Los Angeles and London.

Bylebyl J. J. (1979): 'Galen on the non-natural causes of variation in the pulse', *Bulletin of the History of Medicine* 53, pp. 482–5.

Clay D. (1983): *Lucretius and Epicurus*, Cornell University Press, Ithaca and London.

Cohen H. (1981): 'The evolution of the concept of disease', in Caplan A. L., Engelhardt H. T., McCartney J. J., *Concepts of Health and Disease*, Addison-Wesley Publishing Co., Reading, MA.

Conrad L. I., Neve M., Nutton V., Porter R., Wear A. (1995): *The Western Medical Tradition (800 BC to AD 1800)*, Cambridge University Press, Cambridge.

Deichgraber K. (1930): *Die greichische Empirikerschule*, Weidmann, Berlin (1965 reprint).

De Lacy P. H. (1966): 'Galen and the Greek poets', *Greek, Roman and Byzantine Studies* 7, pp. 259–66.

De Lacy P. H. (1973): 'Galen's Platonism', *American Journal of Philology* 93, pp. 27–32.

De Lacy P. H. (1979): 'Galen's concept of continuity', *Greek, Roman and Byzantine Studies* 20, pp. 355–69.

Dickson K. (1998): *Stephanus the Philosopher and Physician. Commentary on Galen's Therapeutics to Glaucon*, E. J. Brill, Leiden.

Diels H. A. (1905): *Die Handschriften der antiken Ärzte*, vol. I, *Hippocrates und Galen*, Zentralantiquariat, Leipzig (1970 reprint).

Diller H. (1933): 'Zur Hippokratesauffassung des Galen', *Hermes* 68, pp. 167–81.

Dillon J. (1996): *The Middle Platonists*, Duckworth, Bristol.

Dobson J. F. (1925): 'Herophilus of Alexandria', *Proceedings of the Royal Society of Medicine* 18, pp. 19–32.

Dobson J. F. (1927): 'Erasistratus', *Proceedings of the Royal Society of Medicine* 20, pp. 825–32.

Ducasse C. J. (1926): 'Explanation, mechanism, and teleology', *Journal of Philosophy* 23 (reprinted in Feigl and Sellars (1949)).

Durling R. J. (1961): 'A chronological census of Renaissance editions and translations of Galen', *Journal of the Courtauld and Warburg Institutes* 24, pp. 230–305.

Durling R. J. (1993): *A Dictionary of Medical Terms in Galen*, E. J. Brill, Leiden.

Edelstein E. J., Edelstein L. (1945): *Aesculapius. Collection and Interpretation of the Testimonies*, The Johns Hopkins University Press, Baltimore, MD.

Edmunds L. (1972): 'Necessity, chance and freedom in the early Atomists', *Phoenix* 26, pp. 343–57.

Eucken C. (1983): 'Zur Frage einer Molekulartheorie bei Herakleides und Asklepiades', *Museum Helveticum* 40, pp. 119–22.

Evans A. S. (1967): 'Clinical syndromes in adults caused by respiratory infection', *Medical Clinics of North America* 51, pp. 803–15.

Evans A. S. (1976): 'Causation and disease: the Henle–Koch postulates revisited', *Yale Journal of Biology and Medicine* 49, pp. 175–95.

Evans A. S. (1993): *Causation and Disease. A Chronological Journey*, Plenum Medical Book Co., New York.

Everson S., ed. (1991): *Psychology* (Companions in Ancient Thought 2), Cambridge University Press, Cambridge.

Feigl H., Sellars W., eds. (1949): *Readings in Philosophical Analysis*, Appleton-Century-Crofts Inc., New York.

Fleming D. (1955): 'Galen on the motions of the blood in the heart and lungs', *Isis* 46, pp. 14–21.

Frede M. (1980): 'The original notion of cause', in Frede (1987), pp. 125–50.

Frede M. (1983): 'The method of the so-called Methodical school of medicine', in Frede (1987), pp. 2–23.

Frede M. (1987): *Essays in Ancient Philosophy*, Oxford University Press, New York.

Frede M., Striker G., eds. (1996): *Rationality in Greek Thought*, Clarendon Press, Oxford.

Fuchs R. (1894): 'Anecdota medica graeca', *Rheinisches Museum für Philologie* 49, pp. 532–58.

Fuchs R. (1903): 'Aus Themisons Werk ueber die acuten und chronischen Krankheiten', *Rheinisches Museum für Philologie* 58, pp. 69–114.

Furley D. (1989): *Cosmic Problems*, Cambridge University Press, Cambridge.

Furley D. (1996): 'What kind of cause is Aristotle's final cause?' in Frede and Striker (1996).

Galdston I. (1968): 'The decline and resurgence of Hippocratic medicine', *Bulletin of the New York Academy of Medicine* 44, pp. 1237–56.

Garcia-Ballester L. (1974): 'Diseases of the soul in Galen: the impossibility of a Galenic psychotherapy', *Clio Medica* 9, pp. 35–43.

Garcia-Ballester L. (1993): 'On the origin of the "six non-natural things" in Galen', in Kollesch and Nickel (1993), pp. 105–15.

Garcia-Ballester L. (1994): 'Galen as a clinician: his methods in diagnosis', *Aufstieg und Niedergang der römischen Welt* II.37.2, pp. 1636–71.

Garcia-Ballester L. (2002): *Galen and Galenism*, Ashgate Variorum, Burlington, VT.

Gomperz T. (1911): 'Die hippokratische Frage und der Ausgangspunkt ihrer Lösung', *Philologus* 70, pp. 213–41.

Gotthelf, A., Lennox, J. G., eds. (1987): *Philosophical Issues in Aristotle's Biology*, Cambridge University Press, Cambridge.

Grmek M. D. (1991): *Diseases in the Ancient Greek World*, The Johns Hopkins University Press, Baltimore, MD (original French edition, 1983).

Guthrie W. K. C. (1962): *A History of Greek Philosophy*, vol. I, *The Earlier Presocratics and the Pythagoreans*, Cambridge University Press, Cambridge.

Guthrie W. K. C. (1965): *A History of Greek Philosophy,* vol. II, *The Presocratic Tradition from Parmenides to Democritus,* Cambridge University Press, Cambridge.
Hankinson R. J. (1987a): 'Evidence, externality and antecedence: inquiries into later Greek causal concepts', *Phronesis* 32, pp. 80–100.
Hankinson R. J. (1987b): 'Causes and empiricism: a problem in the interpretation of later Greek medical method', *Phronesis* 32, pp 329–48.
Hankinson R. J. (1991a): 'Galen's anatomy of the soul', *Phronesis* 36, pp. 197–233.
Hankinson R. J. (1991b): 'Greek medical models of mind', in Everson (1991).
Hankinson R. J. (1994a): 'Galen's theory of causation', *Aufstieg und Niedergang der römischen Welt* II.37.2, pp. 1757–74.
Hankinson R. J. (1994b): 'Galen's concept of scientific progress', *Aufstieg und Niedergang der römischen Welt* II.37.2, pp. 1775–89.
Hankinson R. J. (1995): *The Sceptics,* Routledge, London.
Hankinson R. J. (1998): *Cause and Explanation in Ancient Greek Thought,* Clarendon Press, Oxford.
Hanson A. E., Green M. H. (1994): 'Soranus of Ephesus: *Methodicorum princeps*', *Aufstieg und Niedergang der römischen Welt* II.37.2, pp. 968–1075.
Heisenberg W. (1930): *The Physical Principles of the Quantum Theory,* translated by Eckart C., Hoyt F. C., University of Chicago Press, Chicago.
Hocutt M. (1974): 'Aristotle's four becauses', *Philosophy* 49, pp. 385–99.
Horne R. A. (1963): 'Atomism in ancient medical history', *Medical History* 7, pp. 317–29.
Hume D. (1748–52): *A Treatise of Human Nature,* Everyman edition, 1961 reprint, J. M. Dent & Sons, London.
Humphreys P. (2000): 'Causation', in *A Companion to the Philosophy of Science,* Newton-Smith W. H., ed., Blackwell, Oxford.
Ierodiakonou K., ed. (1999): *Topics in Stoic Philosophy,* Oxford University Press, Oxford.
Ilberg J. (1889–97): 'Ueber die Schriftstellerei des Klaudios Galenos'. *Rheinisches Museum für Philologie* ns 44, pp. 207–39; 47, pp. 489–514; 51, pp. 165–96; 52, pp. 591–623.
Ilberg J. (1930): 'Wann ist Galenos geboren?' *Sudhoffs Archiv* 23, pp. 289–92.
Iskander A. Z. (1976): 'An attempted reconstruction of the Late Alexandrian medical curriculum', *Medical History* 20, pp. 235–58.
Jaeger W. (1940): 'Diocles of Carystus: a new pupil of Aristotle', *Philosophical Review* 49, pp. 393–414.
Jarcho S. (1970): 'Galen's six non-naturals: a bibliographical note and translation', *Bulletin of the History of Medicine* 44, pp. 372–7.
Jones W. H. S. (1946): *Philosophy and Medicine in Ancient Greece,* The Johns Hopkins University Press, Baltimore, MD (Supplement to the *Bulletin of the History of Medicine,* no. 8).
Jouanna J. (1999): *Hippocrates* (translated by DeBevoise M. B.), The Johns Hopkins University Press, Baltimore, MD.
Kalbfleisch K. (1897): 'Über Galens Einleitung in die Logik', *Jahrbücher für klassische Philologie* Supplement 23, pp. 679–708.

Kidd I. G. (1988): *Posidonius II. The Commentary*, Cambridge University Press, Cambridge.

King L. S. (1963): *The Growth of Medical Thought*, University of Chicago Press, Chicago.

Kollesch J. (1965): 'Galen und seine ärztliche Kollegen', *Altertum* 11, pp. 47–53.

Kollesch J. (1988): 'Anschauungen von den *archai* in der *Ars medico* und die Seelenlehre Galens', in Manuli and Vegetti (1988), pp. 215–29.

Kollesch J., Nickel D., eds. (1993): *Galen und das hellenistische Erbe*, Franz Steiner, Stuttgart.

Kollesch J., Nickel D. (1994): 'Bibliographia galeniana: die Beiträge des 20. Jahrhunderts zur Galenforschung', *Aufstieg und Niedergang der römischen Welt* II.37.2, pp. 1352–1420.

Kotrc R. F., Walters K. R. (1979): 'A bibliography of the Galenic Corpus', *Transactions and Studies of the College of Physicians of Philadelphia* V.1, pp. 256–304.

Kudlien, F. (1962): 'Posidonios und die Ärzteschule der Pneumatiker', *Hermes* 90, pp. 419–29.

Kudlien, F. (1964): 'Hierophilos und der Beginn der medizinischen Skepsis', *Gesnerus* 21, pp. 1–13.

Kudlien F., Durling R. J., eds. (1991): *Galen's Method of Healing* (Proceedings of the 1982 Galen Symposium), E. J. Brill, Leiden.

Lee J. A. L. (1997): 'Hebrews 5:14 and *Hexis*: a history of misunderstanding', *Novum Testamentum* 39, pp. 151–76.

Leitner H. (1973): *Bibliography to the Ancient Medical Authors*, Hans Huber, Bern.

Lieber E. (1979): 'Galen: physician as philosopher. Maimonides: philosopher as physician', *Bulletin of the History of Medicine* 53, pp. 268–85.

Lloyd G. E. R. (1963): 'Who is attacked in *On Ancient Medicine?*' *Phronesis* 8, pp. 108–26.

Lloyd G. E. R. (1964): 'Experiment in early Greek philosopy and medicine', *Proceedings of the Cambridge Philological Society*, n.s. 10, pp. 50–72.

Lloyd G. E. R. (1968): *Aristotle. The Growth and Structure of his Thought*, Cambridge University Press, Cambridge.

Lloyd G. E. R. (1975a): 'The Hippocratic question', *Classical Quarterly* 25, pp. 171–92.

Lloyd G. E. R. (1975b): 'Alcmaeon and the early history of dissection', *Sudhoffs Archiv* 59, pp. 113–47.

Lloyd G. E. R. (1979): *Magic, Reason and Experience. Studies in the Origin and Development of Greek Science*, Cambridge University Press, Cambridge.

Lloyd G. E. R. (1983): *Science, Folklore and Ideology. Studies in the Life Sciences in Ancient Greece*, Cambridge University Press, Cambridge.

Lloyd G. E. R. (1991): *Methods and Problems in Greek Science*, Cambridge University Press, Cambridge.

Lloyd G. E. R. (1993): 'Galen on Hellenistics and Hippocrateans: contemporary battles and past authorities', in Kollesch and Nickel (1993), pp. 125–43.

Lloyd G. E. R. (1996): 'Theories and practices of demonstration in Galen', in Frede and Striker (1996).

Lloyd G. E. R. (2004): *In the Grip of Disease. Studies in the Greek Imagination*, Oxford University Press, Oxford.

Lohmann J. (1952): 'Das Verhältnis des abendländischen Menschen zur Sprache', *Lexis* 3, pp. 5–50.

Long A. A. (1996a): *Stoic Studies*, Cambridge University Press, Cambridge.

Long A. A. (1996b): 'Soul and body in Stoicism', in Long (1996a), pp. 224–49.

Longrigg J. (1993): *Greek Rational Medicine*, Routledge, London.

Lones T. E. (1912): *Aristotle's Researches in Natural Science*, West, Newman & Co., London.

Lonie I. M. (1964): 'Erasistratus, the Erasistrateans and Aristotle', *Bulletin of the History of Medicine* 38, pp. 426–43.

Lonie I. M. (1965): 'Medical theory in Heraclides of Pontus', *Mnemosyne* 18, pp. 126–43.

López Férez J. A., ed. (1991): *Galeno: obra, pensamiento e influencia*, Rugarte, Madrid.

Mace C. A. (1935): 'Mechanical and teleological causation', Aristotelian Society, suppl. vol. 14 (reprinted in Feigl and Sellars (1949)).

Mackie J. L. (1965): 'Causes and conditions', *American Philosophical Quarterly* 2, pp. 245–64.

Mackie J. L. (1974): *The Cement of the Universe*, Clarendon Press, Oxford.

Mackie P. J. (1995): 'Causality', in *The Oxford Companion to Philosophy*, ed. Honderich T., Oxford University Press, Oxford.

Manetti D., Roselli A. (1994): 'Galeno commentatore di Hippocrate', *Aufstieg und Niedergang der römischen Welt* II.37.2, pp. 1529–635 (index pp. 2071–80).

Manuli P. (1993): 'Galen and Stoicism', in Kollesch and Nickel (1993), pp. 53–61.

Manuli P., Vegetti M. (1988): *Le opere psicologiche di Galeno*, Bibliopolis, Naples (Proceedings of the Terzo Colloquio Galenico Internazionale Pavia, September 1986).

Mettler, C. C. (1947): *History of Medicine*, The Blakiston Company, Philadelphia.

Meyerhof M. (1926): 'A new light on Hunain Ibn Ishaq and his period', *Isis* 8, pp. 685–724.

Meyerhof M. (1929): 'Autobiographische Bruchstücke Galens aus arabischen Quellen', *Archiv für Geschichte der Medizin* 22, pp. 72–86.

Mill J. S. (1884): *A System of Logic*, Longmans, Green & Co., London.

Miller H. W. (1952): '*Dynamis* and *physis* in *On Ancient Medicine*', *Transactions of the American Philological Association* 83, pp. 184–97.

Miller H. W. (1960): 'The concept of *dynamis* in *De victu*', *Transactions of the American Philological Association* 90, pp. 147–64.

Miller H. W. (1963): 'The aetiology of disease in Plato's *Timaeus*', *Transactions and Proceedings of the American Philological Association* 93, pp. 175–87.

Moraux P. (1985): *Galien de Pergame. Souvenirs d'un médecin*, Les Belles Lettres, Paris.

Murphy E. A. (1997): *The Logic of Medicine* (2nd edn.), The Johns Hopkins University Press, Baltimore, MD.

Newton-Smith W. H., ed. (2000): *A Companion to the Philosophy of Science*, Blackwell, Oxford.

Nickel D. (1993): 'Stoa und Stoiker in Galens Schrift *De foetuum formatione*', in Kollesch and Nickel (1993), pp. 80–6.

Niebyl P. H. (1979): 'The non-naturals', *Bulletin of the History of Medicine* 79, pp. 486–92.

Nutton V. (1972): 'Galen and medical autobiography', *Proceedings of the Cambridge Philological Society* 198 (ns 18), pp. 50–61.

Nutton V. (1973): 'The chronology of Galen's early career', *Classical Quarterly* 23, pp. 158–71.

Nutton V. (1976): *Karl Gottlob Kühn and his Edition of the Works of Galen*, Oxford Microform Publications, Oxford.

Nutton V., ed. (1981): *Galen. Problems and Prospects*, The Wellcome Institute, London.

Nutton V. (1983): 'The seeds of disease: an explanation of contagion and infection from the Greeks to the Renaissance', *Medical History* 27, pp. 1–34.

Nutton V. (1984a): 'Galen in the eyes of his contemporaries', *Bulletin of the History of Medicine* 58, pp. 315–24.

Nutton V. (1984b): 'From Galen to Alexander, aspects of medicine and medical practice in late antiquity', Dumbarton Oaks Papers, Washington DC, pp. 1–13.

Nutton V. (1985): 'Harvey, Goulston and Galen', in Nutton (1988), pp. 112–23.

Nutton V. (1987): *John Caius and the Manuscripts of Galen*, The Cambridge Philological Society, Cambridge.

Nutton V. (1988): *From Democedes to Harvey*, Variorum Reprints, London.

Nutton V. (1993): 'Galen and Egypt', in Kollesch and Nickel (1993), pp. 11–31.

Nutton V. (1995): 'Roman medicine 250 BC to AD 200', in Conrad et al. (1995), pp. 39–70.

Nutton V., ed. (2002): *The Unknown Galen, Bulletin of the Institute of Classical Studies*, Suppl. 77, London.

Nutton V. (2004): *Ancient Medicine*, Routledge, London.

Oberhelman S. M. (1994): 'On the chronology and Pneumatism of Aretaios of Cappadocia', *Aufstieg und Niedergang der römischen Welt* II.37.2, pp. 941–66.

Pearcy L. T. (1993): 'Medicine and rhetoric in the period of the Second Sophistic', *Aufstieg und Niedergang der römischen Welt* II.37.1, pp. 443–56.

Pearson L. (1952): 'Prophasis and aitia', *Transactions of the American Philological Association* 83, pp. 205–22.

Perry J., Bratman M., eds. (1993): *Introduction to Philosophy* (2nd edn.), Oxford University Press, New York.

Peterson D. W. (1977): 'Observations on the chronology of the Galenic Corpus', *Bulletin of the History of Medicine* 51, pp. 484–94.

Phillips E. D. (1987): *Aspects of Greek Medicine*, The Charles Press, Philadelphia.

Pigeaud J. (1993): 'Les Problèmes de la création chez Galien', in Kollesch and Nickel (1993), pp. 87–103.

Pines S. (1961): 'Omne quod movetur necesse est ab aliquo moveri: a refutation of Galen by Alexander of Aphrodisias and the theory of motion', *Isis* 52, pp. 21–54.

Rawlings H. R. (1975): 'A semantic study of *"prophasis"* to 400 BC', *Hermes*, Einzelschriften, Heft 33, Franz Steiner, Wiesbaden.

Reesor M. E. (1989): *The Nature of Man in Early Stoic Philosophy*, Duckworth, London.

Riddle J. M. (1994): 'High medicine and low medicine in the Roman Empire', *Aufstieg und Niedergang der römischen Welt* II.37.4, pp. 103–20.

Riese W. (1953): *The Conception of Disease*, The Philosophical Library, New York.

Rivers T. M. (1937): 'Viruses and Koch's postulates', *Journal of Bacteriology* 33, pp. 1–12.

Rocca J. (2003): *Galen on the Brain*, E. J. Brill, Leiden.

Ross D. (1995): *Aristotle*, 6th edn. with introduction by J. L. Ackrill, Routledge, New York.

Rothman K. J. (1976): 'Causes', *American Journal of Epidemiology* 104, pp. 587–92.

Russell B. (1917): *Mysticism and Logic*, Penguin Books, Harmondsworth (reprint 1953).

Sarton G. (1927): *Introduction to the History of Science*, vol. I, *From Homer to Omar Khayyam*, The Williams and Wilkins Co., Baltimore, MD.

Sarton G. (1954): *Galen of Pergamon*, University of Kansas Press, Lawrence, KA.

Scarborough J. (1993): 'Roman medicine to Galen', *Aufstieg und Niedergang der römischen Welt* II.37.1, pp. 3–48.

Schacht J. and Meyerhoff, M. (1937): *The Medico-Philosophical Controversy between Ibn Butlan of Baghdad and Ibn Ridwan of Cairo. A Contribution to the History of Greek Learning among the Arabs*, The Egyptian University (Faculty of Arts Publication no. 13), Cairo.

Schlange-Schöningen H. (2003): *Die römische Gesellschaft bei Galen*, Walter de Gruyter, Berlin.

Schlick M. (1932): 'Causality in everyday life and in recent science', Reprinted in Feigl and Sellars (1949), pp. 515–33.

Schopenhauer A. (1847): *On the Fourfold Root of the Principle of Sufficient Reason*, E. J. J. Payne, translator, Open Court Classics, La Salle, IL, 1974.

Schuller S. (1956): 'About Thucydides' use of *aitia* and *prophasis*', *Revue Belge de Philosophie et d'Histoire* 34, pp. 971–84.

Siegel R. E. (1968): *Galen's System of Medicine and Physiology. An Analysis of his Doctrines on Blood Flow, Respiration, Humours and Internal Diseases*, S. Karger, Basle.

Siegel R. E. (1970): *Galen on Sense Perception, his Doctrines, Observations and Experiments on Vision, Hearing, Smell, Taste, Touch and Pain, and their Historical Sources*, S. Karger, Basle.

Siegel R. E. (1971): 'Melancholy and black bile in Galen and later writers', *Bulletin of the Cleveland Medical Library* 18, pp. 10–20.

Siegel R. E. (1973): *Galen on Psychology, Psychopathology, and Function and Diseases of the Nervous System*, S. Karger, Basle.

Singer P. N. (1992): *Galen on the Soul. Philosophy and Medicine in the Second Century* AD, PhD thesis, Cambridge University.

Smith W. D. (1973): 'Galen on Coans versus Cnidians', *Bulletin of the History of Medicine* 47, pp. 568–85.

Smith W. D. (1979): *The Hippocratic Tradition*, Cornell University Press, Ithaca.

Smolin L. (2001): *Three Roads to Quantum Gravity*, Phoenix, London.

Solmsen F. (1957): 'The vital heat, the inborn pneuma and the aether', *Journal of the History of Science* 77, pp. 119–23.

Solmsen F. (1961): 'Greek *philosophy* and the discovery of the nerves', *Museum Helveticum* 18, pp. 159–97.

Souilhe J. (1919): *Étude sur le terme dunamis*, Garland Publishing Inc, New York & London (1987 reprint).

Strodach G. K. (1963): *The Philosophy of Epicurus*, Northwestern University Press, Chicago.

Strohmaier G. (1994): 'Der syrische und der arabische Galen', *Aufstieg und Niedergang der römischen Welt* II.37.2, pp. 1987–2017.

Susser M. (1978): *Causal Thinking in the Health Sciences. Concepts and Strategies*, Oxford University Press, London.

Tecusan M. (2004): *The Fragments of the Methodists. Methodism outside Soranus*, vol. I, *Text and Translation*, E. J. Brill, Leiden.

Temkin O. (1973): *Galenism. Rise and Decline of a Medical Philosophy*, Cornell University Press, Ithaca.

Temkin O., Temkin C. L., eds. (1967): *Ancient Medicine. Selected Papers of Ludwig Edelstein*, The Johns Hopkins University Press, Baltimore.

Urmson J. O. (1990): *The Greek Philosophical Vocabulary*, Duckworth, London.

Vallance J. T. (1990): *The Lost Theory of Asclepiades of Bithynia*, Clarendon Press, Oxford.

Vander Waerdt P. A. (1985a): 'The Peripatetic interpretation of Plato's tripartite psychology', *Greek, Roman and Byzantine Studies* 26, pp. 283–302.

Vander Waerdt P. A. (1985b): 'Peripatetic soul-division, Posidonius, and Middle Platonic moral psychology', *Greek, Roman and Byzantine Studies* 26, pp. 373–94.

Vlastos, G. (1969): 'Reasons as causes in the *Phaedo*', *Philosophical Review* 75, pp. 291–325.

Von Staden H. (1975): 'Experiment and experience in Hellenistic medicine', *Bulletin of the Institute of Classical Studies* 22, pp. 178–99.

Von Staden H. (1991): 'Galen as historian: his use of sources on Herofileans', in López-Férez (1991), pp. 205–22.

Walsh J. (1926): 'Galen's discovery and promulgation of the function of the recurrent laryngeal nerve', *Annals of Medical History* 8, pp. 176–84.

Walsh J. (1929): 'Date of Galen's birth', *Annals of Medical History* ns 1, pp. 378–82.

Walsh J. (1932): 'Refutation of Ilberg as to the date of Galen's birth', *Annals of Medical History* ns 4, pp. 126–46.
Walsh J. (1934–9): 'Galen's writings and influences inspiring them', *Annals of Medical History* ns 6 (1934), pp. 1–30, 143–9; 7 (1935), pp. 428–37, 570–89; 8 (1936), pp. 65–90; 9 (1937), pp. 34–61; 3rd series 1 (1939), pp. 525–37.
Wellmann M. (1895): *Die pneumatische Schule bis auf Archigenes in ihrer Entwicklung dargestellt*, Philologische Untersuchungen, Berlin.
Wittgenstein L. (1961): *Tractatus Logico-Philosophicus* (trans. Pears D. F., McGuinness B. F.), Routledge & Kegan Paul, London.

Index

Abscesses (*apostemata*) 148, 174, 198, 209, 214, 270
Achores 170
Acquired (*epiktetos*) 43
Action (*ergon*), definition of 30
Adenitis (*paristhmion*) 298
Aëtius 85–6, 148
Affection (*pathos/pathema*) 123, 136, 137, 143, 147, 150, 166, 174, 198, 209, 221, 224, 228, 244, 259, 260, 273, 280, 281, 288, 306
   definition of 24–5, 182–3, 184
   relation to symptom 182, 186–7, 211
Agathinus of Sparta 19
Agitation (*klonos*) 193, 195, 274
Akinesia (absence of movement) 187, 190, 269
Alcmaeon of Croton 15, 20, 22, 47
   on disease causation 85–6
Alopecias (*alopekiai*) 192
Alphoi 141, 148, 170, 198, 280
Alteration/assimilation 38
Amblyopia (dim-sightedness) 189, 212, 215, 216
Amentia (*anoia*) 191
Amnesia (*lethe*) 263
Anaesthesia (absence of sensation) 188, 269
Anarmoi onkoi 16, 22, 39, 99, 136, 306
Anasarca 273, 282, 296
Anaxagoras 40, 42, 45
Anomalous *dyscrasia* 169
Anonymus Londinensis 15, 23, 89, 90
   on disease causation 90
Anonymous of Paris 93
Anorexia/dysorexia 226
Apepsia, bradypepsia, dyspepsia 74, 188, 194, 196, 269, 271, 301
Aphonia/kakophonia/dysphonia 190, 239
Apnoea/dyspnoea 190, 226, 231, 232, 239
Apollonius 96
Apoplexy 142, 165, 190, 234, 240, 263
Archigenes of Apamea 19, 104
Aretaeus of Cappadocia 19
Aristotle, general 20, 44, 50, 65, 67, 68, 78, 83, 96, 308, 310

Galen's attitude to 19, 20
   influence on Galen 13–14
   on alteration 38
   on causes 35, 106, 108, 112, 309, 310
   on disease causation 92–3
   on imbalance 39
   on the definition of *dunamis* 28
   on the definitions of state and condition 28
   on *differentiae* 41
   on excretion 42
   on *homoiomeres* 45
   on nutrition 280
   on pores 47
   on sleep 233
Aristotle, works
   De anima 13
   Generation of Animals 43
   History of Animals 40
   Metaphysics 28, 40, 41, 47
   Parts of Animals 46
   Topics 40
Aristotle, spurious works
   Problems 42, 92
Ascites 278
Asclepiades 14, 16, 18, 19, 22, 42, 47, 70, 93, 97, 120, 136, 308
   concept of structure 16, 124, 305, 306
   on constriction and dilatation 72
   relevance for Galen 16
   theory of disease causation 16–17, 98–100, 309
Asclepius 151
Athenaeus of Attaleia 19, 32, 33, 48, 93, 100, 107, 120, 246, 310
   on disease causation 100–1
   on respiration 251
Atomism/Atomists 83, 107
Atrophy (*atrophia*) 151, 192, 279, 301

Bald patches (*ophiaseis*) 192
Bandy-legged (*raibos*) 172
Baryekoïa (hardness of hearing) 52, 189, 215
Belching (*eruge*) 238

Blastema (fleshy excrescence) 276, 277, 291
Boissier de Sauvages, François 78
Borborygmos 199, 249, 287
Boulimia 230
Bradypepsia, see *apepsia*
Breakage (*regma*) 179

Caelius Aurelianus 67
Cancerous sores (*phagedainai*) 170, 272
Cancers (*karkinoi*) 153, 169, 272, 278
Capacity (*dunamis*) 232
  affected by dyscrasias 273–4
  alterative, disorders of 269–70, 281, 295
  attractive, symtoms of 275–7, 281
  authoritative 263
  definition of 28–9, 171
  four capacities 239
  physical 246–7, 249, 268
  psychical 260, 262
  retentive 274–5, 281, 295, 296–7
  separative 261, 281, 295
Cardiac syncope 231
Caries (*teredon*) 178
Catalepsy (*katalepsis*) 191, 231, 234
Cataract (*hypochyma*) 148, 155, 156, 207, 210, 211, 215
Catarrh/coryza 216, 250, 297
Causation, general 82–3
Cause (*aitia/aition*) 310
  definition of 31–2
Causes (effecting) 272
Causes (primary/*per se* and secondary/*per accidens*) 106, 114, 185, 310
Causes (*proegoumenic* and *prokatarktic*) 72, 100, 102, 105, 108, 109, 111, 116, 124, 187, 188, 224, 310
  definitions of 34, 113
Causes (*prophasis*) 115, 116, 124, 310
  definition of 32–3
Causes (*synektic*) 107, 111, 116, 124, 209, 217, 228, 310
  definition of 34–5
Causes of diseases and symptoms 84–5
  excess of cold 164–8
  excess of dryness 168
  excess of heat 160–4
  excess of moisture 168
  of combined diseases 168–9
  proegoumenic causes 5, 147, 163
  prokatarktic causes 85, 163
Celsus 17, 18, 19, 66
  on classification of disease 67
Chalkstones in joints (*poroi*) 148
Chemosis 213
Chokings (*pnix*) 226

Cholerai 275, 281
Chrysippus 14, 31, 38, 310
  Galen's attitude to 14
Classification 307–9
Collapse (*katoptosis*) 230
Coma (*koma*) 165, 190, 191, 231, 233, 234, 301
Condition (*diathesis*) 69, 184, 306
  definition of 27, 182
  as cause of disease 186
Conformation (*diaplasis*) 41
Constitution (*kataskeue*) 69, 184, 306
  definition of 28
Consumption (*phthoe*) 174
Cough (*bex*) 238, 261, 262
Cullen, William 79
Cysts (*melikerides*) 148, 170, 176

Damage (*blabe*) 40–1
Deafness (*kophotes*) 189, 214, 216
Debility (*atonia*) 70, 143–4
Deficiency (*ellipes*) 42
Delirium (*parakope*) 226
Delirium (*paraphrosyne*) 191, 231, 233, 234, 263
Delusion (*phantasma*) 191
Dementia (*morosis*) 191, 263
Democritus 14, 16, 19
Derangement (*paranoia*) 301
Despair (*dysthymia*) 301
Diapedesis 283
Diarrhoea 297
Differentia (*diaphora*) 41–2, 137, 188, 280
  Aristotle on 4
  of digestion 301
  of diseases 5, 69, 140, 152
  of diseases in *homoiomeres* 139
  of diseases in organs 139–40, 148, 152
  of expulsions 200, 289
  of functions 188
  of functions of the soul 188–9
  of health 138
  of respiratory functions 198–9
  of symptoms 5, 187, 188, 197, 274
Dilatation/constriction (*eurutes/stegnosis*) 43, 70, 137
Diocles of Carystus 15, 44, 202
  as Rationalist 93
  on disease causation 93–4
Diogenes Laertius 26, 92
Diogenes of Apollonia 19, 20, 43
Discharge (*ruas*) 151, 156
Disease 136, 147, 185
  causes of 147, 159–60
  classification of in organic parts 71
  combined diseases 152
  definition of 23–4, 186, 306

in relation to symptom 187
of arrangement in organs 177–8
of conformation in organs 172–6
of number in organs 176–7
of size in organs 177
types of in *homoiomeres* 138, 159
types of in organs 138, 144–5, 276, 277, 297
Dislocation
of joints (*exarthresis*) 151
of organs (*exarthrema*) 154, 177, 218
Disorders of movement 238–46
Dissolution of continuity (*lusis sunecheias*) 43–4,
70, 75, 76, 115, 152, 153, 159, 178–9, 206, 214
Distraction (*ektasis*) 301
Distribution (*anadosis/diadosis*) 39–40
Dogmatism/Dogmatics (see also Rationalism)
17, 20, 84, 120, 309
Dropsies (*hydrops/hyderoi*) 192, 198, 273, 274,
296, 300
Leucophlegmatous 278, 296
Dullness (*moria*) 191
Dunamis (capacity) 38, 116
Dysaesthesia (disordered sensation) 187
Dyscrasia/eukrasia 43, 69, 70–1, 75, 76, 79, 100,
113, 119, 135, 141, 142, 143, 144, 159, 161, 197,
199, 200, 206, 211, 214, 216, 234, 243, 251,
263, 269, 272, 277, 285
anomalous (non-uniform) 251, 252, 256
in homoiomeres 297
of uterus 298
Dysenteria 248, 281, 286, 289–90
Dyskinesia (disordered movement) 187, 190
Dyspepsia (disordered digestion) 188, 196
Dyspnoea 226

Ear, disorders of 214–15
Earache (*otalgia*) 189
Echos (ringing sound) 199
Element (*stoicheion*) 47–8, 100, 138
four elements 271
Elephantiasis 114, 141, 196
Elephas 174, 198, 272, 278, 279, 300
Empedocles 19, 89, 92
Emphraxis 16
Empiricism/Empiricists 17–18, 69, 84, 85, 120,
309
Emprosthotonos 142, 190
Enkanthis 151
Entasis 99
Epicurus 14, 16, 136
Epigennema (epiphenomenon) 25, 26, 182, 186
Epilepsy 142, 190, 226, 234, 240, 263, 301
Erasistratus 16, 85, 93, 108, 109
Galen's attitude to 20, 103
on disease causation 97–8, 99, 309, 310

Erysipelas 70, 141, 147, 153, 154, 161, 170, 198,
269, 272, 278
Eye, disorders of 206–14

Fatigue 253, 261, 262
Fatty swellings (*atheromata*) 148, 170, 177
Fever 161–3, 257, 301
bilious remittent 255
tertian 254
Flatulence (*empneumatosis*) 300
Flux muliebris (*rous gynaikeios*) 299
Fluxions 169, 170
Four elements/qualities 15, 19, 24, 66, 306
Four humours 20, 169
Fracture (*katagma*) 152, 218
Freezing (*pexis*) 142
Function (*energeia*) 20, 40, 70, 184, 306
alterative 279
damage of 282
definition of 29–30
involvement in disease 149–50, 185, 197
involvement in symptoms 268
physical 279–82
psychical 262

Galen, general
as a Dogmatist 17
attitude to Aristotle 13
attitude to Chrysippus 14
attitude to Erasistratus 109
attitude to Hippocrates 15
attitude to Plato 11
attitude to schools and other philosophers
19–20
father's influence 7
key terms 30–1
on causal terms 36–7
on causation 17, 64, 85, 102–3, 309–11
on definition 63–4, 77–8
on Empiricism 17, 18
on health and disease 43, 308
on Methodism 19
on Pneumatism 19
on Praxagoras' humours 94
on *proegoumenic* and *prokatarktic*
causes 34
on *psyche* 118
on symptoms 308
on *synektic* causes 107–8
volume of writings 8–9
Galen, works
Ars medica 23, 49
De alimentorum facultatibus 42, 93
De anatomicis administrationibus 13, 219
De atra bile 40

Galen, works (*cont.*)
  De causis contentivis 33, 100, 106
  De causis morborum 33, 34, 43, 44, 48, 99, 103, 106, 112, 116
  De causis procatarcticis 95, 96, 97, 103, 106, 108
  De causis pulsuum 110, 111
  De causis respirationis 9, 110, 112
  De compositione medicamentorum secundum locos 96
  De crisibus 298
  De differentiis pulsuum 41
  De elementis secundum Hippocratem 4, 45, 46, 48, 308
  De facultatibus naturalibus 29, 30, 33, 38, 39, 40, 94, 113, 199, 308
  De libris propriis 9
  De locis affectis 27, 38, 42, 44, 103
  De methodo medendi 4, 9, 11, 21, 22, 24, 25, 26, 28, 29, 30, 33, 34, 40, 41, 44, 45, 68, 75, 76, 78, 103, 104, 105, 155, 298, 307
  De morborum differentiis 22, 23, 34, 39, 41, 42, 43, 44, 45, 47, 67, 68, 76, 276, 305
  De placitis Hippocratis et Platonis 14, 33, 44, 45, 46, 66
  De propriis placitis 118
  De sanitate tuenda 23, 29, 39, 47
  De semine 13
  De symptomatum causis 33, 34, 38, 42, 44, 48, 106, 116, 199, 310
  De symptomatum differentiis 23, 24, 25, 26, 27, 32, 34, 35, 36, 40, 42, 67, 72, 82, 103, 105, 274, 300, 305, 307, 310
  De tremore, palpitatione, convulsione et rigore 48
  De usu partium 9, 13, 37, 39, 40, 41, 42, 45, 49, 103, 110–11
  De veneriis 9
  Quod animi mores 29, 118
  Synopsis librorum suorum de pulsibus 31
Galen, spurious works
  Definitiones medicae 22, 26, 32, 33, 37, 42, 43, 48, 49, 50, 63, 100, 310
  Introductio sive medicus 93, 94, 96, 99
Galenic Canon (Summaria Alexandria) 5, 9–10
Ganglia 170, 176
Gangrenes (*gangrainai*) 170, 198, 272
Gastric syncope 226
Glandular swellings (*bubones*) 161
Glandular swellings (*phugethla*) 141, 161, 170
Gnashing the teeth (*to trizein*) 239
Gnawings (*dexeis*) 195, 300
Gurgling (*trusmos*) 249

Haimodia 104, 217
Hardness of hearing 216
Headache (*kephalalgia*) 189

Health, definition of 21–3, 134–5, 306
Heartburn (*kardialgia*) 189, 226, 230, 300, 301
Heartburn (*oxuregmiodes*) 273
Heat stroke (*enkausis*) 161
Hegemonikon 15, 119–20, 308
  Disorders of function 191–2
Heisenberg, Werner 121
Heraclides of Pontus 16
Hernia
  intestinal (*enteroplokele*) 151, 177
  omental (*epiplokele*) 151, 177
Herophilus 16, 27, 85, 99, 108, 207
  as Rationalist 93
  Galen's attitude to 20
  on disease causation 95–6
Herpes 147, 153, 161, 170, 198, 272, 278
Hiccup (*lynx/lygmos*) 195, 238, 240, 261, 262, 274, 275
Hippocrates, general 18, 19, 20, 43, 78, 211, 308
  as Rationalist 93
  Galen's attitude to 19
  influence on Galen 15
  on blood vessels 165
  on classification 66, 68
  on diarrhoeas 288
  on humours 50
  on melancholia 264
  on pain 220, 221, 252
  on respiration 240
  on rigor 255, 258
  on *tetanos* 224
  on the four qualities 14
  on vision 208
  relation to Chrysippus 14
Hippocrates, works
  Airs, Waters, Places 88
  Ancient Medicine 40, 87, 89
  Aphorisms 88, 292
  Breaths 87, 88, 98
  Diseases II 66
  Diseases III 66
  Humours 88
  Internal Affections 66
  Nature of Man 15, 87
  Prognostic 292
  Regimen 87
  Sacred Disease 86–9
Hippocratic Corpus 15, 32, 66, 86–90, 120
  on disease causation 86
Homoiomeres 13, 39, 42, 45, 46, 48, 68, 69, 70, 71, 77, 107, 112, 113, 115, 119, 124, 137, 139, 141, 144, 152, 154, 172, 196, 200, 206, 209, 210, 214, 272, 274, 291, 306, 308
Horror vacui 97
Hume, David 121

Humour (*chumos*) 50, 76, 94, 100, 113, 228, 247, 258, 260, 263, 271, 277, 299
Hyphaema (*hyposphagma*) 212
Hypochondriasis 264

Ileus 276
Imbalance/balance 39, 70, 95, 135, 306
  of pores 140
Impassible (*apathes*) 40
Indurations (*skirroi*) 141, 151, 174, 209, 214, 218, 269, 291
Inertia (*hesuchia*) 234, 241
Inflammation (*phlegmone*)/inflammatory swellings (*phlegmonai*) 141, 147, 151, 154, 161, 174, 189, 209, 214, 218, 220, 241, 251, 269, 288, 291
Inflation (*pneumatosis*) 194, 195, 274
Innate heat 15, 48, 94, 161, 165, 166, 167, 258
Insomnia (*agrypnia*) 190, 233, 234, 300
Irregularites (*anomalia*) 261, 301
Irritation (*erethrismos*) 234
Ischuria/dysuria 190, 239, 290
Itching (*knesis*) 261–2

Jaundice (*icterus*) 192, 197, 198, 216, 278, 300, 301

Kant, Immanuel 121
Karebaria (heaviness of the head) 300
Kitta (*pica*) 229
Knock-kneed (*blaisos*) 172
Kühn K.-G. 3, 6, 9, 129

Leienteria 194, 248, 273, 275, 281
Leoniceno 10
Leprai 141, 148, 261
Lethargy (*lethargia/lethargos*) 191, 233, 234, 296
Leucippus 14
Leuke/leukai 148, 192, 196, 198, 272, 279, 280, 281
Linacre, Thomas 10, 30
Linnaeus 78
Lucretius 14

Madness (*phrenitis*) 233, 234, 263, 296
Mania 263
Melancholia 226, 231, 264
Methodism/Methodics 16, 17, 18, 22, 42, 69, 70, 84, 99, 120, 308, 309, 310
Mnesitheus 27, 50, 93, 102

Nausea (*nautia*) 300
Nicomachus the Smyrnaean 151
Nose, disorders of 215–16
Numbness (*narke*) 217, 218, 234, 240, 263

Obstruction (*emphraxis*) 42

Oidema (swelling) 141, 151, 154, 214, 269, 291
Olympicus 22, 102
Onkos (mass/swelling) 291, 298
Ophthalmia 154, 155
Opisthotonos 142, 190
Organs/organic structures 115, 124, 137, 172–6, 210, 274, 306, 308
Ostokopos 253

Pain/pleasure 189–90, 220, 260–1
Palpitation (*palmos*) 190, 193, 195, 235, 238, 244, 256, 274
Parakousis (false hearing) 189, 215, 216
Paremptosis 97–8, 99, 109
Parorasis (false vision) 189, 212, 216
Pausanius 89
Perforation (*trema*) 178
Peripneumonia 251
Philistion of Locri 89
  on disease causation 90
Philolaus of Croton 89
  on disease causation 89–90
Philotimus 224, 231
Phlegm 116, 170, 224, 231, 247, 284
Phrenitis (see Madness)
Phthisis (wasting) 114, 151, 192
Plato, general 24, 50, 66, 83, 89, 194, 308, 310
  'demiurge' 13
  Galen's attitude to 19, 20
  influence on Galen 11
  on affections 25, 307
  on classification of disease 66
  on disease causation 90–2
  on health and disease 39
  on imbalance 39
  on pain 221
  on vision 208, 222
Plato, works
  Phaedo 11
  Philebus 221
  Timaeus 11, 66, 90, 220, 221
Plethora 167, 229
Pliny 96
Pneuma 14, 15, 17, 19, 20, 34, 85, 94, 97, 98, 100, 107, 112, 116, 119, 199, 207, 210, 240, 245, 250, 256, 258, 274, 286–8, 299, 301, 310
Pneuma psychikon 119, 212
Pneumatism/Pneumatics 19, 100, 251, 309
Polyuria 249
Pores (*poroi*) 16, 22, 39, 42, 43, 44, 46–7, 70, 99, 135, 137, 144, 153, 159
Praxagoras 13, 15
  as Rationalist 93
  on disease causation 94–5
  on humours 224, 231
Priapism 151, 299

Index

Psorai 141, 261
Psyche (the soul) 118, 188, 259, 269
Pterygium 155, 156, 213
Pus (*puon*) 148
Pustules (*anthrakes*) 147, 153, 161, 169, 198, 270, 272
Pythagoras 92

Qualities 39, 43, 76, 97, 100, 141, 229, 279

Rarefaction (*manosis*) 44
Rasping (*trusmos*) 238
Rationalism (see also Dogmatism) 20, 93, 96
Rigor (*rigos*) 195, 235, 238, 254, 255, 257–8, 261, 262, 275, 301
Rufus 102
Rupture (*spasma*) 179
Russell, Bertrand 121

Satyriasis 170
Scars (*sklerai*) 174
Sceptics 83, 120, 309
Scrofulous swellings (*choirades*) 141, 151
Sebaceous swellings (*steatomata*) 148, 170, 177
Sense perception 37–8
Separation (*apokrisis*) 40
Separation (*ekkrisis*) 42
Sextus Empiricus 18
Shaking (*klonodes*) 190
Shivering (*phrike*) 238, 254, 262, 301
Sleep 232–3
Sneezing (*ptarmos*) 238, 250, 261, 262
Soma and *psyche* 120
Soranus 19, 100, 102
Spasm (convulsion) 142, 174, 234, 235
Spasm (*spasmos*) 190, 193, 195, 238, 240, 256, 274
Spermatorrhoea 240, 299
Speusippus 65
Spinal cord injuries 218
Splashing (*klydon*) 194, 195, 274
Squinting (*strabismus*) 239
State (*hexis*)
    definition of 27–8
Stoics 83, 107, 120, 310
    concepts of 14
Stomach, disorders of 247–8
Stranguria 249, 291
Strato 97
Stretching (*skordinismos*) 238, 261
Subluxation (*pararthresis*) 151
Sunstroke (*ekkausis*) 297
Superfluities (*perissomata*) 113, 229, 260, 270, 277, 281

of digestion 278–9, 288
phlegmatic, bilious and serous 284
Sweats 292–3
Swooning (*leipopsychia*) 230, 260
Sympathetic affection 226, 231
Symptoms 123, 142, 147, 182–7, 192, 306
    classification of 308
    definition of 25–6, 186, 307
    following other symptoms 299–300
    of appetite 192
    of authoritative functions 263–4
    of digestion 192
    of motor functions 190
    of physical organs 192–3
    of separative functions 249
    pertaining to the stomach 226–32
    relation to affection 211
Syncope 292

Teinesmos 248, 290
Teleology 13
Tetanos 142, 190, 225
Themison 18, 100, 102
Theophilus (the physician) 191
Theophrastus, general 68, 78
    on definition and classification 65
Theophrastus, works
    De causis plantarum 44
Thessalus 18, 22, 69, 100, 102
Thucydides 192, 263
Tonsillitis (*antias*) 298
Touch, disorders of 216–20
Tremor (*tromos*) 142, 190, 193, 195, 235, 238, 242, 274
Trusmos 199, 287
Tumours (*phumata*) 141
Typhlotes (blindness) 189, 213, 216

Ulcers (*helke*) 151, 152, 155, 178, 210, 212, 225, 286, 290
    eroding (*karkinos*) see cancer.
Unconsciousness (*karos*) 165, 191, 233, 234
Urinary symptoms (see also *ischuria/dysuria*) 200
Uterus, disorders of 298–9
Uvulitis (*staphyle*) 298

Vomiting 248, 275

Warts (*akrochordones*) 148
Weakness (*arrostia*) 40
Whitlow (*prospaisma*) 230
Wittgenstein, Ludwig 121
Wound (*trauma*) 178, 210

Yawning (*chasme*) 238, 261

Printed in the United States
By Bookmasters